Current
Psychiatric
Therapies
VOL. II — 1962

Current

Psychiatric

Therapies

AN ANNUAL PUBLICATION

VOL. II — 1962

Edited by

Jules H. Masserman, M.D.

Professor of Neurology and Psychiatry, Northwestern University

GRUNE & STRATTON   **NEW YORK · LONDON**

Contents

Preface

THE ENTHUSIASTIC reception accorded the introductory volume of this series has fulfilled the editor's hopes that behavioral scientists everywhere are discarding outmoded dogmas and stereotyped practices, and are seeking for more rational and effective methods for helping the ill and troubled human beings who are their concern. This series is therefore again dedicated to my colleagues in psychiatry, psychology, social service, hospital administration and related fields who have joined in that seeking, and especially to those who have embodied their wisdom in the contributions published herein.

To complete the survey of all branches of psychiatric therapy begun in Volume I, the 35 chapters in the present volume have been arranged in eight Parts dealing with the following topics:
 I. Principles of Psychiatric Therapy; II. Childhood and Adolescence; III. Techniques of Psychotherapy; IV. Treatment of the Psychoses; V. Legal Psychiatry; VI. Part-Time Services; VII. Full-Time Hospital Therapy; and VIII. Psychiatry and the World.
The two volumes thus constitute an authoritative and comprehensive treatise on current practices in the field, and lay a foundation for the reporting of significant advances in future annual editions.

JULES H. MASSERMAN, M.D.,
Editor

Northwestern University
Chicago, January 1, 1962

Roster of Contributors

Frederick H. Allen, M.D., Professor emeritus of Psychiatry, University of Pennsylvania Medical and Graduate Schools.

John H. Beard, M.S.W., Executive Director of Fountain House Foundation, New York, New York.

William Bewley, M.D., Department of Psychiatry, University of California School of Medicine, San Francisco, California.

Walter Bonime, M.D., Associate Clinical Professor, New York Medical College.

Ivan Böszörmenyi-Nagy, M.D., Assistant Professor of Psychiatry, Jefferson Medical College, Philadelphia, Pennsylvania.

C. H. Hardin Branch, M.D., Professor and Head, Department of Psychiatry, University of Utah College of Medicine, Salt Lake City, Utah. President, American Psychiatric Association, 1962-63.

Hilde Bruch, M.D., Clinical Professor of Psychiatry, Columbia University College of Physicians and Surgeons, New York, New York.

Eric T. Carlson, M.D., Instructor in Psychiatry, Cornell University Medical College, New York, New York.

J. F. Casey, M.D., Director of Psychiatry, Neurology and Psychology Service, Department of Medicine and Surgery, Veterans Administration, Washington, D. C.

Ralph T. Collins, M.D., Medical Department, Consultant in Neurology and Psychiatry, Eastman Kodak Company, Rochester, New York.

William R. Conte, M.D., Supervisor, Mental Health, Department of Institutions, Olympia, Washington.

Norman Dain, M.D., Department of History, Rutgers University, Newark, New Jersey.

John C. Ehrmann, Ph.D., Wisconsin State Department of Public Welfare, Madison, Wisconsin.

Henri Ey, M.D., Professor of Psychiatry, University of Paris, Paris, France.

Richard E. Felder, M.D., Atlanta Psychiatric Clinic, Atlanta, Georgia.

Saul H. Fisher, M.D., Associate Professor of Clinical Psychiatry, New York University School of Medicine; Psychiatric Consultant, Fountain House Foundation, New York, New York.

James L. Framo, Ph.D., Instructor in Psychiatry, Jefferson Medical College, Philadelphia, Pennsylvania.

James J. Gallagher, M.D., Professor, Institute for Research on Exceptional Children, University of Illinois, Urbana, Illinois.

Charles E. Goshen, M.D., Director, Community Psychiatric Services, Department of Mental Hygiene, State of Maryland.

Thomas P. Hackett, M.D., Instructor in Psychiatry, Harvard Medical School, Boston, Massachusetts.

Seymour L. Halleck, M.D., Wisconsin State Department of Public Welfare, Madison, Wisconsin.

Gert Heilbrunn, M.D., Clinical Associate Professor of Psychiatry, University of Washington, Seattle, Washington.

Thomas Hora, M.D., Supervising Psychiatrist, Postgraduate Center for Psychotherapy, New York, New York.

Robert C. Hunt, M.D., Hudson River State Hospital, Poughkeepsie, New York.

Clyde J. Lindley, M.A., Special Assistant to the Director, Psychiatry, Neurology and Psychology Service, Department of Medicine and Surgery, Veterans Administration, Washington, D. C.

Thomas P. Malone, M.D., Atlanta Psychiatric Clinic, Atlanta, Georgia.

Sydney Margolin, M.D., Professor of Psychiatry, University of Colorado, Denver, Colorado.

Claude H. Miller, M.D., Psychoanalyst, 7 Park Avenue, New York 16, New York.

Charles Myran, M.D., Psychiatrist, The Veterans' Administration, Chicago, Illinois.

John A. Ordway, M.D., Instructor in Psychiatry, University of Cincinnati, Cincinnati, Ohio.

Martin T. Orne, M.D., Harvard Medical School, Boston, Massachusetts.

Asher R. Pacht, M.D., Wisconsin State Department of Public Welfare, Madison, Wisconsin.

Ernst Papenek, Associate Director, Training Institute for Individual Psychology, New York, New York.

Helene Papenek, M.D., Director, Training Institute for Individual Psychology, New York, New York.

Virginia Patterson, M.A., The Langley Porter Neuropsychiatric Institute, San Francisco, California.

Robert E. Pittenger, M.D., Psychiatric Director, the George Junior Republic, New York, New York.

Leon Salzman, M.D., Associate Professor of Clinical Psychiatry, Georgetown University School of Medicine, Washington, D. C.

Melitta R. Schmideberg, M.D., Director of Clinical Services, Association for the Psychiatric Treatment of Offenders, New York, New York.

Leon A. Steinman, M.D., Hudson River State Hospital, Poughkeepsie, New York.

John H. Vitale, Ph.D., Coordinator, Psychology Services, Menlo Park Division, Veterans Administration Hospital, Palo Alto, California.

Charles William Wahl, M.D., Chief, Division of Psychosomatic Medicine, Department of Psychiatry, University of California in Los Angeles.

John Warkentin, M.D., Atlanta Psychiatric Clinic, Atlanta, Georgia.

Avery D. Weisman, M.D., Assistant Clinical Professor of Psychiatry, Harvard Medical School, Boston, Massachusetts.

Louis Jolyon West, M.D., Professor and Chairman, Department of Psychiatry, University of Oklahoma, Oklahoma City, Oklahoma.

Carl A. Whitaker, M.D., Atlanta Psychiatric Clinic, Atlanta, Georgia.

Jack F. Wilder, M.D., Division of Social and Community Psychiatry, Department of Psychiatry, Albert Einstein College of Medicine, Bronx, New York.

Izrael Zwerling, M.D., Division of Social and Community Psychiatry, Department of Psychiatry, Albert Einstein College of Medicine, Bronx, New York.

Therapy *Sine* Psychotherapy

by C. H. HARDIN BRANCH, M.D.

P SYCHOTHERAPY PRESUMABLY has status as a respectable treatment for illness. This, at least, is the position taken by those who insist that psychotherapy, like other therapies, remains primarily the province of the physician who has a license to treat. Quantitatively, the amount of psychotherapy being performed daily seems to be steadily increasing as more and more psychiatrists complete their training and— at least in the majority of instances—go into private practice where most of their time is spent in psychotherapy with outpatients.

This alignment of psychiatric treatment with the rest of medicine was strongly re-emphasized by Robert H. Felix, in his presidential address to the American Psychiatric Association in Chicago in May, 1961. There is considerable feeling that psychotherapy must subject itself to the same criteria as are applied to any other treatment process if the continued inclusion of psychotherapy as a medical procedure can be justified.

One outstanding difficulty has always been the failure of psychotherapists to provide objective "scientific" validation for the psychotherapeutic process or its results. Nor are patients themselves satisfied with this situation. It has been reported[1] that 65 per cent of the people who sought help for an emotional or "nervous" difficulty, who went to clergymen or physicians felt they found this help, while only 46 per cent of those who visited psychiatrists felt they were helped. On the economic side, it has been repeatedly emphasized by Redlich and Hollingshead,[2] and more recently by Cole,[3] that there is an economic differentiation in the patients who are accepted for psychotherapy. Cole has emphasized that this situation is not the same throughout the country, but there does seem to be reasonable agreement that the lower socioeconomic groups are neither as acceptable for—nor as accepting of—psychotherapy as those at higher levels. Under these circumstances, one has the uncomfortable feeling that the psychotherapist who does not look squarely at these problems places himself rather in the position of the March Hare who defended his use of butter in watch repair on the pathetic ground that "it was the *best* butter, you know."

With this background, it might be useful to look at what seems to me to be some very practical considerations with reference to psychotherapy and the occasions when it would be better to prescribe some other kind of therapy, on the grounds that psychotherapy is not particularly indicated, or is too expensive, or perhaps is not even applicable. Waggoner[4] quotes Munsterberg, as follows:

> Thus, to believe in psychotherapy ought never to mean that we have a right to make light of the other means which, as experience shows, may help toward the treatment of disturbances in the central equilibrium.

It is in the hope that exploration of extrapsychotherapeutic procedures may broaden our approach to illness and thus keep psychotherapy as a treatment procedure, in every sense of the word, that the present chapter is written.

First, it is necessary to take a cold, pragmatic look at therapeutic goals. It is not sufficient for the therapist to take the position that he is going to continue a procedure with the bland assumption that something good will come of it. This casual attitude would not be accepted in medicine and in my opinion is not acceptable in psychiatry. It may well be, of course—as has been repeatedly emphasized—that treatment goals are not the same for the therapist and the patient. The possible objectives mentioned by Garner[5] include: (1) to save from death, (2) to cure, (3) to remove pathologic tissue, (4) to offer symptomatic relief, and (5) to help in rehabilitation. He adds that personal and social values of both the physician and the patient may lead to considerable alteration in these goals. I would modify them thus:

1. *To produce symptomatic relief.* This, although regarded as rather low on the status system, is nonetheless the goal which usually brings the patient to the psychiatrist's office. While admittedly the upper-class patients sometimes come because of dissatisfaction with their internal adjustments, this in itself is a symptom, and the eradication of this symptom is the reason for the initial visit.

2. *The prevention of foreseeable crippling difficulties.* Under this heading might be subsumed those procedures which have to do with adolescent maladjustment problems, some marital difficulties, the psychotherapeutic procedures carried out between recurrent depressions, psychotherapy for the polysurgical patient, and so on.

3. *The improvement of social adjustment.* This could include a multitude of possibilities, ranging from the schizoid and therefore socially maladaptive individual to the person who, because of physical

characteristics or educational or social limitations, is simply unable to relate to his or her fellow men or women.

4. *The eradication of all psychopathology.* This, of course, is a grandiose and completely unrealistic goal, but does justify mentioning because it is sometimes set either by the patient or the therapist.

5. *Rehabilitation.* This involves somewhat different criteria than treatment in general, as rehabilitation experts and geriatricians know only too well. In the treatment of acute illness, the goal is obviously the return of the individual to the level of functioning which he had before this was interrupted by the acute illness. In rehabilitation, the goal is the achievement of the best possible practical adjustment in the light of the individual's obvious—and in some instances—irreversible difficulties.

In the light of these psychotherapeutic objectives, it might be useful to speculate for a few moments on what goals people actually have for their psychotherapeutic ventures. It has been pointed out that the aims of the patients to some extent depend on their socioeconomic level. The lower income bracket people are "resigned and apathetic."[1] Of those who had sought help, 42 per cent complained of difficulty with their marriages, 12 per cent of difficulty with the children, and only 18 per cent of difficulty with "personal adjustment problems." The first procedure in psychotherapy[6] must therefore be an agreement between the therapist and the patient as to what goals will be mutually acceptable, or at least mutually recognized.

The Joint Commission Report states:

> Psychiatrists apparently play a self-limiting role. Tending to regard support and comfort as secondary to therapy, they therefore may be restricted—in the amount of help they can give—to patients who have enough selfawareness to accept the necessity for exploration of their personalities and subsequent re-education.

Since it would appear that "support and comfort" are the things which the patients desire, the psychotherapist and the patient must inevitably find themselves immediately at odds.

It is possible—in fact probable—that the reasons which bring a patient to a psychotherapist are rather different in many instances from those which the patient actually expresses to the psychotherapist or which the psychotherapist assumes to be the reason for the patient's being in his office. When one reviews his practice, he will certainly find a reasonable number of people who are uncomfortable, who are crippled, who are functioning poorly, and who very specifically need readjustment of their personality reactions in order to achieve any degree of successful adaptation to the life situation, but there are others whose reason for being in the psychotherapist's office are not so clear-cut. Yet it is somewhat unusual to find a psychotherapist who will turn away a patient if there is: (1) *a complaint,* (2) *psychopathology, and* (3) *motivation for therapy.*

This is not to be cynical about the psychotherapist's acceptance of such patients, but to point out that it is rare, in my experience, to have a psychotherapist tell a patient "psychotherapy is not what you need; your problems can be better handled by other means."

One of the problems which brings a certain number of patients into the psychotherapist's office is boredom, expressed in one form or another. Perhaps it is simply a lack of satisfaction with one's situation in life, or it may occur in the individual whose internal resources have always been somewhat inadequate and who approaches retirement with no real satisfaction to be gained from his life situation. In the self questioning upper income group, such a person is quite likely to develop somatic complaints which will sooner or later lead him to a psychiatrist's office.

Another yearning, which is perhaps seldom recognized, is the need of individuals for a time for quiet contemplation. Patients have sometimes expressed the feeling that the psychiatrist's office is the one place where there are no pressures and where an individual can, in a leisurely way, discuss thoughts and feelings. The individual who sits quietly in his own home is very likely to be regarded as ill or angry, and only in certain religious situations is this type of quiet contemplation considered to be respectable. As Wordsworth says:

> The world is too much with us. Late and soon,
> Getting and spending, we lay waste our powers.
> Little we see in nature that is ours.

And I believe it was Edna St. Vincent Millay who poetically explained the Bluebeard story by pointing out that the room from which his wives were excluded was actually his attempt to maintain a study for himself. At any rate, it would appear that the quiet of a psychiatrist's office is, for a good many patients, the only relatively serene place they have.

Some patients obviously seek in psychotherapy weapons which can be used against parents, spouses, employers, and others. This kind of patient may be the compensation-seeking individual who blames his difficulties on his job; in the Joint Commission report,[1] this was listed as one of the major causes given for threatened "nervous breakdowns." Such persons may also want to obtain some concession from a spouse or a parent by going through the motions of psychotherapy: e.g., one of our patients said that she hoped, if she kept her appointments regularly, her parents would see that it was necessary for her to have a car in order to keep up her psychotherapy. Or the patient may wish to obtain some agreement by the psychotherapist that other significant individuals are responsible for the difficulty. In any event, these individuals certainly do not have the same goals as those which are customarily set out for psychotherapy.

Perhaps related to this group are those who seek in psychotherapy some sort of status. Some of these may be individuals who think of themselves as artistic and become indoctrinated by their friends in the idea that people who are sensitive and high strung quite often need psychotherapy. The group would include also those who rather resent the fact that a spouse or a relative is receiving this sort of attention, feel left out, and consequently seek help for themselves.

Lastly (the list is by no means complete), there are very many patients who seek in psychotherapy a way of dodging all the responsibilities for their own difficulties. These are the individuals who have the impression that if they continue psychotherapy for a long enough period of time, sooner or later a revelation or a magic resolution of their difficulties will appear out of thin air. For example, we recently saw a lady who had, through one manipulation or another, been able to maintain some six years of psychotherapy in our outpatient clinic without once accepting responsibility for doing anything at all on her own initiative to deal with her life situation. This instance obviously is also indicative of our own dereliction in insisting that she take more responsibility for doing something for herself.

The patient who complains of social inadequacy, for instance, may make no effort to achieve better grooming or more social grace, even though these lie no farther away than the nearest beauty parlor or dance studio. Similarly, the individual who complains of feelings of intellectual inferiority may be more comfortable in shrugging helplessly because of this inadequacy than in improving his own grammar, or reading enough to become at least an adequate conversationalist.

Leaving out of our discussion any consideration of the economics involved, it is, therefore, an occupational hazard for a psychotherapist who has been trained to think loosely that where symptoms coexist with psychopathology, that two plus two plus two equals six, and consequently the patient should be accepted for psychotherapy. Our position is that the coexistence of symptoms and psychopathology does not necessarily mean that there is a cause-and-effect relationship between these two, or that psychotherapy will be effective. It would be better for all concerned—and might conserve precious psychotherapeutic time for those individuals for whom psychotherapy is realistically a desideratum—if the psychotherapist discussed with the patient, and perhaps with other members of the therapeutic community, other approaches to the patient's problem which might not involve psychotherapy, or at the very most, would involve a minimum of time in this area.

Many persons simply need encouragement to go in for changing their life situations on a "do-it-yourself" basis. While we tend to pride ourselves on being an individualistic culture, many people actually need a great deal of stimulation to strike out on their own. This is particularly true of those who have lived in grooves all their lives (one example would be the woman who can think of herself as a wife and mother, but has no concept of herself apart from these roles) ; and once these grooves are no longer applicable to the life situation, they are incapable of self determination. One can, of course, wail at the culture which produces such dependencies, but this is likely to be an unproductive procedure. More useful might be the strong insistence, either instead of or as an adjunct to psychotherapy, that the patient actually makes some moves on his or her own behalf. It might be suggested, for instance, that he improve his intellectual skills by adult education classes, by joining Toastmaster Clubs, or other activities of this sort. One is often surprised first, by the resistance against such a definitive step and second, by the tremendous gratification which sometimes results when the patient is led to do something on his own.

In this connection, the matter of the personal appearance and grooming of the patient is something about which the psychotherapist can sometimes comment most helpfully. In some instances, the advice to improve one's personal appearance, far from being regarded as an unpleasant criticism, may be taken as an indication that the therapist feels the patient is worthwhile. Under these circumstances, it would seem to be approaching the matter from the wrong angle to explore the reasons for the patient's apathy, whereas a firm and friendly encouragement to improve matters in these areas might—as Thorne has pointed out—achieve the same results in considerably less time.

The use of religion as an adjunct has always been a troublesome question. On the one hand, participation in religious activities is so socially acceptable and so widespread that the psychotherapist is quite likely to feel that the reason why the patient has not taken advantage of it must be psychopathologic. However, it did appear, again from the Joint Commission survey,[1] that those people who regularly attended church had in many instances less discomfort than those who did not. Whether or not the encouragement of the patient to realign himself with religious activity would be useful in most cases is an open question, but it would certainly seem that this is something which might be explored with the patient in terms of the real benefits to be derived from alignment with religious groups. In some instances, the alignment with church activities can be very helpful in achieving a better social adjustment, without necessarily paying attention to the theology involved.

Again, the psychotherapist has the occupational hazard of proceeding on the assumption that the individual is neurotically unable to make these explorations for himself, and consequently, the reluctance itself must be the focus of the psychotherapist's attention. All of us occasionally need encouragement to proceed in new and unaccustomed areas, and the psychotherapist can well take the position of a kindly friend in encouraging activities along these lines without bothering about working on the reasons for the reluctance.

SUMMARY

The psychotherapist must not conclude that psychotherapy is necessarily the only therapeutic tool he has at hand, if he is to justify his position as a physician making a sincere effort to treat patients. Ignoring for the moment such therapeutic adjuncts as mechanical and electrical therapies, group therapy and psychopharmacologic therapies, it would appear that careful, thoughtful consideration should be given to the actual goals of the patient and to the reasons for the patient's incapacity. Neither of these may actually be related to the psychopathology found. Furthermore, neither the patient's needs nor the reasons for the incapacity may be subject to attack by psychotherapeutic methods as efficiently as they may be accessible to activities in other, though related, fields. The psychotherapist should be constantly alert to the possibility that psychotherapy is not necessarily the treatment of choice and that satisfactory results can be obtained in some instances by bringing to the patient's attention the community resources available for help in some specific areas. Such an approach would not preclude psychotherapy which might well continue hand-in-hand with these other activities.

REFERENCES

1. Joint Commission on Mental Illness and Health: Americans View Their Mental Health. Report 4. New York, Basic Books, Inc., 1960.
2. HOLLINGSHEAD, A. B. AND REDLICH, F. C.: Social Class and Mental Illness: A Community Study. New York, John Wiley and Sons, Inc., 1958.
3. COLE, N. J., BRANCH, C. H. H., AND ALLISON, R. B.: Some Relationships between social class and the practice of dynamic psychotherapy. Am. J. Psychiat. (In press).
4. WAGGONER, R. W.: The Integration of Therapy. *In:* Progress in Psychotherapy: Social Psychiatry, 5:91. Jules H. Masserman and J. L. Moreno, editors, New York, Grune & Stratton, 1959.
5. GARNER, H. H.: Treatment—review of a medical concept. J. of Am. Geriatric Soc. 9:886, (Oct.), 1961.
6. BRANCH, C. H. H., AND ELY, J. W.: Teaching the principles of ambulant psychotherapy. Am. J. Psychiat. 115:887-91, (Apr.), 1959.

Therapeutic Implications of Diagnosis

by CHARLES E. GOSHEN, M.D.

CORRELATION OF DIAGNOSIS AND THERAPY

CLASSIFICATION SYSTEMS for psychiatric diagnosis developed in a rather piecemeal fashion during the past three quarters of a century, following precedents established by Moebius and Kraepelin. Psychotic disorders were the original subject of these efforts, with the milder and organic disorders being included later. During World War II, the military services adopted a modification of the prevailing system for their purposes, and this was subsequently modified further by other groups, such as the various psychoanalytic groups and the Veterans' Administration. In 1952, the American Psychiatric Association adopted a standardized system of nomenclature which is in general use today throughout the U.S. and Canada.

In psychiatry, the underlying, but seldom acknowledged viewpoint determining the choice of diagnostic terms has been that of the disposition of the patient in question. In other words, the classification systems used have been oriented to the goal of making appropriate sociologic decisions such as: will the patient be institutionalized or not; will he be exempt from or discharged from military service; will he be held accountable for crimes committed; will he be granted a pension; will he be a suitable employee; or will he be a security risk? Ultimately, these questions can be narrowed to one general issue: will he be included or excluded from normal human society? Psychiatrists often complain of the frequency with which this attitude governs the conduct of laymen toward psychiatric patients, but seldom appreciate the degree to which they, themselves, make clinical judgements from the same nonclinical viewpoint.

It is generally conceded that the most scientific grounds for a diagnostic system is one based upon etiology. It would be premature, however, to hope for any widespread acceptance of any given etiologically based system in psychiatry, because of the wide divergence of theoretic viewpoints prevailing. It does not appear to be premature to consider a sys-

8

tem of nomenclature which classifies people into categories which are comprehensive enough to include all and discrete enough to convey significant prognostic and therapeutic implications. Such a system is herein proposed. It foregoes the temptation to invent a new terminology, relying only on a few standard terms which are given definitions of greater sharpness and simplicity.

A good classification system does not begin merely by listing all conceiv-

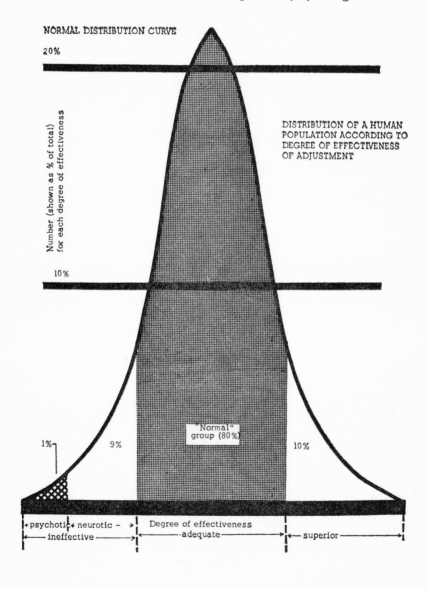

NORMAL DISTRIBUTION CURVE

DISTRIBUTION OF A HUMAN POPULATION ACCORDING TO DEGREE OF EFFECTIVENESS OF ADJUSTMENT

Number (shown as % of total) for each degree of effectiveness

20%

10%

1% 9% "Normal" group (80%) 10%

←psychotic←neurotic→ Degree of effectiveness ←superior→
←——— ineffective ———→ ·adequate·

able categories in the hope that the list will thereby be comprehensive—although this is the way in which the official psychiatric diagnoses have evolved. Instead, a good system begins with the total population involved and divides it into smaller groups according to some variable or set of variables which the members of the population have in common but vary in degree.

Fig. 1 shows a normal distribution curve which will be used as a basis for the following discussion. It portrays the probable distribution of a large, unselected population of our society according to "the degree of effectiveness of adjustment (to society, culture or environment)." This variable is considered appropriate because: (1) each individual possesses some degree of adjustment to his society; (2) individuals vary in degree of adjustment over a wide range, but tend to cluster in largest numbers near a *norm;* (3) those with psychiatric disabilities are most distinctly characterized from others in the sense that they consistently demonstrate a lower level of adjustment, either in the degree of success in making an adjustment or in the degree of effort, pain or sacrifice required to maintain some level of adjustment; (4) within the group of psychiatrically disabled is a continuation of the same distribution over a wide range (it is not an all-or-none issue); and (5) the therapeutic implication involved consists, simply, of the principle of moving an individual from a lower to a higher level of adjustment. Furthermore, this concept implies that there will also exist a small number of people who differ from the large group in the middle levels (*norm*) by virtue of their demonstrating superior levels of adjustment. This implication is, of course, in accordance with what we all know to be true.

Each society establishes standards for levels of adjustment of its members which serve to identify both those few who fall into the upper levels and become, thereby, the leaders of the society, and those who fall into the lower levels, which include the psychiatrically disabled. All societies do not, however, draw the lines separating these groups at the same place. Some, for instance, recognize only very tiny numbers as leaders. Oriental cultures tend to fall into this pattern.

In our American society, the ratio of 10 per cent turns up time after time as the approximate proportion of any group which qualifies either as being superior or inadequate, leaving the "normal" or adequate group as making up 80 per cent of the total. In the military services, for example, there is an approximate ratio of one officer to ten enlisted men. At the other end of the scale, estimates made of the total number of "failures" in our society, including psychiatric problems, criminals, alcoholics, etc. add up to about 10 per cent of the total population. These ratios are not necessarily a product of deterministic factors, but are, instead, a reflection of the capacity of society to provide for, or to "afford," these special groups. Affluent societies can afford larger ratios than deprived societies, and the capacity to afford a larger luxury tends to apply to the numbers of leaders produced. Likewise, as a society develops in respect to affluence, the members of both leaders and the inadequately adjusted tend to increase.

As shown in fig. 1, the lower 10 per cent of the population, in respect to adjustment adequacy, represents the probable size of the segment containing psychiatric problems, while the upper 10 per cent includes the leaders of society whose adjustment levels are superior. Within the "ineffective" group, the same distribution trends continue, with a lower 10 per cent of this group (1 per cent of the total) representing the least effective. This lower 10 per cent, including the 1 per cent subgroup, can be very conveniently regarded, psychiatrically, as equivalent to the psychoneurotic and the psychotic classes of people. No additional subclassification within these groups is necessary to an understanding of the mechanisms underlying these conditions or the therapeutic implications.

Fundamental to any person's degree of adjustment to society is the choices he makes in the pursuit of his life activities. The inadequately adjusted people turn out to be those whose decisions have been irrational in respect to their social and biologic survival. The making and implementation of these decisions make up what we know as "taking responsibility." The way in which people vary in relation to their responsibilities follows the same type of distribution indicated above. We know that most people accept responsibility with a relatively willing attitude, and, as a result, acquire sufficient experience in discharging it that they acquire both skill and confidence in so doing. This "average" or "normal" group will nearly coincide with our 80 per cent of "adequately" adjusted people. In addition, we also know that a few people do much more than this "adequate" amount, and others do much less. Those who do more are the ones who have more than adequately taken responsibility for themselves, and in addition, have assumed and discharged successfully responsibilities for others, thus becoming the leaders of society.

Among those who fall into the lower levels on the responsibility scale are two rather distinct groups. Persons in one group, although disliking responsibility, nevertheless regard it as a necessity. With this attitude they assume responsibilities reluctantly, or accept some but not others, or accept all of them part of the time but not all the time, or carry them out to a minimum degree, avoiding them when they can justify it. These attitudes and practices are characteristic of, and fundamental to, the condition known as "psychoneurosis." As a result of such attitudes these people fail to accumulate enough experience and success to become skillful and confident, and also fail to perform at a high enough level to assure a consistent and adequate level of adjustment.

There is still another quality which may characterize certain people within the group who are antagonistic to responsibility. This second group not only regards responsibility as evil, but also as unnecessary, whereas the psychoneurotic group treat it as a necessary evil. This second group avoids responsibility at every opportunity, even without justification. It is, specifically, this lack of justification which makes this group appear "crazy" to others, and this is the group which coincides with the psychotic group in the classification system proposed. The fact that people can be classified according to their relationship to responsibility in a way which parallels the distribution of people's adjustment levels is not a coincidence. Instead, it is specifically one's type of relationship to responsibilities which determines his mode of making decisions, and therefore his type of adjustment to society, and, from a subjective viewpoint, his sense of success or failure.

Within the concept of the classification system proposed, other factors traditionally regarded as having psychiatric significance (such as organic damage to the brain, mental retardation, etc.) must be regarded as characteristics of the individual's environment with which he is making some kind of adjustment, and not a feature of the adjustment itself. The justification for this assumption lies in the fact that these other factors are extrinsic to the individual's *consciousness,* and though existing within the body constitute external problems which increase the difficulty of adjustment, but otherwise do not predetermine the level of adjustment.

BACKGROUND FOR THERAPY

The logical goal of treatment becomes easily derivable from the proposed classification system, namely: change of adjustment level to higher levels of adequacy. The method of achieving this is also apparent, namely: a change of the decision making process in the individual to higher levels of responsibility. The technique required of the therapist to effect this change is not so simply stated, however, and will almost inevitably demand considerable technical training and skill. Some of the ingredients necessary for success will include:

1. *Cooperation of the Patient:* Without some degree of willing participation on the part of the patient, success is unlikely. Psychiatrists have too often concluded that the failure of a patient to improve must inevitably be due to a defect in the treatment, and do not accept the limitation that success is necessarily dependent, as well, on the patient's cooperation.

   The therapist is not entirely helpless in instituting a promising treatment program when he is faced with an uncooperative patient, however. He has at least two levers at his disposal. In the first place, he might achieve an effective influence on the patient through the agency of some other person. Childhood problems, particularly, lend themselves to treatment by concentrating the therapeutic effort on parents or teachers, thus, in effect altering the environment with which the child has to cope and thereby stimulating the development of a new orientation on the part of the child. Also, alcoholics can often be effectively influenced by working with the husband or wife. The other way by which the uncooperative patient might be approached is through a direct attack on the uncoopera- tive attitude itself. Success in such efforts seems to be determined to a large extent by the degree of patience exhibited by the thera- pist. If an offer of help is made to an uncooperative patient and the opportunity is presented to outline what it entails, in spite of the fact that there may appear to be no immediate acceptance, in a high number of cases it will be found that acceptance does develop later on. It might be many months or years later before the patient acts on the recommendations made, and he might return to another therapist for help, but there is a high likelihood that he will find that the reasonable approach and the interest shown by the original therapist continues to nag at him in spite of his own efforts to discredit or dismiss the need for treatment until he finally becomes willing to give it a trial. Allowing the patient to make his own decision without requiring that he give an immediate answer (which is too likely to be "no") leaves him in a state of indecision, which is more likely to be resolved favorably when the therapist's approach is one of patience.

On the other hand, most patients, in order to have come to the attention of a therapist in the first place (except in the case of committed patients to hospitals) have already demonstrated a certain degree of acceptance of treatment. It is true that their concepts of treatment are likely to be distorted and unrealistic, but their mere presence is evidence of a substantial effort on their part to investigate the possibilities of treatment. In a sense this degree of cooperation already indicates some preparedness to change and much of the success achieved in treatment is founded on this step, for which the therapist can take no credit.

2. *Example Set by the Therapist:* Whether it is the therapist's inten- tion or not, the example he sets for the patient will become the principal message he conveys to the patient. Psychiatric patients are like children, however, in the sense that words alone have little influence on them. Instead, they tend either to rebel against or imitate the examples set for them by significant people in their lives. The therapist is likely to become a member of this class of people, and, as such, will serve as a model toward which, or away from which, the patient will tend to mold his own actions. Like a child, also, both his imitations of and his attempts to be different from the model may be distortions, principally because he is likely to see the form rather than the essence. In time, though, the deeper

meaning behind the external form of behavior does have an influence, so that the patient begins to do *as* the therapist does instead of doing only *what* the therapist does, if therapy becomes successful.

Because the example set by the therapist is so fundamentally important to the outcome of therapy, the level of adjustment of the therapist himself becomes a limit beyond which the patient will not develop. In other words, the therapist cannot teach by example, what he does not know himself.

Certain qualities or attitudes on the part of the therapist are likely to represent very substantial assets in treatment, and may not seem to be very closely related to the technical aspects of psychiatry. Some of these qualities are: self confidence, calmness, good humor, dependability, patience, concentration of interest on the patient to the exclusion of other interests during the treatment sessions, relaxation, and honesty. These qualities tend to establish the nature of the atmosphere in which the treatment takes place, and thereby become essential ingredients of the example set by the therapist.

GOALS OF TREATMENT

In any collaborative effort involving two people, it pays to select those objectives about which there exists the maximum amount of agreement. The good therapist is dedicated to the proposition of helping his patients feel better, but must take the initiative in placing in proper perspective the issue of short-range versus long-range comfort. The patient almost invariably sees his major problem as being that of discomfort, or unhappiness. Accordingly, the therapeutic goals of both therapist and patient can be regarded as having an improved state of comfort or happiness as an end product. This might be the only area of agreement between the two. The therapist can easily see that the patient's current state of discomfort is a byproduct of his failures in meeting the standards of adjustment (success) set by himself and/or society. The patient may not appreciate this, however. As a matter of fact, it can be safely stated that a true appreciation of this would require a degree of maturity (sense of responsibility) which, if present, would have protected the individual from the failures in question.

The appropriate goal of therapy becomes that of attaining successes in place of failures. The greater state of comfort desired by the patient is something the therapist predicts will happen once successes have been attained, or appear to be within reach. Again, the patient and therapist may disagree on what constitutes success. Success in adjusting to society's standards is often interpreted by the patient to mean doing what is expected of him by others, and thus appears distasteful. This is the child's concept of responsibility. Instead, the therapist's needs to demonstrate (by example more than by words) that genuine, satisfying success consists of accomplishing one's own ends, of making one's own decisions, of taking one's own responsibilities and, as long as doing this does not trespass on the rights of others, it will meet the standards of adjustment set by society. To this end, therapy itself must be regarded as something designed to make itself ultimately unnecessary. Self confidence is a quality which the patient generally appreciates to be absent from his own current life. Like a child, however, he is inclined to expect self confidence to come as a result of recognition by others. The therapist needs to demonstrate to him, instead, that it is an attitude which results from the acquisition of skill in self reliance, which, in turn, is derived from experience in assuming responsibility.

METHOD OF TREATMENT

To attain the stated goals of therapy, namely, success in handling responsibility, requires implementation at the level of the decision making processes of the patient. Presenting such a proposal to the patient is very likely to be complicated by the fact that his concepts of decision making are too immature to allow a deep appreciation of its connotations. He is apt, for example, to misconstrue the process of forming opinions as being equivalent to the making of decisions. If we regard opinion formation as the process of categorizing phenomena as "like and do not like," or "being for or against" and, on the other hand, if we regard decision formation as the process of "planning for action," then the two become very different concepts. The patient, childishly, is most often preoccupied with what he likes and what he does not like rather than with what he is going to do. If he is advised to make his own decisions, he will probably construe this to mean getting what he likes which, invariably, becomes the avoidance of responsibility. Such misconceptions must be brought out and clarified in therapy.

The use of thinking processes for the purpose of making responsible, self-reliant decisions is the essential biologic function of mentation, inasmuch as it is the uniquely human mechanism of survival. The use of thinking processes for other purposes is likely to jeopardize survival if done to the exclusion of, or at the expense of, decision-making. Both neurotic and the psychotic persons expend a major share of their thinking time (that is: waking time) in phantasy, which is a non-decision-making, or even an anti-decision-making, process. Therefore, both such persons will jeopardize their survival. Since human survival is inextricably interwoven with social existence, these people will correspondingly hamper their social adjustment. Incidentally, the great concern expressed in many psychiatric and other scientific circles concerning questions such as "the biologic basis of schizophrenia" can be clarified by closer attention to the *biologic function* of intelligence, namely, survival through decision making, rather than the more usual preoccupation with the molecular and cellular mechanisms of nerve cell metabolism.

In short, it can be stated that treatment methodology consists of an alteration of the patient's decision making processes from infantile to more mature, more responsible ways. Such a task is essentially the same as the one confronting the parent and teacher in respect to helping children learn how to grow up. As with the good teacher or the good parent, success of the therapist is most readily assured when this educational process is seen as one which demonstrates by example, not only how to make rational decisions, but the desirability of doing this as well. When the parent, the teacher, or the therapist is able to convey to others that he reaps rewards and satisfactions from making his own decisions, he thereby sets the stage for his child, student or patient developing an interest in following the example. The psychiatric patient has failed to acquire such an interest in the past because of the absence of such examples in his life. Instead, he has been shown that the process of making his own decisions is unrewarding, risky, and likely to expose him to criticism.

OBSTACLES TO THERAPY

Assuming that a patient in question is sufficiently cooperative to present himself for treatment, there still remain substantial obstacles to success, and these obstacles are commonly known as the patient's "resistance." The most difficult part of the therapeutic program consists of convincing the patient that what he wants most (greater comfort or happiness) is achievable through doing what he dislikes the most (responsible decision making). Perhaps physicians are more effective as therapists than non-physicians because this apparent contradiction is something which any patient expects to find in medical treatment, namely, the treatment process itself might turn out to be as painful as the pain which brought the patient to the physician. The apparent, but short-lived, success of pharmacologic means of treating psychiatric problems can be attributed to the fact that such methods are much more closely in accordance with the patient's irrational concepts of what he needs.

Until this point, our discussion of treatment has not distinguished between the neurotic and psychotic, because what has been said applies to both. The question of "resistance" has important differences, however, in the two general categories of patients. Since the psychoneurotic person has previously looked upon responsible decision making as a necessary evil, he has acquired some experience in doing it, but has not found it to be a pleasurable experience. The therapist can profitably demonstrate to him that it has not been the *act* of making decisions which has been painful in the past, but it has been the patient's *way* of doing it which made it painful. Because he took his responsibilities reluctantly instead of willingly, he was deprived of the satisfactions which come from doing something with enthusiasm. Because he fulfilled the minimum number of responsibilities that he could manage to justify, he did not acquire enough skill to develop self confidence. Because many of his efforts were wasted in avoiding responsibilities instead of carrying them out, he worked harder than necessary at the job. Because he often procrastinated, he often ended up being exposed to pressures which were unpleasant. Because he did not plan and prepare for new tasks in advance, he often failed. In short, he misconstrued his painful *way* of handling responsibility as meaning that responsibility is necessarily painful. The therapist can be effective in teaching his patient the significance of these phenomena by helping him understand the importance of each person's individual *way* of doing things as representative of the important differences in people. The therapist, himself, will then present his own *way* of doing things as a more effective, comfortable, method which is, consequently, more apt to yield success and satisfaction. The therapist, of course, can do this only if his way is an improvement over the patient's way.

The psychotic person's "resistance" is more difficult to deal with because much more radical changes are needed in his concepts of responsibility and decision making. Useful parallels can be drawn between the psychoneurotic and the ordinary adolescent on the one hand, and the psychotic and the younger child on the other. The young child does not yet know enough about responsibility to realize that it is a necessity of living. The adolescent knows of its necessity, and has had some experience with it, but has not yet adopted it as the means by which he expects to realize his objectives in life, seeing it instead as something which others require of him. The psychotic and the child are apt to see life simply as one of seeking immediate gratification of wishes with other people either helping or preventing. The psychotic, having failed in these childish objectives has learned to distrust others, and will carry this distrust over to the therapist. His wish for help, when contaminated by his distrust, is likely to take the form of "testing out" the therapist in an irrational and self-defeating way. The process of managing therapy in the face of these traps become the art of treating psychotics, without a mastery of which treatment becomes unduly burdensome to the therapist and unrewarding to the patient.

OUTCOME OF THERAPY

If therapy is seen as the process of moving a patient's adjustment level from a low to a higher point on the distribution curve mentioned before, then there is no definite point at which therapy can be regarded as completed, since any degree of elevation on the scale could be followed by an even higher one. Two different criteria of success might be used, however, with some effectiveness. One criterion could be the mere determination that a change has taken place in the right direction, since change alone is likely to become a process which continues without further therapy. Another measure of success could be the determination that *enough* change has taken place, wherein "enough" is a degree which is regarded as mutually satisfactory to therapist and patient. Concepts such as these do not allow for a measure of "cure" in the same connotations this is used in other branches of medicine. Instead, they come closer to measures of success used in education, wherein there exists a steady continuum in both depth and breath without any endpoint which could be regarded as a state of completion.

Advances in Psychoanalytic Therapy

by GERT HEILBRUNN, M.D.

A T A TIME when the "chemical revolution"[2] exerts an increasingly mechanizing influence on psychiatric thinking, it appears appropriate to establish a statistical baseline for the wisdom of future psychological and/or pharmacologic action. It is salutary that the biologist is preparing for a breakthrough where psychologic methods are of debatable value and that the chemist hopes to find shortcuts where psychiatric measures have proved especially cumbersome and expensive. Questions of primary interest concern the proportions of therapeutic success and failure in correlation with diagnostic categories and methodologic procedure. I have therefore reviewed my clinical, analytic work of the last fifteen years from a statistical point of view.

RESULTS

The present evaluation comprises 44 private patients who had been in psychoanalysis for an average of 424 hours over a period of 3.1 years and at a frequency of 3.4 sessions a week. The inclusion of cases 26 and 29 (table 1), despite their treatment frequency of only two sessions per week was deemed justifiable because the treatment met the traditional analytical standards in terms of total number of therapeutic hours, treatment goal, continuity of transference and working through. Twelve patients had fewer than 300 treatment hours. Termination in eleven of these instances was prompted by hospitalization (1 and 2), increasing alcoholism (37), and patient's choice (24) and a variety of practical circumstances and/or achievement of treatment goals in seven. One patient (32) is still in therapy. The latter nine patients were evaluated as a separate group (table 2, category i) for comparison with category h whose members had comparable diagnoses and a total number of treatment hours above the 300 mark. Since the improvement rates proved almost identical in these two groups, they were finally combined into one (table 2, category k).

To ease the difficulty of clinical evaluation, I applied four simple,

TABLE 1

Case #	Sex	Age	Diagnosis	Total # Of Trmt. Hrs.	Years Of Treatment	Sessions Per Week	Result†	
			PSYCHOTIC DISORDERS, Schizophrenic Reaction					
1	M	35	paranoid type	230	1½	4	U	*
2	M	21	paranoid type	153	1½	1-4	U	
3	F	25	chronic undifferentiated type	641	6	3-5	U	
4	M	34	chronic undifferentiated type (overt homosexuality)	1030	5	5	U	
			PERSONALITY DISORDERS Personality Pattern Disturbance					
5	M	31	schizoid personality	1220	8	4	S	° *
6	M	29	schizoid personality	348	2	4	U	
7	F	40	paranoid personality	403	3	3	U	
			Personality Trait Disturbance					
8	M	21	emotionally unstable personality	560	3½	4	M	
9	F	38	emotionally unstable personality	239	2	3	U	
			Passive Aggressive Personality					
10	M	27	passive-aggressive type	702	4½	4	U	
11	M	31	passive-aggressive type	564	3	4	G	
12	M	40	passive-aggressive type	556	5	3	M	
13	F	26	passive-aggressive type	335	2	4	G	
14	M	34	passive-aggressive type	231	2½	3	M	
15	F	26	passive-aggressive type	197	1½	3	M	
16	F	40	passive-aggressive type (adult situational reaction)	1350	8	4	M	
17	F	30	passive-aggressive type (adult situational reaction)	361	2	3	U	
18	F	32	passive-aggressive type (hysterical trends)	620	5	3	M	° *
19	F	33	passive-aggressive type (hysterical trends)	476	3½	3	M	
20	M	41	passive-aggressive type (Don Juanism)	260	3	3	M	
21	M	27	passive dependent type	375	4	3	U	

†G = great improved   S = slightly improved
M = moderately improved   U = unimproved

No.	Sex	Age	Diagnosis				
22	M	45	passive dependent type	338	2¾	3	S
23	M	40	passive dependent type	308	2	3	S
24	M	34	passive dependent type	199	1¾	3	S
25	F	26	aggressive type	710	4	4	M
26	F	32	aggressive type	317	4	2	U
27	F	32	Compulsive Personality	520	8	3	S
28	F	30	Compulsive Personality	345	3	3	M
29	M	29	Compulsive Personality	336	3½	2	M
30	M	25	Compulsive Personality	320	2½	3	M
			Sociopathic Personality Disturbance				
31	F	26	sexual deviation (homosexuality)	555	5	3	U
32	M	24	sexual deviation (homosexuality)	310	2½	3	U
33	F	30	sexual deviation (homosexuality)	194	1¾	3	G
34	M	40	sexual deviation (homosexuality and chronic alcoholism)	348	3	4-5	U
35	M	33	sexual deviation (sexual sadism)	399	4	3	S
36	M	33	chronic alcoholism	595	4	4	U
37	M	38	chronic alcoholism (emotionally unstable)	220	1¾	4	U
38	M	38	drug addiction	310	2½	4	U
			PSYCHOPHYSIOLOGIC DISORDERS				
39	F	41	Gastrointestinal Reaction (ulcerative colitis, post-op.)	485	3	4	G*
40	F	32	Gastrointestinal Reaction (mucous colitis)	261	1½	4	S
41	M	35	Gastrointestinal Reaction (peptic ulcer)	302	2	3	G
42	M	32	Cardiovascular Reaction (hypertension)	298	2 1/3	3	M
			PSYCHONEUROTIC DISORDERS				
43	F	24	Anxiety Reaction	314	2	4	G
44	F	36	Obsessive Compulsive Reaction	265	3	3	U

*Still in treatment
oTwo analyses

TABLE II

Number of Patients	Diagnostic Category	Range Number of Sessions	Average			Sessions per Week	Results in Percent			
			Age	Number of Sessions	Years in Therapy		G	M	S	U
44	a. all diagnoses	153-1350	32	424	3.3	3.4	14 / 41	27	16 / 59	53
7	b. schizophrenia, schizoid and paranoid personalities	153-1180	31	571	3.9	3.8	0 / 0	0	14 / 100	86
5	c. male homosexuality and addiction	220-595	35	357	2.7	3.8	0 / 0	0	0 / 100	100
12	d. categories b and c combined	153-1180	32	482	3.4	3.8	0 / 0	0	8 / 100	92
27	e. all diagnoses except schizophrenia, schizoid and paranoid personalities	302-1350	32	471	3.6	3.3	18 / 48	30	19 / 52	33
10	f. all diagnoses except schizophrenia, schizoid and paranoid personalities	194-298	34	236	2.1	3.2	10 / 50	40	10 / 50	40
37	g. categories e and f combined	194-1350	33	407	3.2	3.3	16 / 49	33	16 / 51	35
23	h. all diagnoses except schizophrenia, schizoid and paranoid personality, male homosexuality and addiction	302-1350	31	484	3.7	3.3	21 / 56	35	22 / 44	22
9	i. all diagnoses except schizophrenia, schizoid and paranoid personality; male homosexuality and addiction	194-298	34	238	2.1	3.1	11 / 55	44	11 / 45	33
32	k. categories h and i combined	194-1350	32	415	3.3	3.2	19 / 56	37	19 / 44	25

clinical grades which are commonly used in medical statistics. In order to obviate controversy I avoided the term "recovered". The criterion "Greatly improved" (G) was a close runner-up which, together with the following "Moderately improved" (M), may for clarification of statistical survey be considered as one group. The remaining two may also be treated as one, since the degree of the "Slight improvement" (S) was a mere shade above the "Unimproved" (U). Improvement was measured by the degree of lasting amelioration of symptoms through the emotional recognition and control of impulses and the ability to "work and love" at an optimal psychoeconomic level.* The popular and sometimes professional claim that every person benefits from the unique experience of psychoanalysis educationally and/or emotionally was not admitted as too vague and nonspecific. The diagnostic terminology complied with the standard nomenclature of Mental Disorders adopted by the American Psychiatric Association.[3] A standard or nonstandard descriptive adjective was occasionally added in parenthesis.

Table 1 provides statistical data about each patient. At the same time groups were established according to diagnoses and total number of treatment hours. The averages of each group singly and in certain combinations were listed in table 2. Thus I obtained an improvement curve which rose on a percentage scale from zero for the combined groups of schizophrenia, schizoid and paranoid personalities, male homosexuality and addiction (category d) to an intermediate level of 41 per cent comprising all diagnoses (category a) and reached its peak of 56 per cent for category k which included only the symptom and character-neuroses under exclusion of the mentioned zero categories.

I must confess that I find these results confusing and disturbing. My greatest effort in time and energy was spent for the unsuccessfully treated groups of schizophrenic and borderline patients (see table 2). Was it I who failed or was it the patient who did not respond? The literature on the psychoanalytic treatment of schizophrenia contains a number of reports on individual cases who "improved", "adjusted", became "rehabilitated," "returned to the community," etc. Unfortunately, only one[19] of the sources presents a statistical balance sheet. I stress the need of statistics to assess the efficacy of psychotherapy in relation to the established baseline of 40 per cent[16] for spontaneous remissions. According to Scheflen[19] Rosen obtained improvement in four of eight patients treated

---

*With this stipulation we find ourselves in agreement with the five criteria suggested by Knight (12): "symptomatic improvement, increased productiveness, improved adjustment and pleasure in sex, improved inter-personal relationships, and ability to handle ordinary psychological conflicts and reasonable reality stresses".

with 'direct psychoanalysis'. Hoch[11] however, discredited these results, when he attributed improvement to reduction of "some of the anxiety which is behind the symptom" and when he declared "that very few of the numerous claims of cure in schizophrenia have stood up after five years."

I am now in the face of the available evidence compelled to the unpleasant conclusion that my psychoanalytic ministrations prevented the schizophrenic patients from improving spontaneously; or may I assume that this small group happened to include only ill fated cases? Is it permissible to infer from published case descriptions that probably most instances of so-called beneficial therapeutic intervention coincided with a spontaneous remission or improvement which received the psychodynamic halo *post hoc,* not *propter hoc?* Everyone who has had occasion to work in mental hospitals for a number of years knows that schizophrenic patients may improve all of a sudden whether they had cold or warm mothers, painful injections and visitors, total push or no push. It can be argued that psychoanalytic therapy may benefit many a patient who would not have improved otherwise. For convincing proof, however, the statistical burden rests on the claimant.

Whereas the foregoing might understandably induce a skeptic to ask with Auerbach[4] "can schizophrenia be cured by psychotherapy," a similar doubt concerning the analytic treatment of the neuroses would be considered outright blasphemy. And yet the observations from various quarters confront us with startling figures and disquieting perspectives. In a thorough search of the literature for the "Effects of Psychotherapy" Eysenck[6] computed improvement among 760 psychoanalytic cases published between 1920 and 1941 by Fenichel, Kessel and Wyman, Jones, Alexander and Knight, at 44 per cent and that of a tenfold number of eclectically treated patients between 1927 and 1951 at 64 per cent. Comparing these figures with his "baseline estimate of spontaneous remissions of 72 per cent," Eysenck concluded:

> ". . . (these data) fail to prove that psychotherapy, Freudian or otherwise, facilitates the recovery of neurotic patients. They show that roughly two-thirds of a group of neurotic patients will recover or improve to a marked extent within about two years of the onset of their illness, whether they are treated by means of psychotherapy or not. This figure appears to be remarkably stable from one investigation to another, regardless of type of patient treated, standard of recovery employed or method of therapy used."

Stevenson[22] in a recent paper contended similarly that according to several independent sources 40 to 60 per cent of neurotic patients enjoy spontaneous remission "within a few years of the first observation of their conditions." These studies seem to mock at our analytic treatment efforts, reducing them to an academic pastime at best and to an impediment of spontaneous recovery at worst. It appears, however, that definite justification of our endeavours accrues from the observation that in the majority of our cases the neurotic discomfort had prevailed much longer than "two" or a "few" years, which according to Eysenck and Stevenson were required for the spontaneous abatement of the illness. I can affirm *that treatment and improvement were more than coincidental in most of my successfully treated patients since there had been ample time for spontaneous improvement before treatment was begun.* I cannot deny however,—and here we approach the crucial question of the therapeutic process—that consistent with Stevenson's report[22] fortuitous circumstances and life situations facilitated salutary behavioral responses in many a patient. Not only did the average treatment duration of 3.3 years allow for the occurrence of a good many desensitizing and supporting events; this span of time also offered the opportunity for growing maturity and integration.

The Therapeutic Process

What else beyond time and circumstance may have therapeutic import? We do not know precisely and as long as we do not have the answer we do well to be reminded of the question. At this point we believe that psychotherapeutic interaction with our patients draws on three sources:

(1) *The Intellectual:* Traditional concept and treatment aim at freeing the patient from his compulsion to perceive the present in anachronistic terms; relevant interpretations and confrontations attempt to substitute Ego for Id and mobilize adaptation potentials.

(2) *The Affective:* New orientation of appetitive and averse feelings is mediated through the transference and the countertransference.

(3) *The Moralistic Ethical:* As members of a society with a well defined behavioral code the patient fears, placates and emulates the analyst as the sentinel of that code. The analyst reinforces the social conscience indeed through his emphasis on impulse control and sublimation.

From the simultaneous presence of these modalities in the therapeutic situation arises the question of their proportionate influence on the patient. Our ignorance concerning this quantification is not necessarily related exclusively to intellectual insight, emotional catharsis, affective support or altered superego orientation.

Analysis of the transference into its various elements including emphasis on the attendant components of hope[16] and trust[21] proved adjuvant particularly as a spur to intensified scrutiny of the counter-transference. It was Zilboorg who, among others, punctured the myth of "lofty Olympian objectivity presumably heretofore attained by the training analysis," with the analyst's confession to "most of the variations of human frailties and psychological limitations.[23]

Countertransference reflections lent added significance to the question concerning the quantity of the analyst's permissible and/or desirable reaction to his patients' emotional behavior. If the therapeutic process can be defined as action of unknown amounts of reason, affect and ethics through equally undefinable amounts of learning and identification, the therapist must obviously make use of all factions to insure qualitative efficiency, but remain reserved to avoid quantitative blunder. Conversely, a segmented approach creates an artificial vacuum in place of the omitted vector. The analyst who by consistent silence and restraint intends to prevent emotional contamination of the operational field may effect exactly the opposite. The patient may interpret—and not always incorrectly—the analyst's attitude as lethargy, as hostility, as lack of understanding, etc. Only adaptable therapy, brief or extended, can provide the opportunity for corrective intellectual, emotional and ethical experience.[1]

Since analytic therapy is primarily attitudinal in scope, and since the personality of the analyst influences and shapes the face of the analysis, objective norms are but the basic framework to contain the therapist's intuition. Compared with the orderly sequence of a surgical operation, psychoanalysis is a complex procedure. The textbook's phallic, anal and oral chapters and the triple stratification of the personality do not come forth with sectional simplicity but present themselves in obstinate fusion. There is no organized peeling of layers, penetration of structures or repair of mechanisms. There is no uniform routine. At this juncture there is only and must prevail an intuitive ("gifted") appraisal of and disciplined response to emotional, moral and cognitive forces. This regrettable dearth of technical precision cannot be substituted by dogmatic rituals of time and silence. Procedural modifications accrue as a resultant from the analyst's personality and the patient's symptoms. They are as unpredictable as the ultimate prognosis. We accept patients for therapy mainly by more or less educated hunches and embarrassingly often have to revise our initial impressions about their Ego strength, pliability, motivation, and projected treatment time on purely empiric grounds. I recall a number of patients who for various reasons could not follow my urgent advice to continue analysis, and who after 60 or 80 sessions had shown a degree of lasting improvement that any analyst would have gladly and proudly credited to a labor of four or five hundred hours. Conversely I had to intensify treatment to traditional proportions in a comparable number of cases whom I had considered ideal candidates for brief psychotherapy. Posttherapeutic comparisons and evaluations failed likewise to issue reliably guiding criteria for subsequent therapeutic indications and forecasts.

OUTLOOK

As physicians, analysts cannot possibly object to the selective application of so promising a method as brief psychoanalytic psychotherapy with its many advantages over a cumbersome and expensive analytical course. The statistical momentum of modified analytic procedures is still an unknown potential which may reach fuller capacity if and when the intricacies of the therapeutic process are better understood and more incisively administered.[14]

Considering the present therapeutic yield, we can ill afford to turn inert and contemptuous backs on challenging news and overlook technical facilities which might extend therapeutic amenability to now refractory cases. In this respect recent neurobiologic observations may transcend mere academic significance. The localization of numerous pleasure and pain foci in the brains of animals and humans[5, 9, 15, 17, 20] and the issue of memories upon electrodal stimulation[18] may, with future refinement of tools and methods, add topographic accuracy and detailed quantification to the psychiatric and psychoanalytic armamentarium.

A comparable approach may develop from the future use of new drugs which selectively stimulate pleasure systems, blockade pain centers and facilitate recall. Kubie[13] encouraged the study of the effect of psychoactive drugs on conscious and unconscious processes including repression, free association, the transference and others "in the course of psychotherapy of the neuroses and the psychoses, in the private office, in the outpatient department and in the psychiatric hospitals". Undesirable transference complications may actually be turned into therapeutic assets by the vigilant research therapist. Such a blend of the mechanical with the intuitive would bear out Freud when he proclaimed in his last work: "The future may teach us how to exercise a direct influence, by means of particular chemical substances, upon the amounts of energy of the mind. It may be that there are other undreamed-of possibilities of therapy."[8]

Résumé

Our statistical survey including the singularly poor results with schizophrenics, schizoid and paranoid personalities, male homosexuals and addicts adds an uncomfortable question mark to the title of this paper. The answer: Abstaining from ambitious expansiveness and restricted to the psychoneuroses and certain personality disorders, analysis benefits approximately one-half of the cases treated. The long duration of illness prior to treatment exempts these results from spontaneous remissions, but does not detract from the healing power of time and fortuitous circumstances enjoined by the catalytic function of the therapeutic process. The intellectual, affective and ethical forces of that process still depend on the intuitive deployment by the therapist and should not be isolated a priori.

Favorable results with brief analytic therapy have convinced many and should have taught all analysts that analysis is not the exclusive treatment of choice even under the most auspicious conditions. Mass-empirical evaluation must replace guess work and chance as the only presently available indicators. The concern for transference implications can do more harm than a liberal, experimental approach might do good. Drugs, words and electronics will perhaps accelerate the treatment pace, place the analyst in a promising research position and brighten pessimistic clinical prognoses.

REFERENCES

1. ALEXANDER, F., AND FRENCH, T. M.: Psychoanalytic Therapy, New York, The Ronald Press Co., 1946.
2. ALTSCHULE, M. D.: Drug action and psychological function. J. Neuropsychiat. 2:71-74, 1960.
3. American Psychiatric Association: Diagnostic and Statistical Manual: Mental Disorders. Washington, D.C. Committee on Nomenclature and Statistics, American Psychiatric Association, Mental Hospital Service, 1952.
4. Auerbach, A.: A survey of selected literature of psychotherapy of schizophrenia. Appendix 'A' to Scheflen, A. E.: A Psychotherapy of Schizophrenia. Springfield, Charles C. Thomas, 1961.
5. DELGADO, J. M. R. AND HAMLIN, H.: Spontaneous and evoked electrical seizures in animals and humans. In: Electrical Studies on the Unanesthetized Brain, E. R. Ramey and D. S. O'Doherty, eds. New York, Paul B. Hoeber, Inc. (Medical Division of Harper and Brothers), pp. 133-158, 1960.
6. EYSENCK, H. J.: Handbook of Abnormal Psychology. New York, Basic Books, Inc., 1961.
7. FRENCH, T. M.: The Integration of Behavior. Chicago, Univ. of Chicago Press, 1952.

8. FREUD, S.: An Outline of Psychoanalysis. New York, W. W. Norton and Co., Inc., 1949.

9. HEATH, R. S. AND MICKLE, W. H.: Evaluation of seven years' experience with depth electrode studies in human patients. In Electrical Studies on the Unanesthetized Brain, E. R. Ramey and D. S. O'Doherty, eds. New York, Paul Hoeber, Inc. (Medical Division of Harper and Brothers), pp. 214-247, 1960.

10. HEILBRUNN, G.: The Neurobiologic Aspect of Three Psychoanalytic Concepts. Comp. Psychiat. (To be published).

11. HOCH, P. H.: In A Survey of Selected Literature on Psychotherapy of Schizophrenia. Appendix 'A' To A. E. Scheflen, A. Auerbach. Springfield, Charles C. Thomas, 1961.

12. KNIGHT, R. P.: Evaluation of the results of psychoanalytic therapy. Am. J. Psychiat. 98:434-446, 1941.

13. KUBIE, L.: A psychoanalytic approach to the pharmacology of psychological processes. In Drugs and Behavior, L. Uhr and J. G. Miller, eds., New York, John Wiley and Sons, pp. 209-224, 1960.

14. LEVY, N. A.: An investigation into the nature of psychotherapeutic process: A Preliminary Report. In Science and Psychoanalysis, vol. IV, J. Masserman, ed. New York, Grune and Stratton, pp. 125-149, 1960.

15. LILLY, J. C.: The Psychophysiological Basis for Two Kinds of Instincts. J. Am. Psychoanal. Assn. 8:659-670, 1960.

16. NOYES, A. P. AND KOLB, L. C.: Modern Clinical Psychiatry. Philadelphia, W. S. Saunders, Co., pg. 417, 1959.

17. OLDS, J.: Differentiation of reward systems in the brain by self-stimulation technique. In Electrical Studies on the Unanesthetized Brain, E. R. Ramey and D. S. O'Doherty eds. New York, Paul Hoeber, Inc., Medical Division of Harper and Brothers, pp. 17-51, 1960.

18. PENFIELD, W.: The role of the temporal cortex in recall of past experience and interpretation of the present. In Ciba Foundation Symposium on the Neurological Basis of Behavior. Boston, Little, Brown and Co., pp. 149-174, 1958.

19. SCHEFLEN, A. E.: A Psychotherapy of Schizophrenia. Springfield, Charles C. Thomas, 1961.

20. SEM-JACOBSEN, C. W. AND TORKILDSEN, A.: Depth recording and electrical stimulation in the human brain. In Electrical Studies on the Unanesthetized Brain, E. R. Ramey and D. S. O'Doherty, eds. New York, Paul Hoeber, Inc. (Medical Division of Harper and Brothers), pp. 275-290, 1960.

21. SILVERBERG, W. V.: An experiential theory of the process of psychoanalytic therapy. In Science and Psychoanalysis, vol. IV, J. Masserman, ed. New York, Grune and Stratton, pp. 158-171, 1961.

22. STEVENSON, I.: Processes of "spontaneous" recovery from the psychoneuroses. Am. J. Psychiat. 117:1057-1064, 1961.

23. ZILLBOORG, G.: Emotional engagement of patient and analyst. In Science and Psychoanalysis, vol. IV, J. Masserman, ed. New York, Grune and Stratton, pp. 260-270, 1960.

Existential Psychotherapy

by THOMAS HORA, M.D.

BASIC PRINCIPLES

IN HIS 1961 address to the plenary session of the third World Congress of Psychiatry, Jules Masserman* pointed out that anxiety in man is centered around three major concerns: First, his physical integrity; second, his social integration; and third, whether he may be nothing more than a "cosmic triviality."

Existentialism emphasizes the importance of this third concern and points to the fact that it is exactly the capacity for such concern which particularly distinguishes man from all other living creatures. Therefore any attempt at understanding man must of necessity take this special "gift" of human consciousness into consideration.

Existential psychotherapy therefore views man primarily from an *ontic perspective*.[1] It considers man's harmony or disharmony with existence as of primary significance and views pathology as a manifestation and consequence of man's failure to be that which he truly is.

Since the objective of existential psychotherapy is the *"dis-covery" of the authentic individual*,[2] it follows quite understandably that the primary qualification of the psychotherapist must be his own freedom from artificiality, technicity and preconceived theoretic dogmatisms. (Including existentialism as mere philosophy.)

This does not mean that he must be uninformed and untrained. To the contrary, he must be so familiar with most schools of thought as to remain unhampered by a tendency to cling to any particular frame of reference for a subjective sense of comfort, security and guidance. It can be said therefore that existential psychotherapy requires freedom from technical concerns. (Somewhat like a good musician might be while playing, say, Bach.) *Transcendence of the need for technique* makes it possible for a genuine encounter to occur between doctor and patient.

---

*This address (cf. Current Psychiatric Therapies *1*:216-218, 1961) also contained a critical review of phenomenologic-existential concepts—ED.

Encounter is a special feature of the doctor–patient relationship in existential psychotherapy. Its essential spontaneity and lack of structuring makes it possible for the patient to reveal his mode of being-in-the-world without premeditation or interference on the part of the physician. The physician in turn, being free of the encumbrances which theoretical and technologic considerations tend to pose, is enabled to perceive "what really is" phenomenologically. Having thus perceived that which reveals itself, he is able to "shed light" on it.

This activity is not so much interpretative as *phenomenologically eluci-dating* (phaos = light, apophansis = statement, language).

The perspective of the existential psychotherapist is neither objective nor subjective, neither personal nor interpersonal. It is rather *trans-personal.*[3] This requires a capacity for cognitive transcendence to be realized both by the therapist and patient.

Cognitive transcendence means that the therapist's and patient's concern is with the truth as it reveals itself *through man.* For *man does not produce truth, he manifests it and is defined by it.*

The capacity for cognitive transcendence is realized through a process of *freeing the mind of its epistemic prison.* Which means that the liberation of consciousness from ingrained categories of thought becomes an important aspect of the existential therapeutic process.

In the course of existential psychotherapy patient and doctor partake again and again in the experiential realization that truth liberates, understanding (i.e. seeing) transforms and love heals. Consequently, the essential concerns of the doctor and patient are: *understanding (i.e. seeing) of truth as it emerges within a climate of love.*

Significantly enough, patients initially find it most difficult to be truly concerned with the above aspects of life, even though they quite readily pay lip service to them. Tacitly, however, they tend to consider these issues idealistic and somewhat irrelevant to practical existence, well being and mental health.

However, in the course of the therapeutic process it becomes quite evident that love, understanding and truth are fundamental and essential issues of existence because the unfolding and realization of human potentialities hinges upon them. The loving state of consciousness enables the mind to realize its optimum cognitive potentialities. Understanding makes it possible for man to commune meaningfully with his fellow man. Truth in turn liberates man from his past and makes him fully available for the present.

From what has been said until now it may be justly deduced that

existential psychotherapy is neither causalistic, historical, genetic, etio-
logic nor teleological. It is mainly *epistemologic*[4] in its focus. Which
means that it seeks to benefit man through the optimal unfoldment of his
cognitive capacities.

In the course of this therapeutic process the historical, causal, genetic
and teleologic aspects of individual human existences tend to emerge
into consciousness spontaneously and are taken cognizance of implicitly
rather than explicitly.

> "On ne guérit pas en se souvenant
> mais on se souvient en guérissant."
> (One does not heal by remembering
> but one remembers as a result of healing.)

As mentioned above, existential psychotherapy is viewed as a *process
of cognitive unfoldment.* Aspects of the patient's authentic individuality
which are hidden, covered up, obstructed, undeveloped become gradually unveiled, liberated from the fog of pretensions.

For everyday life proceeds largely in the realm of inventions; that is,
everyday life is not really lived but "conducted" along routine preconceived lines and assumptions of what "should be" and what "should not
be." Mental assumptions tend to become more important than reality
and human consciousness tends to be hampered by them in its cognitive
function. The process of dis-covering the authentic being consists of uncovering, *dispelling the "inventions"* which mask and cover the truth of
what really is.

The existential therapist's characteristic attitude expresses the principle
of "letting-be." (Not to be confused with leaving alone.) *Letting-be*[5]
is the open-minded wakeful receptivity to that which reveals itself without interference.

It is the manifestation of *reverence and love* in the process of paying
attention to understand the truth of what really is from moment to
moment. Letting-be may seem trivial, yet it is actually the most difficult
aspect of existential psychotherapy, as most trainees will readily admit.
While leaving alone is an interpersonal act, "letting-be" is neither an
act nor interpersonal. It is a state of consciousness.

Wakeful receptivity is a mode of human functioning which eludes
both the categories of activity and passivity. It is neither active nor
passive. Wakeful receptivity is the precondition for understanding to
happen. For understanding cannot be produced.

Understanding is a cognitive event. That which is understood needs
no interpretation. It speaks for itself. Human suffering and despair are
mostly conditioned by deficiences in man's capacity to understand. The

discovery of the true nature of understanding often relieves man of his tragic inclination to pride himself arrogantly on discursive knowledge, and to confuse explanations or interpretations with true understanding. The very understanding of the nature of understanding tends to transform man and make him more humble. The "open mind" is attained through the experiencing of the closed mind. The open-minded wakeful receptivity to the truth as it reveals itself in the encounter between therapist and patient proceeds in the here and now of the *absolute present*.

For most patients, however, the present is to a great extent but a reverberation of the past, for they tend to be time-bound. To be the "captive of time," i.e. to have a problem of *temporality* means to be hampered in one's freedom to respond to what truly is because of the habit of evaluating the present in the light of the past and the conjectured future. For most patients the words of Ecclesiastes (3:15) have much validity:

> "That which hath been is now,
> and that which is to be hath already been."

For the therapist in turn, the final sentence of the same quotation carries the therapeutic message:

> "And God requireth that which is past."

To be free and in harmony with the flux of life, man must cease clutching at the past. He must become open, receptive and fully *responsive (responsible) to the present*.

Since ontology views man as a "translucent medium of Existence,"[6] there follows one basic and essential difference in its definition of the summum bonum, the optimal good. Whereas the prevailing concern of our culture is with man's successful "functioning" in order to master the world (through conquest), the existential view is that man can become complete (whole—holy—healed) only by finding a way to live in reverent, loving harmony, i.e. *at-one-ment with the world* of which he is inescapably a part.

Consequently, the prevailing concern of existentialism is the realization of the *loving mode of being-in-the-world*. The realization of at-one-ment and love as a mode of being-in-the-world tends to relieve man from problems of *spatiality*. The term spatiality is related to the fact that the subject-object dichotomy requires human consciousness to take into account space as an existential coordinate. Consequently, spatial aspects of life situations may at times assume problematic character, as in agoraphobia, in some compulsion neuroses, or psychotic distortions of body-image and space perception, etc.

The reader may at this point ask: And what about transference, counter-transference, resistance, dream interpretation, libido, psycho-sexual development, unconscious conflict? What about nosology and differential diagnosis, psychodynamics, symbolism, genital primacy? What about psychic mechanisms, infantile amnesia, ego psychology, archetypes, conditioned reflexes? What about neurophysiology, psychopharmacology, etc.?

The answer concerning these questions is that while the sum total of part phenomena never adds up to a whole, and while the whole of man can never be understood in parts, nevertheless the thorough study of the part aspects of man seems warranted and necessary. Existential psycho-therapy does not reject the part phenomena. Interestingly enough, when viewed in the broader context of Existence, these phenomena tend to assume new and somewhat different meanings. In actual therapeutic practice, however, they seldom require explicit utilization. As far as the patient is concerned, the therapeutic process is a *holistic and primarily epistemological—existential experience.*

The realization of harmony with Existence, i.e. *ontic integration* does not fail to be reflected in favorable social adaptability as well as improved organismic-biological function. Healing is a manifestation of Existence. *Medicus curat, Natura sanat.* The physician treats, but Nature heals.

The Therapeutic Process

The psychotherapeutic session is a segment of life. Life is an event in time. Existence is manifested through man somewhat like light which becomes visible while passing through a translucent medium. Man partakes in existence. He does not cause it to be. Should he, however, fancy himself as the "maker" or "master" of existence, he will invariably run into conflict with the fundamental order of things. He will find himself in disharmony with the ontologic conditions of existence.

Thinking in terms of "techniques" of psychotherapy or of "doing" psychotherapy poses a similar problem, for it fails to take into considera-tion the fact that existence is an *event.* The idea of "managing" or "handling" cases in psychotherapy represents an objectification which violates the essence of man as an existential phenomenon. Since man is never just a "case", psychotherapy—strictly speaking—cannot be "done."

Psychotherapy, as life itself, is an event in time. It is a process. In the psychotherapeutic situation, as in all human encounters, patients appear not only as samples of various psychic mechanisms or disease entities but, above and beyond that, as people with specific ways of experiencing and cognizing life, specific ways of responding to stimuli, and specific ways of responding to deep stirrings of inner potentialities which demand realization within a *limited but unknown time span.*[7]

The event of the existential encounter however, as already mentioned above, is phenomenologically characterized by a *transcendence* of the temporo-spatial coordinates of existence.[8] Which means that in the existential encounter itself the experience of the passage of time and the awareness of separation between subject and object are absent.

Phenomena are manifestations of existence. Man's awareness of the phenomena is obscured and limited by his strivings to impose his will upon what is. The pursuit of what "should be" tends to make man unaware of the phenomena as they occur. Therefore, a therapeutic process cannot be conducted, intended, managed; it must be *allowed to occur.*

The essence of existential communication[9] lies in its nonteleological character. In the light of this the concept "free association" reveals itself to us as a misnomer containing a double contradiction. First, it is not free because it is *intended* to be free; second, it is not free because it serves a *purpose.*

To understand himself man needs to be understood. By being understood he learns to understand. When two people share in understanding, they experience *communion.* Communion is that union which makes differentiation possible. Man becomes an individual through participation. By losing himself in participation, he finds himself as a Presence. For individuals are wholly similar and wholly different at the same time —just as mosaic pictures may contain similar stone fragments but be entirely different in their overall design.

In the moment of being understood patients experience communion, that is, they experience a release from *epistemic isolation.* The subject–object dichotomy between patient and therapist melts away. This is in marked contradistinction to being given an interpretation which is often experienced as an accusation, an attack, or even condemnation.

When striving and intending are recognized as self-defeating therapeutic attitudes, there is a tendency to conclude that passivity might be a desirable one. This, however, is a mistake since striving to be active and striving to be passive are the same. This points up the futility of the perennial disputations between the so-called active therapists and the adherents to the traditionally passive approaches. The issue is neither activity nor passivity, neither directiveness nor non-directiveness but *awareness,* that is, being in a *condition of wakeful receptivity and responsiveness to the phenomena.* This condition of being is vitiated by striving and intending, evaluating, judging, categorizing, pigeonholing into conceptual schemes and psychodynamic patterns. Freud, interestingly enough, wrote about this problem quite clearly:[10]

> "For as soon as attention is deliberately concentrated in a certain degree, one begins to select from the material before one; one point will be fixed in mind with particular clearness and some other consequently disregarded, and in this selection one's expectations or inclinations will be followed. This is just what must not be done, however; if one's expectations are followed in this selection there is danger of never finding anything but what is already known, and if one follows one's inclinations anything which is to be perceived will most certainly be falsified."

Freud recommended the attitude of "free floating attention." It is of great significance that his recommendation was interpreted as passivity. This is easily understood, however, if we consider our propensity to dualistic thinking.

Heidegger speaks of "letting-be." He describes letting-be as a relationship in which all that is can reveal itself in the essence of its being. *Essence* is the inner potentiality of something existing. *Truth* can only reveal itself under conditions of freedom. *Freedom* is letting-be; therefore, *the essence of truth is freedom.*[11]

Letting-be must not be mistaken for quietism, passivity, nondirectiveness or leaving alone. The concept of letting-be means affirmation of the existence of another person. It connotes an attitude which favors the free emergence of the inherent creative potentialities of all. Letting-be expresses a therapeutic attitude of the highest ethical order inasmuch as it refrains from treating the patient as an object of exploration and manipulation, but relates itself to the patient as an *existent* in an affirmative and perceptive way. Affirmation of a person's freedom to be what he is, is an act of love. Love is reverence. Being with a person in the spirit of letting-be makes it possible to comprehend this person in a transjective, that is, experiential way. The experience of being thus understood is therapeutically beneficial in itself.

The existential psychotherapist does not try to "do" psychotherapy, *he lives it.* He meets his patient in the *openness* of an interhuman existential encounter. He does not seek to make interpretations, he does not evaluate and judge; *he allows what is to be, so that it can reveal itself in the essence of its being, and proceeds to elucidate what he understood.* In contrast to the interpretative approach this is a "hermeneutic," that is, clarifying mode of *being with* a patient (Binswanger[12]).

Nonevaluative awareness of what is leads to an understanding of the patient's mode of being-in-the-world with an elucidation of the implications for his existence. Complete understanding of one's mode of being tends to bring about a shift in world view, that is, a changed attitude toward life. Change occurs the moment man can see the totality of his situation. *Change is the result of expanding consciousness.* It is to be emphasized that contrary to general belief, man cannot change himself. Change happens to man. Darkness cannot be removed from a room. It vanishes when light enters.

It seems therefore useless to claim or to aspire to cure patients. Healing occurs through a meaningful shift in the world view of an individual, brought about through genuine understanding of the structure of his existence. As already mentioned, understanding is an event which happens in the openness of the existential encounter. Understanding is a modality of cognition which constitutes the essence of love. *This love is a condition of being in the presence of which constructive events have the freedom to occur.*[13]

Thus the existential psychotherapeutic process can be described as a meeting of two or more beings in openness and wakeful receptivity to *what is,* leading to a *broadening of consciousness* through revealment of that which hitherto has been obscured. The broadening of consciousness and capacity to see what is, bring man into harmony with life. Personality integration becomes an expression of ontic integration.[14]

The existential therapeutic action is neither operational nor explorative, nor reconstructive, nor interpretative, nor directive nor non-directive; it is experiential and hermeneutic, that is, clarifying. Since it is *phenomenological-transcendental,* that is, since the mode of cognition is such that the subject-object dichotomy is transcended, the so-called psychic mechanisms of transference, countertransference, projection, introjection, identification, resistance, empathy, etc. lose much of their significance. The patient participates as a total human being, not as ego, id and super-ego. He is an existent in encounter with an other. His relationship with the therapist is expressed by Buber[15] as "mutual spiritual inclusion," as "intersubjectivity," by Marcel[16] by Heidegger[17] as "being-in-the-world-as-transcendence," and by Rogers[18] as "total presence," which he describes as total organismic sensitivity to the other person. From our standpoint, however, as mentioned above, the nature of the therapeutic relationship could best be characterized as *transpersonal.*

The therapeutic process moves in the temporality which is absolutely real and that is the eternal present. The present contains the past. The proper elucidation of the present reveals the past. This, however, is only a by-product and is of secondary significance.

The capacity to be aware of the experiential impact of the environment upon one and vice versa tends to open up *a dimension of consciousness* which leads to a growing understanding of one's own structure of being-in-this-world or failing to be-in-this-world because of various defensive attitudes and strivings. As one patient put it: "I can feel myself standing in my own way. I understand how isolated and lonely I am."

The experiential awareness of one's own defensiveness converts the meaning of the defenses from comfort to obstacle and impediment. The moment one experiences one's own defenses as impediments, they tend to fall away. The moment one experiences one's own strivings and avidity as sources of stress, anxiety and conflict, one becomes aware of their self-defeating nature.

The ontologic essence and existential meaning of a communication or dream are to be found primarily in the experiencing of its basic existential climate and only secondarily in its symbolic content. A young man reported the following dream:

"I was surrounded by wasps. I tried not to bother them in the hope that they might not bother me. I tried to remain as immobile as possible. When one wasp settled on my eyelid, I was seized with panic and didn't dare to move lest it would sting me through the lid and reach my eye (i.e., "I"). I felt in a real jam. Had I moved, I would have gotten stung. Had I not moved, I would have gotten stung anyway. The anxiety was unbearable. Just at the point where I couldn't stand it any longer, I woke up."

The elucidation of the meaning of this dream lead to a realization on the part of this patient that defensiveness is seldom warranted, whether it is active or passive. He concluded that the best solution is to wake up and understand that what we are mostly defending are our preconceptions, i.e. dreams about ourselves. Defending one's dream is just more dreaming.

One patient was so sensitive to coercive and demanding people that she habitually reacted to them with breathing difficulties, depressions and states of depersonalization.

Having understood her reactions to be of defensive character, she made a surprising remark: "I wish I were a glass window pane!" At first it was not clear what she meant. But from that day on she began to let-go of her defensivenes and began to allow coercive stimuli to pass through herself somewhat as light passes through a window pane. She remained perceptive of the nature of the stimuli, but having ceased to defend herself against them, became immune to them. Interestingly enough, some time later, when reminded of her strange remark, she said: "A window pane is really a good symbol for a human being. It is brittle, easily destroyed, yet enduring. Its function is to be translucent, to shed light. The cleaner it is the more invisible it is, and yet the more light it sheds. The dirtier it gets, the more "ego" it acquires; the more visible it becomes itself the less light it sheds."

Cognition and consciousness are fundamental criteria of mental health, and along with authenticity of being, they constitute the central issues in existential psychotherapy.

One patient whose prevailing attitude toward the therapist was provocatively hostile, having realized after a while the futility of his strivings, changed his attitude to a friendly, ingratiatingly cooperative one just to discover to his surprise that it made no difference in what manner he was striving "to get at his therapist." For as long as he was striving to be good or bad, to agree or disagree, to oppose or cooperate, he had a closed mind. His state of consciousness was such that his cognitive faculties were impaired.

In contradistinction to the traditional psychoanalytic interest in the content of unconscious motivation and its historical context, existential analysis points to the epistemological problem which arises as a result of the mind's tendency to attach itself to mental images and motivations in general. In other words, here the content of the mental preoccupation, or attachment, or striving is secondary. The primary issue is the disturbance of consciousness which results from it.

For as man is, so is his cognition; and as man's cognition is, so is he.[19]

BIBLIOGRAPHY

1. HORA, THOMAS: Ontic perspectives in psychoanalysis Am. J. Psychoanal. 19: (No. 2) 134-142, 1959.
2. BINSWANGER, LUDWIG: Der Mensch in der Psychiatrie Pfüllingen, Guenther Neske, 1957.
3. HORA, THOMAS: Transcendence and Healing, J. Existential Psychiat. 1: (No. 4) 501-511, 1961.
4. ———: Epistemological Aspects of Existence and Psychotherapy J. Indiv. Psychol. 15: (Nov.) 166-173, 1959.
5. HEIDEGGER, MARTIN: Gelassenheit. Pfüllingen, Guenther Neske, 1959.
6. ———: Sein und Zeit. Tübingen, Max Niemeyer Verlag, 1953.
7. MINKOWSKI, EUGÈNE: Le Temps Vécu. Paris, J.L.L. d'Artrey, 1953.
8. ———: Encounter and Dialogue. Paper read at the International Congress of Psychotherapy, Barcelona, 1958.
9. HORA, THOMAS: Existential Communication and Psychotherapy Psychoanal. 15: 1957.
10. FREUD, SIGMUND: Collected Papers, vol. 2. London, Hogarth Press, 1924.
11. HEIDEGGER, MARTIN: Existence and Being. Chicago, Regnery, 1949.

12. BINSWANGER, LUDWIG: Grundformen und Erkenntniss Menschlichen Daseins Zürich, Max Niehans Verlag, 1953.
13. HORA, THOMAS: Spiritual Love and Mental Health. Paper read at the World Congress of Mental Health, Paris, 1961.
14. ——: Ontic Integration. Paper read at the International Congress of Psychotherapy, Barcelona. 1958.
15. BUBER, MARTIN: Between Man and Man. Boston, Beacon Press, 1955.
16. MARCEL, GABRIEL: The Philosophy of Existence. London, Harvill, 1948.
17. HEIDEGGER, MARTIN: Sein und Zeit. Tübingen. Max Niemeyer Verlag, 1953.
18. ROGERS, CARL: Persons or Science? A Philosophical Question Am. J. Psychol., 1955.
19. HAAS, WILLIAM S.: The Destiny of the Mind. New York, Macmillan, 1956.

PART II

Child Psychotherapy

by Frederick H. Allen, M.D.

T HE BASIC characteristic of childhood is the dependency upon the parental figures from whom the child differentiates himself and emerges as a separate but related human being. Emotional problems emerge out of this growth process, even where the child has been organically damaged. Therapeutic efforts will be built on this foundation and our knowledge of the nature of the psychologic growth process will be incorporated into it.

Adult and child, acting on and reacting to each other, giving a living quality to this universal relation wherever the human drama unfolds. In its early phases the parent, usually the mother, is the giver, the child the taker. This is the dependency feature from which emerges the normal shifts as the child, who in using what is given, starts on the road to self development. This individuating process is always one of differentiation with other living or human beings. The *I* and the *You,* always separate and different, come into a functioning relation to each other.

Three basic movements emerge as parent and child interact on each other in this process: The first is the movement away from the maternal figure. Birth with biologic separation is a total separating event. Following this, the psychologic reunion with the maternal figure occurs as it is clear the child cannot live as a separate person. But the early moving away occurs as he becomes aware of being a person apart from the mothering figure. He can move about, he can manipulate objects, he can perceive the presence and absence of the giving person. He can do things on his own as he reaches out to satisfy his basic needs.

From this first movement emerges the second—the moving toward or the reuniting process—so essential because of the dependency element. The separating movement arouses anxiety in some degree. The child feels alone and the positive values of this feeling is that it motivates the second movement toward the object from which he feels separated. He discovers he is a separate person but wishes to reunite himself with the those upon whom he is dependent. This is beginning of the balance so essential in these two primary movements.

Early in this process emerges the third movement—the oppositional or the anti-movement. The child is not a passive organism and reacts against restrictions of his body movements, against delays which leave him hungry, etc. In fact, he reacts in varying degrees against the necessary organizational efforts of the adult. He learns also to yield and gradually balance is established.

So many if not all the behavioral problems, which necessitate therapeutic intervention, emerge as these three movements get out of balance and dilute the normal values of each in relation to the others. The unseparated child clinging to the mother, the remote and isolated child who has few rewards from his affectional relation to the parent, the rebel who asserts against the outer world—all represent an imbalance and a hiatus in the normal growth process. Anxieties beyond the capacity of the child to master becomes the dominant, emotional tone.

This preamble to a discussion of psychotherapy with children lays the foundation for a new and unique growth experience which therapy should provide. Building the structure on this sound understanding is essential. Child psychiatry, as this specialty has evolved, has become family centered with the focus of concern on an emotionally disturbed child. This has happened because the structure has been built both on understanding the nature of childhood and the dynamics of family interaction. The child is a dependent organism and needs the support of the adult figures as he moves in an unsteady way to becoming a person. He is vulnerable to stress, to parental uncertainties and anxiety. He is responding to his own internal needs. While striving for individuality the child at the same time discovers he is awakening in a world of other people who guide and influence the kind of individual he becomes. Here is the universal conflict between the need to maintain individuality and the need to become a related and social being. From this basic conflict arise many of the problems in the parent/child interaction that opens the need for psychotherapeutic intervention.

Psychotherapy with children has many unique characteristics. An important one is that a child does not initiate the process. He is impelled into this by significant adults, usually the parents, who are concerned about the child and who seek help. They open the therapeutic door and in doing so, discover the part they will need to play in sustaining what they have started.

Every parent, in making a tentative move to seek psychiatric help for a child, has some anxiety and doubt about this decision. In this first phase, they need help to bring their feelings into the period of planning with those who are providing help. This is the parent-centered phase and is designed to help the parents test out the validity of their first move. They must be aided to bring into the open their doubts and misgivings and to feel that the problem they describe in their child warrants going ahead with this plan. They learn the part they will need to take after the child is included and to discuss how they can prepare the child. The decision to go ahead may be made in this first interview, but in most instances the parents need time to digest what took place and to return for a second conference before the child is included.

Where the child lives with both father and mother, it is important that both participate in this first phase. The therapeutic process is then geared to the family realities and the role distortions among father, mother and child are more clearly defined and brought into the open. Fragmentation, so commonly found in families with an emotionally disturbed child, can be accentuated if the planning involves only one parent. For example, the mother may take the full responsibility for initiating the helping process on the assumption that the father has no interest or is even opposed to seeking psychiatric help. To proceed on such a basis can distort further the family drama and isolate the father from an experience which aims not just to help the child but to restore a balance in the family reality with the father, mother, and child finding new values in their interacting roles. Achieving this is the ultimate goal of psychotherapy with children.

An essential element in enlisting parents in a therapeutic program for a child must be based upon a positive foundation. Their participation in this program is needed not just because of their involvement in the child's emotional problem, but more because they are so important in helping the child to gain a new balance, both in himself and in his relation to them. They are the important persons in a child's world and need to feel this in a therapeutic program. While many may feel their job is completed by turning the child over to a psychiatrist, they must realize that they are needed to nourish what gains the therapist can bring about in the child. To isolate the child's experience from the day-to-day realities they provide would be a fairly sure way of minimizing those values and defeat the basic purpose of the experience to bring about a new family climate in which the child could grow.

This is the essence of the more positive approach to the parents. They come expecting to be blamed and are ready to defend themselves in one way or another. Many fathers stay away because this is their concept of clinical help. However, so many fathers enter the clinical program when they can feel they are needed. For many fathers this is a new concept, particularly in the many families where they have been kept on the side lines and allowed a minimal participation in the growing up of the child.

The fact that parents have asked for help is in itself evidence of some strength and responsibility, although this may be disguised by the many conflicted feelings parents have toward themselves and toward the child. The swirl of these feelings become focused around the fact that they are concerned enough about the child to ask for help. This is the starting point, and those who work with the parents must never lose sight of this fundamental fact.

Just as the growth process is one of differentiation with the emergence of the self pattern of the child, so the therapeutic process provides an unique growth experience for the child. In this unique setting, the child participates in a variety of ways: sometimes in silence, other times through verbal communication or through acting out his disturbed feelings. He may use available material to dramatize the nature of his emotional problems while, at the same time, telling his therapist how he feels about this new relation into which he has been impelled. Important content is brought out by the child as he begins to communicate. He reveals the nature of his anxiety and fears, his hostile feelings toward significant adults, his negative feelings, etc. Content and process come into a new relation to each other. The dichotomy between fact and feeling is also partially bridged in these early hours. For example, a fearful child may verbalize what he is afraid of—this is fact—but in the process of revealing, he is being helped to have a beginning experience in mastering the fear engendered by being propelled in a new experience. What he reveals and the new opportunity provided by the therapist, provide the dynamic that gives the therapeutic potential.

Throughout, a child creates its own realities not unlike those of everyday life against which he may be reacting. He has his regular time with the same psychiatrist, limited to an hour and adhered to. The child may seek to control these boundaries and his aggressive reactions bring out both feelings and action. He meets limits on action but has complete freedom to express his feelings. He can use available material but he is not allowed to destroy it. These limits are not for restrictive purposes but more to define the boundaries. They have dynamic values in that the child's efforts to control bring out much of this feeling. He has the opportunity both to assert and yield, and to use and feel the strength of his therapist who stands steady in face of the child's swirling conflicts.

Phases of Therapy

Psychotherapy with a child has three phases, all interwoven but having fairly well defined characteristics: the beginning phase, the reorganizational phase, and the ending phase. Throughout each, the three basic movements described earlier are in evidence in this new and unique experience. These are the toward, the away, and the against directions. The differentiating process involved in each contains the dynamic and the impact of this new experience modifies the ongoing reality of the child in his family.

The Beginning Phase

Introducing the child into the plan is a recognition by all concerned that he has a part in creating his emotional disturbances. He is not regarded as a nonparticipating victim of external influences. He is not a pawn but a reactor, and can bring about change.

Children are prepared for this first visit in a variety of ways. With many, this is done sensitively and realistically by the parents; others come with inadequate or confused preparation. Irrespective of how this has been explained to the child, one element always is present: he is being exposed to a person who is going to help him. Every child organizes himself against being changed, although the oppositional direction is overtly acted out with some, and well disguised with others. He may move in almost totally, and thus neutralize the assumed power of this new force; or move away into a corner and refuse to communicate, or be openly hostile thus disguising his anxiety. He may state his problem with the assumption that this person will take over and correct the situation, or he may deny having any difficulty. In a variety of ways he reacts with his own feeling to this new experience and in reacting he is engaged in a beginning relation that has a potential for being helpful.

In this beginning phase important things happen both for the child and for the therapist. For the child, he finds a person interested in the way he feels, who helps him to express being afraid, hostile, withdrawn, etc. For the therapist, this beginning phase provides an important diagnostic opportunity. He sees the child as he is and not just the person described in a variety of ways by the parents. Here is a living entity. The therapist is able to get impressions about the degree of accessibility, what the child presents as his own problem, and the way he can express feeling engendered by this new experience. The therapist observes how the child leaves the parent to come with him and how he returns to the parent at the end of each session. In a variety of ways, the therapist gets a tentative diagnostic picture, while opening the door to a therapeutic journey which may follow.

In the early phases of the process, the child will perceive the therapist as he has other adults in his life—hostile, possessive, benevolent, etc. He will project on the therapist both what he expects, what he wishes, and what he fears him to be. The child will invest him with the magic to cure without having to do anything himself. The therapist will both allow and help the child to test out these preconceptions, but will maintain his own integrity and not become the projection. While the child tries to make him be the good or the bad parent, the therapist remains himself and thus provides a new, differentiating experience for the child.

From the beginning phase, with its diagnostic and therapeutic values, emerges a plan for sustaining what opens up in this period. This plan is based upon the physical condition of the child, the evaluative studies by the psychologist, the child's capacity to form a relation to the psychiatrist, and the parents' commitment to go ahead. All are factors in determining both the nature of the child's problem and the mode of proceeding. Important shifts in the family and in the child can be evaluated at this point and, in many instances, new directions are noted which are important determinants. In less severe cases, they acquire a new grip on the situation and decide to go on their own. But here we are concerned with the clearer indications that a more sustained process is needed and agreed upon.

The tempo of that which follows is geared both to the severity of the problem and what is realistically possible. In clinic practice, it is common to set up a plan for weekly appointments. More frequent interviews may be needed, but it is important that a definite schedule be agreed upon, with child and parents having separate and wherever possible concurrent appointments, since much of the family-centered emphasis gets clouded when the child comes at one time and the parents at a different time. The integrated plan of concurrent but separate interviews is more feasible in clinic practice where the team plan allows the parents to work with one staff person, usually the social worker, and the child with his therapist, usually the psychiatrist.

The primary emphasis throughout is on the experiential values of the relationships that unfold for the child and his parents. All three reveal a great deal of their troubled past but the process of revealing to those who symbolize a new direction, is the important element that brings them into the new and present. The therapist who is sensitive to the uses the child makes of him will be aware of signals that indicate the child is moving out and is approaching the final and in many ways the most important phase, the one of ending.

As indicated earlier, the uniqueness of this relationship is that it is begun with the goal of ending it. In the beginning, the child experiences anxiety about leaving the parent and embarking on a new and unknown course. In the final phases he frequently feels anxiety about leaving his therapist. Just as he struggles in one way or another the impact of the new experience, he will struggle in a variety of ways against its termination and resuming his day-to-day living without this specialized help. In the beginning, he has the experience of mastering this anxiety; in the end phase he has the same experience but with a new sense of values about himself. He learns that a change has taken place within himself and that he has been a participant in bringing this about. At the beginning, he projects on the therapist the power to change him. In the end phase, he has the opportunity to own his part in bringing about the change. As one ten year old girl said in her end phase, "At first, I thought you were going to cure me of my fears. Then I discovered I had to do something myself." She did.

Therapy for a child and his parents helps them to move away from a troubled past in which all have been caught. It can open the door to new values in which the important roles each must fulfill are more clearly interwoven. Where therapy has achieved this, the family becomes one in which each member has gained a new sense of individual values.

If therapy ends with this real quality, it has achieved its real. It will have been more than digging into the past, revealing the pains and struggles of a child's life. It will have been more than a mechanistic experience with emphasis on what was wrong. It will have been what all therapy should be: a meaningful human experience with a person who, from the beginning, was concerned with postive values and with providing an opportunity for a child and his parents to affirm them.

Educational Methods with Brain-Damaged Children

by JAMES J. GALLAGHER,* PH.D.

BACKGROUND

IN THE PYRAMIDING DEVELOPMENT of cognitive processes in childhood, a loss of a fundamental building block in the earlier years is liable to have important consequences in terms of failure of future abilities to develop normally. Much credit for stimulating interest in the problems of brain-injured children should go to such pioneers as Strauss, Lehtinen, Werner, Bender, and Kephart. The Strauss syndrome consists of *perceptual distortions* in which the child shows figure-ground problems, is unable to reproduce geometric designs or rotates and reverses the designs in space, and perseverates. These perceptual difficulties are combined with *conceptual lability* in which the youngsters seem to lack the necessary control to draw an effective boundary line around a concept. These aberrations in cognitive processes are often accompanied by *hyperactivity* and *distractibility*. However, there are many children with unmistakable neurological injury who do not show this syndrome and for whom special educational methods of a different sort need to be devised.

EDUCATIONAL DIAGNOSTIC INSTRUMENTS

Despite impressive gains made in neurology in recent years, the educational planning for the child must still be based upon its intellectual skills and behavioral traits rather than the particular organic injury. Table 1 lists some diagnostic instruments useful in such planning.

Despite the advances made in testing, some diagnostic questions seem to be settled best through methods that could be labelled *diagnostic teaching*. For example, if a child is having difficulty in using sounds as cues in reading, the teacher might present the child with some sound blending

---

*Institute for Research on Exceptional Children, University of Illinois

TABLE 1

Educational Diagnostic Tests for Organically Injured Children

Test	Task Involved	Disabilities Involved
Werner—Strauss Marble Board	Reproducing geometric patterns on a board with different colored marbles.	Perceptual orientation and approach. Perseveration.
Graham-Kendall designs Ellis figure designs	Reproduce, by memory or copying, various geometric figures.	Perceptual orientation and approach. Perseveration.
Syracuse Visual Figure Background Test	Tachistoscopic presentation of common objects embedded in a structured background.	Figure-ground problems.
Kephart Perceptual Survey Rating Scale	Extensive battery of a variety of perceptual motor tasks.	Identify most types of perceptual difficulties, particularly those relying on motor skills.
Illinois Test of Psycholinguistics	Nine subtest obtain information on ability to use Channels of communication (auditory, visual, motor, vocal); Levels of organization (Representative, Automatic); and Linguistic processes (Decoding-Association-Encoding)	Identify special problems in the development and use of language.

exercises. If the child seems to respond and learn quickly through this approach the sound blending lessons are expanded and made more complex. If the child balks or fails, then other sample lessons designed to attack the deficiency in a different way are tried until a proper avenue of approach is found.

SENSORY PROBLEMS

If there is a distinct impairment in the visual or auditory channels, then it is obvious that a certain amount of incoming data is going to be decoded incorrectly or not at all. Where it is not possible to correct one of these defects the method of training is the obvious one of channeling most of the tasks through the unimpaired sensory modality. For example, the child who is hard of hearing would be in serious difficulty if he were taught reading through the use of phonics, even if other children without a similar handicap might be doing very well under such instruction.

Set Problems

In some cases of brain-injured children, it has been observed that a considerable impairment has been suffered by the child's attention mechanism. Thus, the child is equally as receptive to the song of the bird outside of the window as he is to the book lying in front of him, or to his own thought processes. For example, a child asked to name all the articles of clothing he can think of may respond . . . "Shoe . . . my little sister

Table 2

Potential Difficulties Due to Organic Injury and Educational Methods to Meet Them

Area	Problems	Educational Methods
Sensory	Sensory Impairment (blindness, deafness)	Utilize sensory channel least impaired.
Set	a. Poor Attention Distractibility Hyperactivity b. Poor Motivation (Disinterest)	a. Reduce irrelevant sensory stimuli. Use teacher-pupil relationship to direct attention. b. Use "success" as an enhancer of self-concept and builder of interest
Decoding	a. Figure-ground differentiation b. Rotation and Orientation Problems	a. Emphasize cues separating figure from ground. Reduce distractive cues. b. Guide the child in proper direction with additional directional cues.
Integration	a. Language impoverishment b. Inaccurate or distorted	a. Introduce large numbers of verbal labels on items in which the child is familiar. b. Building of classes of relationships. Show the multitude of classes to which one object can belong
Encoding	a. Expressive speech problems b. Motor difficulties c. Perseveration	a. Remedial speech education. Encourage oral communication b. Remedial muscle training and exercise c. Introduce a variety of tasks to break the sequence or pattern.
Feedback	a. Inaccurate evaluation of own performance	a. Give tasks requiring self evaluation under close tutoring and direction. b. Urge child to verbalize his perceptions of self performance in training sequences.

has shoes . . . She had a birthday party . . . I will be six on my birthday . . . I want a bike for my birthday." The present author (1960) has suggested that, from an educational point of view "if the damage lies in the attentional system, then possible modifications of this system should bring quick perceptional learning. If the damage is in the associational networks, then other areas must take over the function of the damaged area and that is a slow and lengthy process."

If the problem is one of distractibility (Table 2), then the method of choice of handling the child is (1) to limit the stimulus value of the irrelevant environment or (2) to utilize the personal relationship with the teacher to have the child pay greater attention to his own performance. All unnecessary pictures and decorations in the classroom, including shiny and ornamental jewelry worn by the teacher may be removed, the windows in the classroom may be made semiopaque, and a screen may provide a more limited environment when necessary. Later, when rapport is better established, the teacher may ask the child to listen to his own performance and check himself when he gets off the track. A greater emphasis is now being placed on teacher methods to control distractibility, hyperactivity and excitability.

Effect of Prior Failure

By the time that the brain-injured child has become the object of special educational concern, he may already have had unfortunate educational experiences. Persistent failure usually brings about a withdrawal reaction on the part of the child. The attentive *set* so necessary to effective information processing has been disturbed. It is therefore important to avoid initial failure by arranging the lessons so that the child experiences a "bath of success" until he acquires confidence. The combination of task success and teacher approval can provide a source of satisfaction that sustains the child through the more difficult periods ahead when he must face frustration without destructive avoidance behavior.

Parents and teachers may extend a neurologist's statement that the brain damage is irreparable to the incorrect conclusion that the behavior caused by the injury *is also irreparable.* But a consistent, firm, and intelligent regime of training can turn a disorganized child of indifferent attention into a pliable and happy child who is eager to learn to the limits of his abilities, even though the basic neurological insult cannot be repaired.

DECODING PROBLEMS

One of the most useful of the information processing skills is the ability of normal individuals to focus attention on a central figure in a situation and to thrust irrelevant details into the background. While we usually think of the visual area when we discuss figure-ground problems, there seems to be analogous function in the auditory channel also. There is considerable research evidence to the effect that many brain-injured children do show disturbance in this area.

The preferred remedy is to aid the child in discriminating foreground from background stimuli by placing greater emphasis on the important figure. For example, if one sees a picture of two men against a pastoral scene, the normal individual will concentrate his attention upon the figures to such an extent that the picture becomes almost three dimensional in character, with the human beings in the foreground. The child who does not automatically see this differentiation can be aided by placing the important or foreground material in strong outline or in a different and striking color.

Orientation

Another important perceptual problem of some brain-injured children seems to be rotation and orientation difficulties, most evident in the reversal of numbers and letters. Although these problems occur in normal children around kindergarten or first-grade age, they seem to disappear rapidly with continued practice in the construction of these perceptual forms. However, brain-injured children must be guided by using additional directional cues. For example, if the child is continually producing a backward figure three, he can be presented with a series of dots that he is to connect to form a proper "3". It is necessary to supervise closely the child who has orientation problems so that the teacher can catch quickly any errors or mistakes the child is making and prevent the hardening of incorrect habits. Although such problems have often been considered decoding errors, new evidence suggests it may be more of a motor association difficulty.

CORTICAL INTEGRATION PROBLEMS

If an early brain injury results in a memory bank of distorted perceptual images, it is likely that the relationships that are identified during later scanning will come back as inaccurate or distorted, with predictable confusion and conceptual looseness. The general remedial planning as shown in table 2 is based upon two separate procedures. If language impoverishment seems to be the basic difficulty, the method of choice is to introduce large numbers of verbal labels for items in the child's environment with which he is already familiar. The second major area of concern in developing conceptual facility is the proper building of classes of relationships.

Some brain-injured children have difficulties seeing the perceptual boundaries as in the figure-ground problem, whereas others have trouble in seeing the boundaries of classes of concepts. If one asked a child to pick out objects from a number of pictures which had to do with transportation, the child might select a car, a horse, a train and a table!—thus showing a looseness of conceptualization and a blurring of conceptual boundaries. A large number of exercises of classification with the child identifying the essence of the concept can serve to emphasize the relationships in the child's memory. This, in turn, will cause the child to handle incoming information more effectively in the sense that it will now be associated with more clearly defined relationships through the integrative process.

Encoding Problems

These difficulties deal with the ability of the individual to communicate with others and are generally reduced to two major areas, as shown in table 2: *oral expression* and *motor performance*. In terms of oral difficulties, there may be problems involved in the speech mechanism itself or in the cortical areas which direct speech. If the latter is true, we have a condition of expressive aphasia, and the remedial techniques for this condition are complex and painfully slow. If the child has cortical injury in the expressive areas of speech, it might be more useful from an educational standpoint, in order to prevent the complete retardation of perceptual and conceptual development, to have his encoding activities concentrated in the motor sphere. Thus, the individual should express himself through writing, drawing, play-acting, etc. In the case where it is more a problem involving the speech mechanism itself, the educational method of treatment is to obtain some remedial speech training for the youngster and also to encourage oral communication as much as possible. This encouragement is particularly important since one of the standard reactions of children to speech problems is to become mute and to be unwilling to express themselves orally. This results in limited practice of language and delayed language development.

In the case of *motor difficulties* the youngster may obtain remedial muscle training and orthopedic exercises designed to strengthen the impaired limbs. Motor difficulties are educationally important since they interfere with perceptual-motor practice and the possible benefits that such practice together with the feedback process could produce.

Perseveration

This can be observed in children who, when asked to reproduce a series of numbers or letters, produce the first letter and continue on that letter without regard to the new stimulus. So also, a child fresh from aggressive play on the playground persist in such activity in the classroom. The educational method of choice, as indicated in Table 2, is to avoid presenting such a child with series or sequences of drill-like activities, but instead to introduce a variety of tasks, one of which follows quickly upon the other, in order to break up this reverberating circuit of behavior. One cannot stress too strongly the importance of having a very small group of children to deal with in order to counteract effectively some of the more difficult and pervasive perceptual-motor habits.

Feedback

In the process of completing a given task or exercise an individual has a large amount of sensory information fed back to him, concerning his own performance. The degree to which he is able to use this information to modify his performance is, to a large extent, his degree of adaptability. Thus, a child when asked to reproduce a triangle may start to reproduce it upside-down. His ability to look at the drawing and see that he is doing something wrong and then correct it would be one measure of the effectiveness of his feedback mechanism. Similarly, the ability to see the effects that one is having upon his surroundings and companions and to modify one's behavior accordingly is another indication of how effectively an individual is able to utilize his feedback mechanism. The problem most often encountered in using this mechanism is an inaccurate evaluation of self-performance. The individual will say, "Yes, I have done well," when the information returned to the individual by his own performance should clearly indicate that he has done poorly.

The educational methods utilized to handle such a problem involve setting the child tasks which require a certain amount of continuous self-evaluation under close supervision. One highly useful recommendation in this regard is to urge the child to verbalize his own perceptions of self-performance in a given training sequence. This serves the purpose of also controlling attention difficulties since the individual must maintain a constant attention in order to give a continuous verbal description of his performance.

The recent more generous influx of money for educational research has increased the probability that more effective educational procedures will be developed in the near future.

REFERENCES

BENDER, LAURETTA: Psychopathology of Children with Organic Brain-Disorders. Springfield, Ill., Charles C Thomas, 1956.

CAPOBIANCO, R. T., AND FUNK, RUTH: A comparative study of intellectual, neurological and perceptual processes as related to reading achievement of exogenous and endogenous retarded children. Syracuse, N. Y., Syracuse Univ. Res. Inst., 1958.

CRUICKSHANK, W. M., BENTZEN, FRANCES, RATZEBURG, F., AND TANNHAUSER, MIRIAM: Teaching Methods for Brain-Injured and Hyper-Active Children. Syracuse, N. Y., Syracuse Univ. Press, 1961.

GALLAGHER, J. J.: A comparison of brain injured and non-brain-injured mentally retarded children on several psychological variables. Soc. Res. Child. Developm. 3:1-79, 1957.

——: The Tutoring of Brain-Injured Mentally Retarded Children: An Experimental Study, Springfield, Ill., Charles C Thomas, 1960.

KEPHART, N. C.: The Slow Learner in the Classroom. Columbus, Ohio, Charles E. Merrill, 1960.

KIRK, S. A.: Early Education of the Mentally Retarded. Urbana, Ill., Univ. of Illinois Press, 1958.

STRAUSS, A. A. AND LEHTINEN, LAURA: Psychopathology and Education of the Brain-Injured Child. New York, Grune & Stratton, 1947.

——: AND KEPHART, N. C.: Psychopathology and Education of the Brain-Injured Child, vol. II. New York, Grune & Stratton, 1955.

The George Junior Republic

by ROBERT E. PITTENGER, M.D.

T HE BODY of knowledge and practice relating to adolescence has been
growing, and increasing attention has been paid to milieu or
environmental factors in treatment and in education. The George Junior
Republic serves as one point of convergence of these interests. The
Republic is a residential setting for teenage boys and girls with problems
of sufficient scope or magnitude to warrant the use of resources away from
home. This paper will present the concepts and practices which make it a
significant laboratory 1) for observing a long standing, extraordinary
milieu therapy program, 2) in which some psychiatric insights can be
contributed and applied and 3) where psychiatric influences on milieu and
educational training can be studied.

The Junior Republic is an educational community and residential treatment center which stresses student–patient responsibility. Founded
in 1895, from the outset it has been a community which provides the
teenager with all the problems and challenges of the ordinary community,
plus the unusual advantages of a specialized educational and treatment
program. It is housed in twenty-four scattered buildings on nine hundred
acres of open country in the Finger Lakes region of central New York
state. The staff of 97 full-time and 10 part-time employees serve 185 boys
and girls, from 13 to 21 years of age.

The Junior Republic is modeled on adult society. Its young "citizens"
have a degree of authority for the governing of their own conduct, and
of responsibility for their own maintenance,[1] which to our knowledge is
unparalleled in American child care homes, hospitals or schools or
in adult treatment centers.

Their codified laws have been passed at monthly town meetings,
presided over by their duly elected officials. The regulations of their
various governmental bureaus and departments are enforced through
their own police and through their highly sophisticated court system. In
this they have the support, as a matter of policy, of the members of

the staff, and they have also the support of traditions well established at the Junior Republic.

Most of the young "citizens" go to school for half a day and have work experience the other half.[2] They are paid in Republic currency in both areas, on a graduated scale, in keeping with the quality of their performance. It is with these earnings that they pay for services such as board and room, support their government through taxation, pay for luxuries (e.g., cigarettes and snack bar items) and "redeem" packages from home. They learn to live within the limitations they set for themselves. The token currency they use has for them the reality that U.S. money has for adults, for the consequences of their having or not having it are very real.

The young person admitted to the Junior Republic experiences three important shifts in focus:

(1) Because of the self-government, his rebellion, distrust or misunderstanding against authority shifts from adults to peers. He experiences the authority of contemporaries whom he has voted into office, and of laws which he has helped to pass in "town meetings." Thus, too, the adult becomes freer of the need to be *the* authority and can be the young person's ally, aid and counsel.

(2) The requirement that the young people earn what they need, besides teaching them the realistic meanings of money and of their own work for it, frees them from some of the cultural pressure to be ambivalently grateful for an unearned "dole" from parents. The economic system operates to provide intrinsic reenforcement for behavior which is socially acceptable in the community.[3]

(3) The Junior Republic, through all of the subinstitutions of which it is comprised, impels the young person to self study. In the cottage, on the job, in the group-constituted Magistrate's Court and elsewhere, the demand is made of the "citizen" that he take responsibility for his own performance; that is, that he understand it and that he act upon his sharpening self-assessments. He learns by doing and observing the effects of doing.

The young "citizens" are referred to the Republic because they had not functioned well, often from homes that did not foster growth and development. The Junior Republic excludes young people diagnosed as psychotic or as suffering from organic damage to the nervous system; the prospective young "citizen" must be sufficiently strong and well organized to permit him to use what the community has to offer. Beyond this, the Junior Republic throughout its history has welcomed and worked with young people with whom the ordinary community has not known how to deal or with whom the community has failed to deal— youngsters who have engaged in a broad range of socially unacceptable behavior, i.e., school failure, personality conflicts, truancy from home or school, auto theft, sexual deviation, withdrawal, etc. For those adolescents whose defensive postures have taken a form which is destructive to society and to themselves, the Junior Republic has provided more flexible, socially acceptable and individually rewarding methods for the young person for dealing with his problems.

After they come to the Republic of course many, indeed most, of the young people continue to misbehave to one degree or another. The Republic, in contrast to other institutions and communities, can absorb this behavior and still continue to work with the youngster. If, for instance, a boy cannot perform academically, he may for a while cease to attend classes (not possible in most schools) through the action of a guidance committee; but he will continue to be in and a part of the community, simply spending more time on the job than previously, the entire experience of the Republic being seen as educational. Or, a girl who misappropriates property belonging to cottage mates may be sentenced by the court of her peers to a term in government custody (which places the young citizen on certain social restrictions, and requires that she do extra work). This will have its unpleasant aspects for her, but it involves neither rejection (expulsion) by the community nor protection from the social impact which her behavior has on the peers and adults in the community. As examples of other significant moves, a citizen may change jobs, either because he decides to quit or because he's fired by his employer; or he may change his residence, again, either of his own free will or at his houseparents' request. The mode of functioning will vary, but there *is* always a way.

There are, to be sure, limits in the services which adolescents can render to their peers. For this reason, as part of the Junior Republic's structure, there are services rendered by professional staff members known as social doctors. They may come from disciplines of social work, psychology, guidance or psychiatry. Social doctors are charged with the overview of a citizen's total program. They may act to enforce participation or remove a youngster partially or completely from those facets of the Republic program to which the citizen is unable to adapt as a free member in the community.

The *social doctor's* function with Republic citizens is based on the concept that many of the major problems with which the adolescent struggles are essentially social illnesses. The social doctor with his overview of the citizen's use of the various aspects of Republic life is a consultant to the houseparent or employer. He corresponds with home and/or referral agencies on behalf of the citizen or the Republic to interpret the educational–treatment program in process. The social doctor may see the citizen regularly, but informally, or in direct consultation with the citizen in casework, counselling or therapy. There are multiple possibilities of service but also real limitations. For the citizen there are protections of civil rights in the Republic similar to those in adult society. The social doctor cannot usurp functions of the houseparent or employer, nor can he legislate or govern. Any staff member may offer his advice to a citizen or government official. Whether or not the citizen elects to follow this advice, his accomplishment and reputation in the community are determined by his own actions. Similarily, a houseparent, employer or social doctor gains his reputation by his decisions and, while it is appropriate to listen to advice and counsel, a citizen or a staff member alike may modify his reputation by being unduly swayed by others and unable to act on his own decision in areas of his own responsibility.

Special Services within the Republic provide additional environments for boys and girls incapable of functioning adequately in important areas of the Junior Republic community living. Since 1948, the Junior Republic has operated a special residence for boys and, since December 1958, a special residence for girls. In essence, this is a treatment resource within the Republic which is itself in its broad aspects a treatment center for troubled adolescents. The special treatment area within the Republic is integrated within and congruent to the Junior Republic. The youngsters referred to it include the following types known in every community and also within the Republic:

(1) Those who are unable to make wise choices and decisions to the extent that they persistently endanger the peace of the community or themselves, e.g., the rebellious, defiant, openly acting-out person.

(2) Those who present no disciplinary problem but who are unable to take advantage of the developmental opportunities available to them in the community, e.g., the nonrelater, the isolate, the underachiever academically, the overconformer.

(3) Those who are baffled by the complex community life and who are unable to make or follow through on decisions or meet appropriate levels of responsibility as citizens, e.g., in dress, work or cottage behavior.

We think of the Treatment Center as (1) a program which for a time frees a youngster of the necessity for making decisions which he cannot make competently and comfortably, and (2) a program of training which takes as its point of departure the actual maturity level of the youngster, and by slow degrees leads him to accurate perceptions, to foresight, to ability to plan, and to the persistence in endeavor which will enable him to live effectively and comfortably in a free society.

We lay stress upon the *integration* of the Treatment Center with the community-wide program of the Junior Republic. It is a matter of deep conviction that, as necessary preparation for life, the treatment and training of the adolescent in residence must include social experiences of the type which he will encounter when he returns home. It is very easy to institutionalize people; we have no wish to do this. That is why we stress that the Special Services' job (as well as that of the entire George Junior Republic) is not to teach the citizen how to live in the Special Services, but how to live in society. Young people in Special Services, live together, work, attend classes and have their recreation as a group, apart from others. They follow closely scheduled routines from the time they get up to the time they go to bed. The theory behind such a program and an observation about it, is that the structure here frees a youngster from the necessity for making minute-by-minute decisions, and thereby frees him to think about other things.

This program permits youngsters work at which they can be kept under constant supervision. It is important here that the youngster should participate in the experience of work, rather than in verbal debate about it. It is important that the work should have reward in measurable accomplishment and in the knowledge that the task is truly useful. Based on assessments (shared with them) of work and participation they are paid in Republic currency. They are therefore, still responsible pay-as-you-go citizens within the community. To the degree deemed necessary, they are each assisted in accounting and in the handling of their financial affairs congruent with the economic system of the Junior Republic. The citizen is allowed and encouraged to participate fully and progressively in one after another aspect of the non-Special Services program.

From his day of admission, throughout his stay at the Republic, a citizen is invited to a full participation in citizenship. He learns from observing himself and others in the process of accepting and participating in mature adult ways within the community. He also learns from the observation of adults the variety of ways in which they carry on their participation in various aspects of the Republic program. Failure to succeed in carrying out jobs, responsibility and citizenship can be quite as educational as the observation of those who are conducting their lives in a way that would be generally regarded as acceptable. He learns, early in life, that the community gets what it deserves in government— at the local level. Because here, as adults do in the community outside, he votes his beliefs, and if he votes "wrong" he must live with what were his convictions. He can lobby, complain and persuade to seek change and he will have the opportunity to change the government at election time.

No single area is *the* place where learning takes place. In the Republic it is observed to take place in various relationships and situations meaningful to the citizen. This is true to some degree in any setting. It is our impression that this is particularly true in a setting in which: (1) real authority is delegated to the citizen for a mature participation within his community; (2) his participation can be measured in very real monetary terms for himself in the way society in general allows; and (3) the general focus of the entire environment is on the study and development of the individual and his participation in the community.

REFERENCES

1. PITTENGER, R. E. AND MARTINEAU, P.: Some Notes on the Authority Structure and the Responsibility of Adolescents in the George Junior Republic. *Read:* American Psychiatric Association Divisional Meeting, New York City, November 1959. J. Nerv. Ment. Dis. 133:4, 1961.
2. MARTINEAU, P.: The Work Program in Education and Therapy at the George Junior Republic. Freeville, N. Y., Junior Republic Press, 1958.
3. KUBIE, L. S., AND CLUETT, J. M.: The Junior Republic; An Interpretation. Freeville, N. Y., Junior Republic Press, 1955.

The Anaclitic Factor in the Practice of Medicine

by Sydney G. Margolin, M.D.

With regard to the functions of the brain and their effects on pathophysiology, emotions and affects are of paramount importance. Inasmuch as most of the functions of the body participate more or less in the psychophysiology of emotions and affects, it is apparent that both the quality and quantity of any given affect will interact with these body functions. Accordingly, the following two principles may be stated:[3]

1. Affects, moods, or emotions are psychophysiologic states which tend to augment or decrease pathophysiologic states.

2. The interaction of physiologic doses of pharmacologic agents with certain affects may be synergistic or antagonistic. As a result, the effect of a drug may be thereby decreased or enhanced beyond dosage–response expectations.

In the light of these two principles, the controlled ability to influence affects or their properties provides a powerful means of modifying pathophysiology and the response to given doses of drugs.

The psychology of affects is not supported by a satisfactory or generally accepted theory. There are certain features, however, which are clearly verifiable and demonstrable. These are as follows:

1. Affects are invariably accompanied by a variety of physiologic manifestations. These are not necessarily the same for all individuals.

2. For a given individual, however, the psychophysiologic patterns of an affect tend to be grossly characteristic, subjectively and objectively. Nonverbal affective behavior is readily comprehended.

3. Affects are pleasurable or unpleasurable, the former associated with a sense of wellbeing, the latter with a sense of disease.

4. Affects are related to the manifestations and derivatives of bodily needs and to their gratification or reduction. It is in this area that a psychologic theory of affects fails us. In the human being, the psychic representation of infantile bodily needs develops into a complex elaboration of entero-exteroceptive perceptual and executive mechanisms, under the influence of a mental apparatus for regulating and acknowledging the needs and the modes of gratification.

5. The affective transformation of the needs, gratifications, entero-ceptive and exteroceptive perceptions of bodily parts and substances into radiating signals, signs and symbols does occur. Thus affects and their associated psychophysiologic functions can be psychologically influenced by recognizing and gratifying the needs of patients. This can be done directly in terms of elemental body needs or in the sense of "higher nervous activity," i.e., through sensory and verbal representations of the needs and their reduction.

6. A bodily need that can no longer be deferred compels direct elemental gratification. Somatic illness lowers the threshold for deferral of the need reduction by "higher nervous activity". That is to say, a physically ill patient is psychophysiologically prepared for more or less direct solutions of his needs. Ontogenetically speaking, this represents a regression to the infantile modes of need satisfaction.

The sick patient can be regarded as seeking to delegate certain perceptual, integrative and executive functions of his own personality to that of the physician. Where this effort is successful and reinforced by the physician, the latter becomes psychically represented as an extension or as an instrument of the patient's own being. This state of affairs seems to be one of the essential features of the relationship that exists between a gratifying mother and her infant. From this point of view, the conclusion is justified that a state of psychologic and social regression has been iatrogenically intensified.

Associated with this iatrogenic regression is the fact that when an individual falls ill, he tends to regress for other reasons as well. For example, he becomes dependent upon his environment for help and for the external maintenance of those capacities which are decreased by his illness. This regressive reaction to disease is adaptive in that it permits an attitude of dependency which in turn favors constructive external help. A third source of regression also of varying degree may be inherent in the character structure of the particular patient. That is to say, he may have latent or clinically overt psychopathology. Hence, the resultant pattern of regression is derived from the three sources—the inherent personality of the patient, the adaptive reaction to disease, and the response to the physician. These regressive tendencies appear to be the nature of the patient's participation in the "art of medicine" situation.

ANACLITIC THERAPY

The methods of observing the characteristics and properties of patient reactions and of patient–physician interaction consisted essentially of planned modifications of the timing, duration, and intensity of the factors in the treatment situation. Over a period of time these experimental steps and maneuvers formed into a plan of comprehensive management which was designated as "anaclitic therapy." The term "anaclitic" is borrowed from Freud who used it in two senses: first, to designate the dependency of infantile instinctual needs upon certain ego functions and, second, to identify some special qualities in the infant's relationship with its mother.[2] With usage the term has been enlarged in its meaning, so that it now also applies to the general period of early infant life when anaclitic relationships are first established. For example, the term "anaclitic depression" used by René Spitz refers to a special kind of infant depression characterized by varying degrees of apathy to bodily and interpersonal needs and to their gratification.[7]

The term "anaclitic" was chosen, first, because of its historical connection with Freud; second, because of its meaning; and, third, because it emphasizes the psychoanalytic frame of reference in terms of which this investigation was formulated and the empiric observations were systematized.

Anaclitic therapy has been described elsewhere as:

> . . . a commonsense approach consisting of kindness, tolerance, indulgence, allaying of anxiety by any available trial and error means, demonstrative friendliness and reassurance, deliberate omniscient and omnipotent behavior of the doctor for the purpose of enhancing confidence in him, total somatic care in terms of nutrition, medication, hygiene and agreeable environment. The deliberate induction of insight into the unconscious mental processes of the patient is not attempted.
>
> The therapist assumes a role of total permissiveness and all discipline or compulsory formalities are dispensed with to the greatest possible extent. Instead of formal, scheduled daily visits the therapist seeks out the patient wherever he is several times a day. The guiding principle of this frequency is analogous to that of the "demand feeding" schedule of infants. Physiological needs of hunger, thirst, the excretory functions, fondling, rest, sleep, and play are anticipated and indulged. Food may be prepared and served by the therapist, usually in the form of high caloric milk mixtures. It is available on demand and often is given to the patient by his therapist. The patient is touched and handled, areas of pain and discomfort are massaged and stroked. The therapist is actively comforting and reassuring with an attitude of omniscience and

omnipotence. He is available to the patient at all times. The activities of nurses, attendants, family—in fact, all personnel—and the administration of somatically directed therapy are represented as being under the direct control and supervision of the therapist.

To summarize in psychologic terms the principles upon which anaclitic therapy is based, it can be said

1. That the pleasure principle is emphasized rather than what might be called the reality principle.

2. Maximum expression of affects is encouraged and accepted as indications for adaptive and corrective responses on the part of the therapist. The latter seeks to decrease this psychophysiologic behavior not by suppressive exhortation, but by dealing with the need associated with the affect. Thus, the patient is maintained in that state of psychophysiologic equilibrium which follows the continuous gratification of needs.

3. Every effort is made to allay anxiety and its somatic analogue, pain.

4. These physical and emotional gratifications are offered continuously without any indications that they were requested or required by the patient, and despite his ambivalence, phobic reactions, anxiety, hostility, and guilt.

As experience grew it was realized that this latter principle could not be stressed strongly enough. It was learned that communication between the patient and the therapist in the anaclitic relationship, as with the mother and her infant, is essentially nonverbal and consists for the most part of responses to cues, signs, signals, and symbolic manifestations. The verbalization that does occur is generally limited to basic or elemental bodily or emotional needs such as food, fluids, physical discomfort, and the presence or absence of the therapist or of his activities, in short, to basic concepts. There were many indications that even when the profoundly regressed patient's language was less concretistic, the symbols used tended to be heavily associated with self references of a need–gratification nature.

This experimental magnification of several aspects of the therapeutic intentions and activities tended to induce correspondingly magnified reactions in patients. Two of the responses arrested attention as possible active ingredients in the therapeutic artful interaction between patient and physician. One was the process and state of regression. The other was affect, viewed as a psychophysiologic state.

With regard to regression, the continuous active gratification of the patient's latent or suppressed wishes, regardless of what he manifestly seems to demand, reinforces the patient's tendency to endow the physician with the attributes of omniscience and omnipotence. Questioning a patient as to his desires instantly put a limit to his regression and determines his prevailing affect. A decision is demanded and the patient is obliged to modify his wishes in accordance with his capacity and desire for reality testing. Thus, the patient's fantasy of the therapist's omniscience is more or less restricted by reality. Moreover, the patient's wishes are obscured by value judgments (expectations of pain or pleasure) of the therapist's attitudes in order to avoid unpleasurable affects such as guilt and anxiety. In short, the patient is obliged to retain his more matured (though not necessarily healthy) ego functions rather than regress to infantile ego activities.

The compounded regression normally is progressively given up as the signs and symptoms of physical disease begin to subside. At this time the patient may develop reactive attitudes towards the physician's previous supportiveness and towards his own deep seated wishes for continued regressive gratifications. Regardless of whether these take the form of "flight into health" or hypochrondriacal preoccupations, it is the patient's premorbid personality that is involved in this reaction. The physician's art, however, takes these manifestations into account by his intuitively directed timing of the change of "pleasure principle" into "reality principle."

The anaclitic factor is most clearly revealed in the successful management of those relapsing and remitting, often intractable, diseases with high mortality or morbidity. Here the regressive factors are generally quite intense. Even during the periods of remission, the patient is only relatively well, for there is an underlying tissue pathology, a fatalistic expectancy of relapse and persistent sense of dependency on medical care. The prevailing mood and affect in the remission phase can be regarded as a psychophysiologic state in which the vectors of organ functions oppose those of the pathophysiology. The most common antecedent for a relapse is change of the prevailing mood into one in which the affects of depression are persistent and dominant. The epiphenomenal psychophysiology of this reactive depression has an augmenting effect on the latent or manifest pathophysiology.

The discussions of the antecedent circumstances of relapsing diseases often tend to become polemic, even where there is no real disagreement.[3a] For example, in a long term study of a patient with a gastric fistula, it was learned that the complex variations in gastric physiology could not be correlated with the subject matter and verbal content of mental activity. To the extent that the physiologic findings were classifiable, these varied with broad categories such as affective states and defense mechanisms.[6] Similarly, the varying life situations which provoke depression have in common the very broadly interpreted concept of loss or separation. It is obvious, however, that the actual events, or their representations, that are classifiable as loss or separation, are infinite in number and do not contain the kind of pathogenic specificity associated with an allergen or infectious organism. To continue this analogy, the depressive reaction is comparable to the allergic reaction in that any one of innumerable specific precipitating circumstances combine with bio-genetic and psychogenetic predisposing factors and result in non-discriminating allergic or psychophysiological states. The physician and psychiatrist can not infer the specific allergen or loss. To put it another way, not all allergens result in allergic reactions and not all losses or separations lead to a depression.

SUMMARY

1. The investigation of the "art of medicine" by the method of exaggerating selected elements of the patient–physician interaction, indicates that the "anaclitic factor" may be an effective component. The "anaclitic factor" is the physician's ability to support a patient's regressive reaction to his disease and to gratify the needs appropriate to the regression.
2. Affects, moods or emotions are psychophysiologic states which tend to augment or decrease pathophysiologic states.
3. The interaction of pharmacologic agents with certain affects or emotions may be synergistic or antagonistic.
4. A patient reacts to his disease, to his treatment, and to his physician with manifest psychological, cultural, and—for want of a better term— physiologic regression. Where the regression is not manifest there are obvious pathologic efforts of the patient to obscure it.
5. By means of iatrogenically induced regression it is possible to bring about new affects or mood states.
6. The bodily functions which are psychophysiologically excited or inhibited by the regression or the defenses against it either increase or oppose the pathophysiology of the disease.

REFERENCES

1. DINGLE, HERBERT: History of Science and the Sociology of Science. Scientific Monthly 82:107, 1956.
2. FREUD, SIGMUND: On Narcissism: An Introduction; In Collected Papers, vol. IV. London, Hogarth Press, 1934.
3. MARGOLIN, SYDNEY G.: On Some Principles of Therapy; Am. J. Psychiat. 114:1087-1096, 1958.

3. (a) ——: p. 1096.
4. ——: Psychotherapeutic Principles in Psychosomatic Medicine; Wittkower,
    E. and Cleghorn, R., eds. Philadelphia, J. B. Lippincott Co., 1954.
5. ——: Genetic and Dynamic Psychophysiological Determinants of Pathophysi-
    ological Processes: *In* The Psychosomatic Concept in Psychoanalysis;
    Deutsch, F., ed. New York, International Universities Press, 1953.
6. ——: The Behavior of the Stomach during Psychoanalysis; Psychoanalyt.
    Quart: 20:349-373, 1951.
7. Spitz, René. Anaclitic Depression: In The Psychoanalytic Study of the
    Child, vol. II. New York; International Universities Press, 1953.

Activity in the Psychotherapeutic Process

by HILDE BRUCH, M.D.

IN CLASSIC PSYCHOANALYSIS, the therapist has been likened to an "inactive" blank mirror who reflects the patient's productions and becomes the object of his transference reactions. Occasionally, he will give interpretations to help the patient become aware of unconscious meanings and associations. If the therapist is directive, outspoken and elaborate in confronting the patient with such interpretations, his approach is called active.

Doubts about the effectiveness of the classic model of psychoanalysis have been raised in many quarters. Extending the psychoanalytic approach to the psychoses demanded considerable changes in technique. Sullivan,[11] who in 1931 reported on extensive psychotherapeutic experiences with schizophrenics, pointed out that the passive mirror-like attitude of the classic psychoanalyst was not conducive to a favorable outcome. He conceived of the role of the psychiatrist as that of a "participant observer" who investigated in collaboration with the patient, the vicissitudes of his early development. Whitehorn[12] stated that therapy is most effective when the doctor succeeds in *evoking* the patient's resources and activities, and that improvement in a schizophrenic patient is more likely to occur when the physician aims at assisting the patient in making more constructive use of his assets rather than focusing on psychopathology. Fromm-Reichmann[8] points out the usefulness of letting the patient—as far as possible—uncover the meaning of his own communication. Lidz and Lidz[10] observed that schizophrenic patients can achieve self esteem only through the realization that their own desires and impulses count, that their beliefs and opinions can have value as a guide to living. The therapist who presumes to know all the answers plays into the patient's belief that somebody else knows the way and will care for him magically. This is coupled with the patient's desire that the therapist also *need* him. Clarification of what the patient is saying is best carried out in a manner that can be followed step by step by the patient rather than through interpretation.

In this communication, the awakening in the patient of awareness of his own psychological effectiveness will be considered as the *decisive, active* factors in the therapeutic process. The need for this emphasis was recognized in the treatment of patients suffering from severe eating disorders, in whom it became apparent that indocrination with psychodynamic formulations stood in the way of their recovery. They may recite the psychodynamics of their illness in great detail and often sound as if they had devoured and literally incorporated every psychoanalytic interpretation that had come their way—yet underlying disturbances remained unrecognized and uncorrected. In the continued study of obese and anorexic patients, an implicit error became apparent: namely, that psychoanalytic preoccupation with conflicts and motivation had excluded from the therapist's awareness the importance of other factors. It was recognized that these patients, like schizophrenics with distorted body images, suffered from disturbances in the perceptual and conceptual field. They were unclear about the nature of their feelings and thus unable correctly to identify bodily sensations and emotional states.[1, 2, 6, 9]

These clinical observations led to the conclusion that from birth on two basic forms of behavior must be differentiated: behavior that *originates* in the child, and behavior *in response to* stimuli from the outside. This distinction applies to the *biologic* as well as the *emotional* and *interpersonal* fields, with a wide range of individual variations in every aspect. It is essential that a child receive *appropriate* response to behavior initiated by himself. Only when this is forthcoming can he develop an adequate sense of autonomy, initiative and trust in his own functioning.[3]

The observations underlying such theoretic constructions were made when the therapeutic approach was changed from an interpretative to a fact finding one, with minute attention to the contradictions and distortions in the patient's recollection of past and current events. This detailed inquiry was supplemented by interviews with the parents to elicit their attitude toward the child and their concepts of child care. In this way it could be recognized that confirmation of child-initiated behavior had been deficient in respect to physiologic and psychologic needs. For example, in patients with eating disorders, such as bulimia or refusal of food, experiences conducive to learning properly to perceive and identify the signals indicating nutritional needs had been inadequate. Invariably there was evidence that other aspects of child-initiated behavior had been disregarded.[4]

For these reasons, a treatment technique with direct focus on helping a patient become aware of self-initiated feelings, thoughts and behavior was developed and used in the supervision of the residents at the New York State Psychiatric Institute. The approach proved to be effective in patients with phobias, obesity, anorexia nervosa and other psychosomatic conditions, in which traditional psychoanalysis and other forms of therapy had been unsuccessful.

Illustrative is the case of an eighteen and a half year old young man, here called Eric. At the age of 12, he had developed the symptoms of anorexia nervosa. He received psychotherapy and had several hospitalizations for the medical study of his severe weight loss—at times as a life saving measure. He also spent six months on the psychosomatic service of another hospital. His two previous therapists, each of whom had been in contact with him for approximately three years, gave extensive reports on their own experiences. They had proceeded according to psychoanalytic principles, interpreting the underlying unconscious meaning and motivation of his negativistic and argumentative behavior, and of his peculiar eating habits. In spite of all the efforts expended on his behalf, Eric weighed 49 pounds and was 59 inches tall at the age of 18. Skeletal maturation and puberal development were correspondingly delayed.

Eric appeared moderately depressed, but was well oriented in all spheres and seemed to be of fairly good intelligence with a normal range of information. Usually he would refuse to eat; this alternated with episodes of voracity which were followed by vomiting. He expressed his resentment by continuous criticism of every rule and regulation, by making sarcastic demands for privileges, and rejecting all personal contact. His relationship to his first therapist was tenuous at best, then openly hostile. His therapist described as Eric's greatest skill his knack to "divide and conquer."

When, after five months, a change of therapist was decided on Eric refused to see his new therapist and signed himself out of the hospital. There was only one difficulty: he knew that both his parents did not want him to come home since he had ruined their life and they did not want what little there was left completely destroyed. When his mother had heard that he had gained some weight, her reaction had been: "But I had been led to believe that there was no hope."

In several supervisory sessions Eric's developmental history and his behavior in the hospital and in psychotherapy were evaluated as expressions of conceptual and perceptual disturbances, and of inadequate experiences for developing a proper sense of self effectiveness. Possibilities of establishing rapport aimed at permitting the development of initiative and autonomy were formulated. The need to outline for him the areas of defective self awareness was recognized. This had to be done without further lowering his self esteem. The therapist let him know that he recognized under the bristling facade of negativism the patient's fear of admitting his impotence and ineffectiveness, even to himself, and that he respected him for this struggle.

Having declared his intent to leave the hospital, though knowing that his parents did not want him home, Eric had no place to go and was forced to withdraw his letter of signing out. This he refused to do for fear of losing face on the ward. His new therapist helped him to recognize that this concern was insignificant in comparison to the much greater issue, namely that the hospital represented his chance of getting well. His sensitivity to the reactions of others revealed that the real problem was that he did not value himself enough, was not aware of his real needs and was willing to sacrifice himself to secondary considerations. By repeating in many variations, in a matter-of-fact, undoubting way, that his doctor valued his life and respected his right to help—even though Eric himself did not seem to do so—he gradually acknowledged that he had basic rights of which he had not previously been aware.

Gradually, the patient expressed active interest in finding out what had gone wrong during his childhood. It was Eric who defined his early feelings that he was the property of his parents, that his mother always "knew how he felt" and decided "what he needed," that his own feelings had never been considered, and that he had not even been aware of them. Treatment was devoted to the continuous pursuit of such discoveries by the patient, permitting him an increase in "feelings of competence by discovering incompetence."[7] The therapist acknowledged the patient's right to feel discomfort about the restrictions of the hospital or other unpleasant events, but also defined for him that an organization needs rules and regulations.

The bizarre eating habits were also approached with this factual attitude, in contrast to the interpretations by his previous therapists who had pointed out to him the self-destructive, punitive and cannibalistic significance of his not eating and self-induced vomiting. This type of comment was strictly avoided. Like other patients of this type, Eric felt that his whole life had been directed by his mother. Interpretations signified to him the painful re-experience that again somebody else knew more about him, his feelings and inner functioning than he himself did. Instead, simple definite statements about the need to eat were made repeatedly. Like many anorexic patients he would declare: "I do not need to eat", or "why should I be bothered and go to the dining room." There was only one reply: "here I disagree—every organism needs food."

For a period he was observed during mealtime, a fact that greatly annoyed him. This again was handled with a factual statement: "It is our obligation as physicians to know *how much* and *what* you eat." Gradually he learned the simplest of all associations: Food is eaten to fulfill nutritional requirements. Everything else, (e.g., the way he had misused it in a frantic effort of self assertion and defiance, or in magical and self destructive ways) constituted his individual distortions that did not alter the basic fact that food was necessary for the maintenance of health and strength. Finally he rebelled against this excessive objectivity: "Don't you think it is important that we find out why I stopped eating?" Now it was *he* who on his *initiative* explored the many motivational aspects that had determined his abnormal behavior.

To give one example: He was quite elaborate in describing the weight scale as his "enemy," the symbol of an outside agency that would give him away, and would reveal his weaknesses. "I am frightened by the scale; *they* always weighed me. It was always somebody else's business. If I lost, my mother blew her head off. If I gained *they* were so proud. Logically I can see it, that it really isn't the scale, but I have the feeling that *I am* getting *evaluated by it.*" At that time he had become quite aware that he had never felt in control of his own life and his biologic functions or thoughts, feeling and aspirations. As he began to accept responsibility for himself he expressed increasing concern about his short stature. This was mingled with the guilt that he himself had ruined his body and his chances for growth. He was afraid of receiving endocrine treatment, that things would be put into his body that were "not natural for me," and that would *force him* to grow. However, in contrast to his previous negativistic attitude he cooperated with extensive physiologic examinations so that an endocrine treatment program could be outlined.

Considering the long standing severe illness of this young man, and the hopelessness expressed not only by himself and his family but also by his physicians and the hospital, improvement was rather rapid. Decided changes became apparent within four or five months. It is now more than two years since the therapy was changed with the direct focus on the deficit in his initiative and the lack of trust in his own mental activities. During the second year of treatment he worked for six months as a messenger boy in a complex organization, where he was given increasing responsibility and learned to deal with a variety of people. When he decided to go to college he prepared himself by systematic reading and other efforts to develop sustained working habits. He has since made a good beginning in college and was able to carry five courses during the first year. For the past eight months, he has been living at his parents' home, is no longer conspicuous in his eating habits and has maintained a stable weight (115 pounds, 62 inches, beginning puberal development). Work with his parents was not extensive, but some re-evaluation of their attitudes was possible. Eric can now face —without becoming unduly involved— his mother's overconcern and her tendency to dominate everybody's life.

In this presentation only two aspects of the initiative-stimulating therapy were described: first, the use of authoritative simple statements as to basic facts of life, knowledge of which these patients have failed to acquire under the confusing conditions of their early development; and second, the continuous alertness to any behavior, expression, thought or feeling, originating in the patient. These were acknowledged and reenforced when they were appropriate, and examined for possible errors and misjudgments when they were unrealistic. It was also useful to draw the patient's attention to the way he used language to disclaim participating in his own life,[5] and to sensations indicating bodily needs.

In all therapy, as the patient becomes aware of and corrects certain aspects of his conceptual confusions, and as he achieves a degree of confidence in his ability to make discriminating observations and judgments, he is ready to approach and analyze the more complex psychodynamic problems dealt with in analysis. His fantasies and dreams, his realistic and unrealistic expectations and disappointments, his feelings and affect in relation to the therapist, can then be explored. With emphasis on the patient's own initiative and trust in his own psychologic functioning, he will be able to use constructive interpretations as hypotheses that need to be examined, verified or disproved. With this approach, there is less danger of treatment deteriorating into resistance and intellectualizing, since the whole emphasis is on helping the patient become an active participant in the therapeutic process.

BIBLIOGRAPHY

1. BRUCH, H.: Conceptual confusion in eating disorders. J. Nerv. & Ment. Dis. 133:46, 1961.
2. ——: Perceptual and conceptual disturbances in anorexia nervosa. Psychosom. Med. (in print).
3. ——: Falsification of bodily needs and body concept in schizophrenia. Arch. Gen. Psychiat. (in print).
4. ——: Transformation of oral impulses in eating disorders: A conceptual approach. Psych. Quart. (in print).
5. ——: Some comments on talking and listening in psychotherapy. Psychiatry 24:269, 1961.
6. BURNHAM, D. W.: Misperception of other persons in schizophrenia. Psychiatry 19:283, 1956.
7. COHEN, R. A. AND COHEN, MABEL B.: Research in psychotherapy: a preliminary report, Psychiatry, 24, suppl. 46, 1961.
8. FROMM-REICHMANN, F.: Principles of Intensive Psychotherapy, Chicago, Univ. of Chicago Press, p. 127, 1950.
9. HOFFER, A., AND OSMOND, H.: A card sorting test helpful in making psychiatric diagnosis, J. Neuropsychiat. 2: 106, 1961.
10. LIDZ, RUTH W., AND LIDZ, T.: Therapeutic considerations arising from the intense symbiotic needs of schizophrenic patients. *In* Psychotherapy with Schizophrenics. A Symposium, Intern. Univ. Press, 1952.
11. SULLIVAN, H. S.: The modified psychoanalytic treatment of schizophrenia, Am. J. Psych. 11:519, 1931.
12. WHITEHORN, J. C.: Goals of Psychotherapy, p. 4 in Research in Psychotherapy, edited by Eli Rubinstein and Morris B. Parloff. Washington, D.C., Amer. Psychol. Assoc. 1959.

Psychotherapy and Hypnosis: Implications from Research

by Martin T. Orne, M.D.

Introduction

IN THIS CHAPTER,* we shall discuss the implications for psychotherapy of some hypotheses that have derived from our research on hypnosis. Our primary research efforts have been concerned with the essential nature of the hypnotic process rather than with its therapeutic application. However, hypnosis and psychotherapy have a common necessary characteristic: the presence of a significant interpersonal relationship capable of altering boundaries of consciousness. The focus of our discussion here will be that in view of both phenomena being analogous in certain basic regards, the problems seen in the study of psychotherapy may well closely parallel those encountered in hypnotic research.

Research In Hypnosis

One of the first problems to arise in our study of hypnosis was that although the phenomenon apears easy to describe, any one description does not hold up in the light of historical perspective. Mesmer,[1, 2] traditionally has been given credit for rediscovering hypnosis. At his seances or *baquets,* without any specific suggestions to the effect, patients had hysterical fits, subsequently lapsed into sound sleep, and later awakened relieved of their symptoms. Although in a sample of several thousand subjects, we have never observed behavior of this type, Mesmer seems to have been able to produce it solely by silent passes

*This paper was condensed from a contribution to the Symposium on "Persuasion, Persuasability and Psychotherapy," American Psychiatric Association Annual Meeting, Chicago, 1961.

The work reported here was supported in part by Public Health Service Research Grant M-3369, National Institute of Mental Health.

I wish to thank Professor Richard Jung and Miss Emily F. Carota for their comments and criticisms in the preparation of this paper.

and the structure of the situation. The description of hypnosis in Coué's[6] work presents considerable contrast. Familiar as the originator of the phrase, "Every day in every way, I am feeling better and better," Coué also employed hypnotic techniques, but his patients were cured without going to sleep or even closing their eyes. These are only two of the many examples of the variability in historic descriptions of hypnotized subjects' behavior.

Naturally a hypnotist may, by appropriate cues, modify the behavior of a subject in hypnosis. However, we are describing here how the hypnotized subject acts in the absence of specific instructions. Today we tend to see a fairly consistent pattern of behavior: the subject's eyes are closed, his voice is low and often childlike, he tends to respond only to cues from the hypnotist, and if requested to perform an action, he does it slowly. Clearly, Mesmer's, Coué's and our present description of hypnosis differ markedly. What could account for such variability in different authorities' reports of the behavior 'characteristically' accompanying the hypnotic state?

It seemed reasonable to hypothesize that *the behavior which a subject will manifest upon going into hypnosis is a function of his concept of how a hypnotized subject should behave.* For an empiric test of this hypothesis, we needed to find an item of behavior which could plausibly be associated with hypnosis but which in fact had *never* been observed to occur spontaneously. We finally decided upon "catalepsy of the dominant hand." The phrase sounds somewhat scientific and evokes in college students vague memories of stutterers, tests of hand dominance, etc.; but although catalepsy is often observed in hypnosis, when it occurs, it is of all limbs, never of one alone.

The experimental procedure consisted of my giving identical lectures on hypnosis to matched sections of an introductory psychology class. However, one section's lecture also included demonstration of the new item. Two members of the section served as 'volunteers' for this demonstration. Unbeknownst to the class, these students had been previously hypnotized and given a posthypnotic suggestion to manifest catalepsy of the dominant hand. In the class demonstration, along with well known phenomena, this characteristic was casually pointed out as typical. An experimenter, 'blind' as to which lecture had been given to each subject, hypnotized in random order volunteers from both sections. Catalepsy of the dominant hand was found to occur *only in the section which had received the lecture demonstrating it as a typical characteristic.*

The implications of this study are far-reaching. It suggests that we have no uncontaminated data about the behavior which is characteristic

of hypnosis, per se.† Probably most, if not all, of the behavioral manifestations of hypnosis can be understood in terms of the subject's previous
knowledge and the cues transmitted during the induction process. It is
entirely possible to conceive of the "typical hypnotic state" as, for the
most part, a historically developed artifact occurring along with a process,
the *essential* behavioral manifestations of which are little known. The
basic process, without the gross behavior which is so variable, might
be called the "essence of hypnosis." This has been the real focus of our
research interest.

The problem of recognizing which elements ascribed to hypnosis
are artifactual is extremely difficult for any individual working with the
instrument. The nature of hypnosis is such that *any* expectation the
hypnotist entertains may unwittingly be communicated to the subject
who then acts in a way that demonstrates the validity of the expectation.
Thus, we have the potentiality for the occurrence of self-fulfilling
prophecies without the investigator becoming aware of his own role in
their fulfillment. It is necessary to get outside of the immediate interaction in order to recognize and isolate the effect of these variables.

In experimental research with hypnosis the gross variability of the
phenomenon persists. Here, too, the subject will behave in accordance
with his perception of the experimenter's expectations. The subject does
not respond merely to verbal suggestion, but rather to the totality of
the situation from which he actively attempts to ascertain what behavior
is desired. The totality of cues which communicate the hypotheses or
wishes of the hypnotist—including the implicit and non-verbal cues from
the experimenter and cues provided by the experimental procedure itself
—we have termed the *demand characteristics of the experimental situation*. What demand characteristics are perceived will vary with the
subject's prior knowledge. Thus, in the same experiment differing demand
characteristics may be perceived by different subject populations. These
will, under some circumstances, be the major determinant of a subject's
behavior. For example, suppose we test a medical student for the Babinski
sign, then regress him to the age of three months and again test the
Babinski sign. The very procedure itself clearly communicates to the
subject that we expect a plantar extension rather than a plantar flexion
because we are dealing with a medical student population which has
at its ready disposal the knowledge that a three month old infant exhibits
an extension. This expectation would not, however, be communicated
if the population consisted of national guardsmen.

---

†Since it is practically impossible to find 'naive' subjects, there seems little
prospect of obtaining such data, short of cross cultural and historical studies.

Experimental findings which are a function of demand characteristics may or may not be replicable depending on whether the replication provides the same cues. However, it is clear that unless the effect of the demand characteristics of the experiment can be determined, it will be difficult to make ecologically valid[5] inferences, i.e., valid generalizations from the experiment to real life situations. Much of our work therefore has been concerned with the development of techniques which permit the study and isolation of the demand characteristics factor.[11]

Briefly, three major approaches are possible: (1) to manipulate the demand characteristics purposefully; (2) to study what demand characteristics are perceived by investigating what the subject believes the purpose of the experiment to be; and (3) to study the effect of the demand characteristics by including a control group which participates in the experiment but which, instead of being subjected to the experimental or independent variable, receives only a 'dummy' treatment.

The common practice of telling the subject a fictitious but plausible reason for an experiment is an example of Approach 1, manipulating the demand characteristics. This is effective only insofar as the subject actually *believes* what he is told. Approaches 1 and 2 both require that the experimenter determine in each instance what the subject's actual beliefs were in the situation.

However, the procedure of inquiring into the subject's perception of an experiment after it is over has inherent factors which make obtaining a valid report difficult. College students know that they are supposed to be ignorant about those aspects of an experiment which are not specifically explained to them and that too much information about a study would disqualify their performance as subjects. The eventuality of disqualification runs counter to their motives for participating in psychologic studies, i.e., contributing to scientific research and investing time meaningfully. They therefore often respond with, "I don't know," to questions about their perception of the purpose of experimental tasks. For similar reasons the experimenter is equally motivated not to obtain such information, as he no more than the subject wishes to waste his time and exclude a subject's performance. As a result he may all too easily accept the initial, "I don't know," and the interlocking motivations of subject and experimenter will thus lead to a pact of ignorance. If the experimenter does not accept the initial denial but acts under the impression that the subject may know more than he is telling (much as would be done in a therapeutic situation), he will find that most subjects are able to verbalize specific hypotheses about the experiment which may or may not coincide with the experimenter's. A better approach still is to have, instead of the experimenter, a different member of the research group perform the inquiry. Using this approach, we have found that subjects' beliefs about the experimenter's hypotheses may be better predictors of what the subjects actually did in the experiment than their reports of what they thought they had done.[12]

Approach 3 consists of a procedure which attempts to maintain the demand characteristics of the situation, in fact to maximize the subjects' response to them, but to eliminate the variable to which the experimental result is usually attributed. One example of such a procedure involves the use of simulating subjects. Subjects who fail to enter hypnosis during repeated sessions are told that they are to simulate hypnosis for the hypnotist. They are further informed that successful simulation is possible, because although the hypnotist will know that some subjects are simulating, he will not know which ones. Subjects are warned that if the hypnotist catches on that they are simulating, he will terminate the experiment. *Under these motivating circumstances, simulating subjects are able to manifest a pattern of behavior almost indistinguishable from the real hypnotic pattern.* Moreover, for this group the independent variable is eliminated: these subjects do not have the subjective alteration in experience which distinguishes the hypnotic state. Simulators must of necessity base their behavior on the demand characteristics of the situation rather than have it determined by hypnosis.

In this type of design the hypnotist must be 'blind' as to the true status of the subject in order that subtle nonverbal communications remain constant for both groups. The real-simulator model is intimately related to the double-blind design employed in certain types of psycho-pharmacologic experiments. The use of simulating subjects makes possible an extension of the blind design to experiments where it cannot be concealed from the subject whether he is to receive an experimental or placebo (dummy) treatment, yet at the same time the hypnotist cannot discriminate between the groups of subjects. *Such a design then enables us to distinguish between those items of real subjects' behavior which may be due to the experimental or independent variable and those which may well be produced simply by the context of the situation or the demand characteristics of the experiment.* That is, the items of behavior that are produced by simulating as well as by real subjects have a conceivable explanation solely in terms of the demand characteristics of the experiment. It is also possible though that in the case of the real subjects, another mechanism is responsible for their production. Further research is necessary to prove which of these alternative explanations is responsible for the effect.

In our research it soon became apparent that the hypnotist's behavior is in many ways as remarkable as the subject's. A characteristic which

The Hypnotic Relationship

seems to accompany all attempts at successful hypnotic induction is that the hypnotist acts in a manner which clearly demonstrates his expectation that the subject should behave as a "hypnotized subject." Furthermore, it is characteristic that the hypnotist responds to his own suggestions by behaving as though *the subject is actually experiencing the content of the suggestions.* This aspect of hypnosis might be characterized as a *folie à deux* and can perhaps be most clearly seen in hypnotic age regression where the hypnotist talks in a manner appropriate to a child as he induces the phenomenon.

We have been filming hypnotic sessions in order to analyze the subject–hypnotist interaction in more detail. In some of this research we have used both real and simulating subjects with the hypnotist being unaware of their true status. In one instance, the hypnotist had become mistakenly convinced on meeting a subject that he was a simulator. In the interaction that ensued, the subject, who usually entered deep hypnosis easily, failed on this occasion to do so and became quite hostile towards the hypnotist who, while giving suggestions as usual, failed in the light of his mistaken impression to play a truly convincing complementary role. Thus, "good hypnotic technique" turns out to be appropriate participation by the hypnotist in the suggestions that he is giving.

For the hypnotic phenomenon to take place, it is necessary that both the subject's and the hypnotist's expectations about each other's role are met appropriately. Subject and hypnotist tend to exhibit standardized behavior, each readily understanding the role of the other. In order for the hypnotist to alter the interaction away from the typical appearance of hypnosis it is necessary for hypnotist and subject to reach implicit agreement as to different roles. It appears that not only is the subject's behavior largely a function of his expectations pertaining to the nature of hypnosis but also the hypnotist's behavior is largely determined by his own expectations about the role of hypnotist. It is of course extremely difficult for a hypnotist in the situation to recognize the extent to which his behavior is determined by his own expectations and by the subject's expectations. Therefore, certain shared expectancies are often viewed as characteristic, necessary aspects of the hypnotic interaction whereas, actually, the primary determinant of these may well be a historical accident.

Hypnosis and Psychotherapy

The real problem in the appropriate utilization of hypnosis as a therapeutic tool may lie in the aspect of hypnosis which emphasizes the therapist's control* over the patient, thus leading to a *folie à deux* of the hypnotist's omnipotence and the subject's powerlessness. It is necessary for the therapist to enter into this aspect of the relationship and at least minimally to act out the *folie à deux,* but at the same time he must maintain sufficient objectivity to recognize that he does not actually acquire the power that the patient ascribes to him. This is perhaps one of the explanations why thoroughly competent therapists, reporting on isolated uses of hypnosis, usually during their wartime experiences, describe attempts at treatment which violate their own very excellent knowledge of psychodynamics. Somehow they seem to get caught in the interaction process and seduced into attempting to compel a patient to change in a manner which is blatantly incompatible with the particular patient's personality structure. Obviously, such an endeavor cannot succeed. In every instance of hypnotherapy where we have had the opportunity of exploring what actually took place, it has been clear that the basic psychodynamic mechanisms operating were in no way altered or suspended because the patient entered hypnosis.

The therapist who becomes caught up in the fantasy of omnipotence will inevitably find serious complications in treatment efforts and the patient's reactions will often demonstrate an underlying recognition on his part that the therapist's powers have only been ascribed and are in fact very limited. Perhaps in psychotherapy (without the use of hypnosis as a tool) the opposite kind of *folie à deux* exists. That is, the therapist will often deny any attempt at control or interest in the patient's behavior or progress. He will insist on his powerlessness to affect the patient, and both he and the patient may operate under the shared illusion that the patient totally determines the content of treatment. The most extreme formulation of this position was put forth in Rogers'[15] original statement of nondirective therapy.

Certain aspects of hypnotherapy are of further interest insofar as they shed light on psychotherapy in general. Differences between psychotherapy and hypnotherapy are usually ascribed to the fact that the latter utilizes hypnosis as an adjunct in treatment. It is entirely possible that

---

*In point of fact, no rigorous experimental evidence is available to show any increase of control when hypnosis is induced over that already inherent in the context of the relationship prior to the induction of hypnosis. Thus, even without hypnosis, experimental subjects will carry out actions such as removing a coin from fuming nitric acid with their bare hands, which would seem to be outside of the range of behavior that can readily be elicited from a waking subject. Because the range of behavior that can be elicited from the subject (i.e., the social control inherent in the relationship), is not ordinarily tested, we are struck by an apparent increase in control which may be erroneously ascribed to hypnosis.[13]

many of the differences could be explained rather on the basis of a different set of mutually shared expectations about the process of treatment.

For example, since Freud[4] the statement has become well known that unconscious material is more readily available in hypnosis than otherwise. It is not clear, however, to what extent this clinical fact is due to hypnosis *qua* process and to what extent this may be a function of the shared belief that hypnosis allows the individual to experience and verbalize material otherwise too threatening. In hypnotherapy, being in hypnosis may represent to the patient a time when the therapist will accept responsibility for the patient's thoughts, words, and actions. (Similarly, in psychotherapy, lying on the couch may legitimize for the patient thought content not otherwise available.) Further, being awakened from hypnosis (or getting up from the couch) clearly marks the ending of the period and indicates when the patient must again observe the usual social amenities. Although we are not implying that hypnosis may not also cause differences in modes of thinking, we are suggesting that certain explicit expectations about hypnosis (and analogously the couch in psychoanalysis) may in part explain the availability to consciousness of material apparently otherwise unacceptable.

Another aspect of hypnotherapy and hypnoanalysis that must be examined in the light of a mutually-shared-expectations hypothesis is the belief that the use of hypnosis in these methods of treatment leads to more rapid progress; indeed it is felt that hypnoanalysis permits accomplishment of the same essential goals in a fraction of the time. [3, 17] However, we know that the length of analysis can vary and in fact that in recent years it has tended to become progressively more lengthy. The increasing length for the period required to complete analysis has been attributed to changing orientations regarding its goals. However, it is possible that both shortening analysis by employing hypnosis or lengthening it in order to achieve more goals may be more plausibly and simply viewed in terms of certain shared expectations of certain therapists and patients about how long analysis should take. To what extent shared expectations may affect the rate of progress and the actual length of treatment is an empirical issue.

Earlier in this chapter it was pointed out that although hypnosis appears easy to describe, little is actually known about its *essential* characteristics. We should now like to draw a comparison between this aspect of hypnosis and psychotherapy in general. Frank[7, 8] has documented the observation that no evidence is available demonstrating the effectiveness of one method of therapy over another, or that there is any increase in effectiveness of therapy over faith healing. Analogous to hypnosis, the phenomena of psychotherapy vary widely in appearance: different methods lead to similar outcomes and may indeed have similar essential characteristics even though these characteristics are not clear. So long as therapist and patient have mutually shared expectations about the nature of the therapeutic process and about their roles, typically predictable interactions can take place. These interactions may indeed have so much uniformity that universal characteristics can be inferred, which may nonetheless be epiphenomenal. That is, many aspects of psychotherapy which appear to be essential may appear so because of shared expectations and these may be determinants of the therapeutic outcome. This hypothesis would help to explain such findings as those of Hollingshead and Redlich[9] supported by more recent studies [10, 16] that lower class patients are not generally taken into psychotherapy, and when they are, they do not profit so greatly as do middle and upper class patients.

If we view mutually shared expectations about therapy as essential for the therapeutic process to take place, it would follow that the group which has the least exposure to such expectations would be the group most difficult to treat. Since education is highly correlated with the overall rating of social class, it would follow that those individuals who have had the least acquaintance with the expectations of therapy would be the lower class patients. Further, this group has probably not had contact with many doctors other than medical practitioners. Given that their expectations as to how a therapist behaves is as a practitioner, they would expect that they as patients should talk about symptoms. The therapist, on the other hand, expects his patient to talk about feelings, and the relationship is complicated from the onset by both psychiatrist and patient failing to meet each other's role expectations. Since initial contacts to a large extent determine future contacts, it is easy to recognize why this factor might crucially interfere with the therapeutic process. While we recognize that other factors are also significant—i.e., different group identifications, backgrounds, aims and experiences—between therapists and lower class patients, our central hypothesis would predict that the different expectations of the lower vs. the middle and upper class patients would in and of themselves largely determine the course of treatment.

With increasing education through mass media of communication reaching all levels of society, we may find that lower class patients become progressively more accessible to insight therapy, as the role expectations for psychotherapy become more widely known. Thus, education may lead to greater accessibility for psychotherapy of larger proportions of the population. At the same time, however, as in the case of hypnosis where the subjects' expectations are so widely distributed that we cannot find naive subjects, the more knowledge that is distributed to all segments of the population, the more difficult it will be to explore the essential characteristics of the psychotherapeutic interaction in the absence of well defined expectations on the part of the patient.

Deriving from our mutual-expectations-hypothesis, it is possible to devise an empiric test as to whether lower class individuals can be made more accessible to psychotherapy by acquainting them in detail with what is expected of them in treatment and what they are to expect of the therapist. Our prediction is that such an educational procedure would greatly facilitate treatment of the lower class group.[14]

CONCLUSIONS

In this paper we have applied to the phenomenon of psychotherapy some hypotheses that arose from our current research on hypnosis. Whether or not there exists a valid analogy between the therapeutic process and the hypnotic state, the specific hypotheses may be potentially fruitful in inquiries about the nature of the therapeutic process. Any conclusions about their validity will, of course, have to await concrete results of research. Some of the methodologic considerations and tools which we have developed to deal with problems in the study of hypnosis may be useful in testing similar hypotheses about psychotherapy.

REFERENCES

1. BINET, A. AND FÉRÉ, C.: Animal Magnetism. New York, D. Appleton & Co., 1888.
2. BORING, E. G.: A History of Experimental Psychology (2nd ed.) New York and London: Appleton-Century-Crofts, Inc., 1950, pp. 116-133.
3. BRENMAN, MARGARET, AND GILL, M. M.: Hypnotherapy: A Survey of the Literature. New York, International Universities Press, 1947.
4. BREUER, J., AND FREUD, S.: Studies in Hysteria. (Re-issue of 1895 ed.) J. Strachey, (transl.) New York, Basic Books, Inc., 1957.
5. BRUNSWIK, E.: Systematic and Representative Design of Psychological Experiments, with Results in Physical and Social Perception. (University of California Syllabus Series No. 304) Berkeley, Univ. of Calif. Press, 1947.
6. COUÉ, E.: Self Mastery through Conscious Auto Suggestion. A. S. Van Orden (transl.). New York, Malkin Publishing Co., 1922.
7. FRANK, J. D.: Persuasion and Healing: A Comparative Study of Psychotherapy. Baltimore, The Johns Hopkins Press, 1961.
8. FRANK, J. D., GLIEDMAN, L. H., IMBER, S. D., STONE, A. R., AND NASH, E. H.: Patients' expectancies and relearning as factors determining improvement in psychotherapy. Amer. J. Psychiat. 115, 961-968, 1959.
9. HOLLINGSHEAD, A. B., AND REDLICH, F. S.: Social Class and Mental Illness. New York, John Wiley and Sons, Inc., 1958.
10. LIEF, H. I., LIEF, V. F., WARREN, C. O., AND HEATH, R. G.: Low dropout rate in a psychiatric clinic. Arch. Gen. Psychiat. 5, 200-211, 1961.

11. ORNE, M. T.: The demand characteristics of an experimental design and their implications. Paper read at the Symposium on the Problem of Experimenter Bias, Amer. Psychol. Assoc. Convention, Cincinnati, 1959.

12. ——: The nature of hypnosis: artifact and essence. J. Abnorm. Soc. Psychol. 58, 277-299, 1959.

13. ——: Antisocial behavior and hypnosis: problems of control and validation in empirical studies (in press).

14. ——, AND WENDER, P. J.: Anticipatory socialization for psychotherapy. (To be published.)

15. ROGERS, C. R.: Counseling and Psychotherapy. Boston, Houghton-Mifflin Co., 1942.

16. ROSENTHAL, D., AND FRANK, J. D.: The fate of psychiatric clinic outpatients assigned to psychotherapy. J. Nerv. Ment. Dis. 127, 330-343, 1958.

17. WOLBERG, L. R.: Hypnoanalysis. New York, Grune and Stratton, Inc., 1945.

Modern Techniques of Adlerian Therapy

by HELENE PAPANEK, M.D. AND ERNST PAPANEK, ED.D.

FIFTY YEARS have passed since Alfred Adler broke with Freud and Freud's group and began developing his own theory of Individual Psychology. These fifty years have been a stormy period for the newly emerging sciences of psychotherapy, dynamic psychology and psychiatry, a period of much questioning and criticizing, theorizing and experimenting, inventing of new names for old observations, formulating of new theories for old knowledge. Many of the concepts of Individual Psychology—inferiority complex, life style, social feeling, the holistic and finalistic approach—have not only survived but have become an integral part of our thinking and vocabulary. Adlerian propositions are especially important in the fields of psychotherapy and education.

PSYCHOTHERAPY

Each psychotherapeutic school attempts to find "the psychological conditions which are both necessary and sufficient to bring about constructive personality change."[1] All schools agree on three things: first, the therapist must promote a "therapeutic relationship" between himself and the patient; second, the therapist must "understand" the patient; and third, the patient must learn to "understand himself" better.

From the Adlerian viewpoint the relationship between patient and therapist is understood as an interactive one; the two people involved exert a constant and mutual influence on each other. If he is to help, the therapist, from the very first session, should show a warm, active, and genuine interest in his patient. Because of the patient's fears and distortions, his behavior in the therapeutic situation will inevitably pass through many stages of dependency and rebellion, irrational distrust and irrational hope. The therapist's attitudes are based on his understanding of what Adler called the patient's "private world," that is, the idiosyncratic pattern of percepts and concepts which the patient has been developing since childhood. His partly intuitive, partly intellectual knowledge of his patient's phenomenologic field enables the therapist to respond even to neurotic behavior with genuine fellow feeling and empathy. The therapist's attitudes, though consistent with his *own* personality, will change in response to the patient's expectations and demands.

The therapeutic relationship combines an acceptance of the patient as he is with a mild, firm, steady pressure toward change, this by sometimes gratifying the patient's needs and wishes, at other times depriving him of such gratification and explaining the social necessity for these frustrations. This mixture of security and challenge, essential in psychotherapy and education, promotes and helps develop adequacy and social feeling in the child as well as in the adult.

In observing the patient, the therapist is interested not only in his fears, frustrations, distortions, complexes and symptoms. There must be an evaluation of the patient's assets, his adaptive strength, the genuineness of his desire for change, the extent to which he has been able to develop his own innate capacity for cooperation and social usefulness. The therapist's awareness of the patient as he is *and* as he can "become"[2] gives hope and encouragement to the patient and clarifies the purpose of the therapeutic relation: to help the patient to help himself through his own potentiality for cooperation, autonomy and creativity.

The therapist's understanding of his patient's *life style* and his openness to the latter's communications create an atmosphere of closeness between the two, which gives the patient a salutary experience of the possibility of mutual relatedness and the satisfaction derived from it.

Characteristic of Individual Psychology is the holistic approach: it strives to understand behavior as derived from a unique, self-consistent individual personality structure. In psychotherapeutic practice, this means that the therapist must be attentive to details and sensitive to the cues that can be gleaned from the patient's behavior and verbalizations, which he must combine into a meaningful whole. Four types of observation are regarded as especially important for the creative reweaving of the fabric which constitutes the life style:

(1) *Early recollections:* Conscious memories from childhood demonstrate that the child makes an active choice out of the multitudes of daily events, considering some incidents particularly important and worthy to be remembered. What these memories are, whether pleasant or unpleasant, whether the child participates actively or passively, what sort of role each person plays, etc.—all these are characteristic of the child's and adult's apperceptions and expectations. In other words, early recollections are to be used as a projective test.

(2) *Family constellation:* An understanding of interaction patterns

and dynamic group forces in the original family, parents and siblings, contributes to the reconstruction of the matrix from which the adult has formed his picture of "reality."

(3) *Dreams:* "The supreme law of both life-forms, sleep and wakefulness alike, is this: the sense of worth of the self shall not be allowed to be diminished. The so-called conscious and unconscious are not contradictory, but form a single unity, and the methods used in interpreting the 'conscious' life may be used in interpreting the 'unconscious' or 'semiconscious' life, the life of our dreams."[3, 4]

(4) *Behavior and the therapeutic situation:* The therapist can use verbal and nonverbal communication for direct and immediate observation of life style and purpose.

Historical and genetic formulations may account to some extent for the origin of life style and motivations, but they cannot explain the persistence of neurotic behavior and symptoms. Unadaptive behavior must be understood as an adjustment to "reality" as perceived and misinterpreted by the patient in accordance with his insecurity and fears, and as the way of living he has chosen in an attempt to compensate for them.

This approach, the explanation of persistence of neurotic symptomatology by exploring its purposefulness, gives useful therapeutic leverage in unlocking the static feedback mechanism of early experiences which have created a vicious circle of distorted apperceptions that lead to behavior motivated by irrational anxiety which in turn discourages any attempt to correct faulty expectations and conceptualizations.

Interpretations which explain neurotic behavior by emphasizing the patient's past with its "traumatic" influence may offer a perfect rationalization for continuing neurotic behavior. Patients can use these explanations as a justification for inadequate or asocial behavior, since it is "determined" by the past. Emphasis on the past, therefore, can perpetuate and strengthen neurotic attitudes, whereas emphasis on the future implies the existence of a free will. If the patient understands that his own suffering and the damage to others resulting from his neurotic life style will also continue, then he can change to a more constructive life upon acquiring a new understanding of how to do this. The appeal and exhortation to the patient, "You don't need this neurotic behavior, you don't need this or that symptom any more," actually works if and when in the course of analysis, with the help of the corrective experience of the therapeutic relationship, the patient's self image has changed. To be able to change, the patient needs motivation and strength. The latter increases with the lessening of inferiority feelings; the erroneous conception of the helpless self changes to the conception of a more adequate self; when you are no longer afraid you meet with a new openness toward yourself and others.

Group Psychotherapy

Since the concept of social interest (*Gemeinschaftsgefühl*) is of such pivotal importance in Adlerian thinking, the group as a social situation is considered a logical, highly effective tool for understanding and treating abnormal behavior patterns.[5]

The therapy group must be cohesive and democratic to provide security with peers through the experience of cooperation, mutual identification and belongingness; but it must also provide security in relation to authority by affording the possibility of challenging, criticizing and rebelling against the authority-figure of the therapist. But cohesiveness and equality are not the only therapeutic factors, nor are they easy to achieve with insecure individuals who use relationships mainly to protect themselves and who are afraid to relate mutually and trustingly. Members are prone to envy, resentment, anger toward one another. These feelings should be expressed freely, even if this would seem to threaten the unity of the group. The wholeness of the group is not to be preserved at the expense of the individual; each person has the right and the obligation to express his positive and negative feelings. Learning and restructuring of the life style can take place only through open communication and free interaction between members.[6] By observing each other realistically, the patients achieve greater clarity and correctness in their mutual understanding.

From the holistic viewpoint, this therapeutic development can be described as interaction between the unity and wholeness of the individual and that of the group. Even if each person must first experience his own irrationality or impulsivity before attaining a higher level of integration and maturity, this will not destroy the group. Each incident exemplifying this interaction helps to socialize the patient and, at the same time, to enrich him and the group.

The structure of the therapy group, its values and norms, must be clearly different from and healthier than those the patient experienced in his own family. Just as these past experiences led to the neurotic life style, it is corrected, frequently even without the patient's awareness, when he is forced through the pattern of the group Gestalt to assume a new role. Concomitant individual and group therapy is often indicated in order to mobilize a rigidly fixed neurotic life goal which the patient has been trying to achieve by establishing a static neurotic interaction with other group members.[7]

A brief case history may serve to illustrate some of these Adlerian principles:

Leonard, 35 years old, a lawyer, started therapy because of tenseness, gastro-intestinal and other psychosomatic complaints of many years duration, and marital problems. As the oldest child and only son he had become the pawn of his parents, who fought constantly and blamed each other for their poverty. His mother neglected him except when he was ill.

Leonard's life style hinges on deep feelings of insecurity, for which he sought relief by a whiny compliance and a demanding passivity. Hidden under these attitudes and revealed in his dreams, was a deep resentment and the striving toward a goal of male strength which would enable him to take revenge on his torturers: his mother who had victimized him, and the boys who had teased him because he didn't dare to fight back. But Leonard also found a healthier way to compensate for his inferiority complex in sports, athletics and intellectual achievement. He chose for his wife a very attractive but extremely neurotic girl who had been even more deprived than he. Her personality, similar to his, was even more pathologic, with excessive demandingness and severe psychosomatic symptoms. At the beginning of their marriage this constituted a background against which he could feel healthier and stronger, but later on it only increased his anxieties and aggravated his symptoms.

Individual sessions revealed Leonard's life style in a few months because he felt quite happy in a dependent relationship in which the therapist had to take care of him. Psychosomatic symptoms disappeared and he became more assertive on his job. His relation to his wife became worse, with increased mutual demandingness and estrangement. They stopped having sexual intercourse. Both talked about divorce but were afraid of it. Leonard was very much attached to his 5 year old son and could not think of leaving him.

Group therapy slowly mobilized the patient's neurotic pattern. He came to find great satisfaction in helping others, though at first he would quickly become impatient when other group members did not show him enough appreciation by improving rapidly. His life goal of "male strength" was frequently expressed in petulance and gruffness, but he could hardly ever give open vent to rage or anger. This restraint, in the therapist's opinion, was not only the result of his sense of insecurity and weakness. His genuine good nature and social feeling made it impossible for him to be cruel or destructive either to group members or to his wife. His genuine involvement in the group process and with all his co-patients, whether they liked him or not, and his eagerness to understand himself and others contributed a great deal to his gradual rehabilitation and re-education. His efforts to gain attention by being sick or whiny ceased and he learned to help his wife with the firmness, warmth and understanding she needed.

MILIEU THERAPY

A step away from the one-to-one therapeutic relationship of patient and therapist and from group therapy is what is often called "milieu therapy,"[8] since it has been developed mainly in residential treatment centers for disturbed or delinquent children or young adults. The "milieu" per se is not considered to be the therapeutic factor, just as the group per se, without the therapist in the leading role, is not considered group therapy. In an understanding, non-threatening, moderately challenging and moderately competitive, accepting and cooperative environment, the child has a chance to learn that his conception of a hostile world—which he thought he had to fight—was wrong. Here he can gain new perceptions that are less biased, and can find new incentives and motivations for tolerating more frustrations, for making positive choices, for assuming responsibility.

THE THERAPEUTIC INSTITUTION

The most extensive and intensive milieu therapy can, of course, be carried out only in special institutions.[9, 10] Thus, institutional care has an important place in child treatment and is not just an emergency tool. Institutions are not substitutes for the family and should not imitate the family. They should not have "cottage parents," but trained counsellors or "educators." The children's community is the right instrument for helping the kind of children who are so untrained emotionally or socially that they cannot fit into private family life, their own or that of a foster home. The institution offers a structured yet flexible environment where the young patients, by being understood, advised, and helped, and by getting another chance at trial and error without the deathly fear of failure, can broaden their personalities and their social interest; here they will learn that they can win social acceptance.

This type of institution must endeavor to provide a healing environment, which enables the child to acquire education, re-education and therapy, and to practice a healthy and constructive way of living before returning to his previous social surroundings. In this process understanding and "permissiveness" are only a preliminary stage; reorientation and re-education will often dictate that the child shall experience the consequences of his actions, with constructive help.

"Need for punishment," "social anxiety," or even a heightening of the "sense of guilt," when not carefully interpreted and guided, are not constructive factors in therapy or education. They may sometimes be helpful in preventing further wrongdoing when more ethical, emotional or intellectual motivations for rightdoing cannot be immediately attained.

Concepts of belonging are without meaning if they are not closely interrelated with, are not derived from, or do not lead to social and psychological responsibility. Many children, and grownups as well, when prevented from taking a responsible place in the community, overcompensate for their feeling of social and emotional inferiority by "acting out" in neurotic or delinquent fashion. In therapy as well as in education, we succeed only if we are able to win the cooperation of those whom we want to educate or re-educate. Group meetings "to talk it out" are the mainstay of community education. Highly successful also are weekly general assemblies of all the children and the staff, conducted by the director. These assemblies, partly different in setup and method from group therapy for adults, serve two main purposes:

(1) The working out of tensions in a large group, the airing of general hostilities and discontents, the constructive shaping of group sentiment and opinion, the settling of group complaints—all as first steps in socialization and cooperation in and with the community.

(2) Gradual education in democratic community procedure, free speech, respect for the opinions of others, courageous and disciplined opposition to them, organized election of representatives and committees, understanding of and purposeful cooperation with the administration and staff.

(3) Children, like all human beings, enjoy working and achieving mastery over materials and handling tools, until misuse, wrong interpretation and misguidance corrupt their attitudes. They like to contribute by their work to the good of the community and to their own well being. They must have the opportunity to contribute to community needs by working without payment, and to earn money by additional work. Work and worker should never be dishonored by being forced to work as a punishment.

Education must develop the child's innate desire for mastery and his potentiality for social living—out of many innate potentialities—so that they grow together steadily from the very limited social interest of the infant in his mother, father and siblings, to a constantly increasing social interest in his peer groups, school community, local community, occupational groups, town and nation, to an ultimate interest in the welfare and progress of mankind and his own individual contributions to it. "In the stream of evolution there is no pause. The goal of perfection draws us onward."[11]

A. H. Maslow[12] has tried to classify our basic needs, as motivating forces, in a hierarchy, starting with physiologic needs, safety needs—which would correspond to our feeling of security—belongingness, love needs, esteem needs, and the need for what Kurt Goldstein calls self-actualization.[13] Lower needs must be satisfied before prepotent higher needs can emerge to motivate behavior, "since the gratified needs are not active motivators." Where the lower needs—which Maslow also calls the more selfish ones—remain unsatisfied, the individual may not be interested in the higher.

One of the remedial therapists at the Wiltwyck School for delinquents[14] argued the matter of learning to read with a boy but could not convince him that there was any good reason to do so. The boy was planning to become a gang leader and would not need such skills. The therapist then asked him what he would do if a very important message came to him from a member of his gang and he could not read it, to which the boy replied that he would hand the message over to another member of the gang to read for him. "But what would you do," the therapist persisted, "if it was a very confidential message that no one else should see?" "All right," the boy capitulated, "let's begin." And he did begin, soon learned how to read and write and forgot all about his false motivation. Having satisfied the lower need of security—not to be forced to hide the fact that he considered himself too stupid to learn—he could step up a grade in the hierarchy of motivations.

Our schools have not done too bad a job of helping to develop scientific knowledge and technology. Where our schools have failed badly is their ethical and social teaching, because it has not been based on an experience of social interest and loyalty constantly widening from family and tribe, from community and nation to mankind. The artificial limitation of loyalty and social interest makes it impossible to educate children to a truly broad social interest.

REFERENCES

1. ROGERS, C.: J. Consult. Psychol. 21:2, 1957.
2. ALLPORT, GORDON W.: Becoming. New Haven, Yale Univ. Press, 1955.
3. ANSBACHER, H. L. AND ROWENA R.: The Individual Psychology of Alfred Adler. New York, Basic Books, 1956.
4. Ibid.
5. PAPANEK, H.: Changes Effected by Group Psychotherapy, Evaluated by Projective Tests. Internat. J. Group Ther. 10:446, October 1960.
6. ———: Psychotherapy Without Insight: Group Therapy As Milieu Therapy. J. Individ. Psychol. 17:184, Nov. 1961.
7. ———: The Hysterical Personality in Combined Individual and Group Psychotherapy: A Case Report. Internat. J. Group Psychother. 12, 1962.
8. PAPANEK, E.: In-Service Training of Educators for Maladjusted Youth. Proceedings, Fourth Congress of the International Association of Workers for Maladjusted Children. Lausanne-Paris, 1958.
9. ———: A New Approach to Institutional Care for Children. In Essays in Individual Psychology (Edited by K. Adler & D. Deutsch), New York, Grove Press, pp. 139-152, 1959.
10. ———: Das Kinderheim, seine Theorie und Praxis im Lichte der Individualpsychologie. Acta Psychotherapeutica 4:53, 1956.
11. ADLER, A.: Der Sinn des Lebens, Vienna, Ralph Passer Verlag, 1933.
12. MASLOW, A. H.: Motivation and Personality. New York, Harper, 1954.
13. GOLDSTEIN, K.: The Organism. New York, American Book, 1939.
14. McCORD, W. AND J.: Psychopathy and Delinquency. New York, Grune & Stratton, 1956.

Countertransference: A Therapeutic Tool

by LEON SALZMAN, M.D.

I N ESSENCE, Freud defined transference as the process whereby individuals react to one another on the basis of previous experiences, anticipations, expectations, and stereotypes. Historically, the confusions and distortions in the patient's imagery were of prime importance to the psychiatrist in the therapeutic process. In recent years there has been a renewed interest in the effect of the therapist's counterdistortions on the therapeutic process. These responses, called countertransference, are obviously the same phenomena taking place in the therapist rather than in the patient.

In a letter to Ludwig Binswanger in February, 1913, Freud wrote, in referring to the problem of countertransference:

> It is one of the most difficult ones technically in psychoanalysis. I regard it as more easily solvable on the theoretical level. What is given to the patient should indeed never be a spontaneous affect but always consciously allotted and then more or less of it as the need may arise. Occasionally a great deal, but never from one's unconscious. This I regard as the formula. In other words, one must always recognize one's counter-transference and rise above it; only then is one free oneself. To give someone too little because one loves him is being unjust to the patient and a technical error. All this is not easy, and perhaps possible only if one is older.

As we belatedly recognize that the therapist's responses are inevitable and not accidental elements, we are forced to explore their role in the therapeutic process and to discover ways of utilizing them to best advantage.

Our theories about the therapeutic process will determine the significance and emphasis of the technical maneuvers we employ. For example, when the theory involves a revivification of early experiences, we will encourage regressive maneuvers designed to achieve this. Lying down and facing the wall or ceiling rather than the therapist, coupled with long silences, tends to enhance the patient's infantile attitudes and feelings. When we assume that mental disorder is the result of a distorted

94

libidinal development, we naturally focus our main attention on the history and process of sexual development.

When therapeutic rationale is based on the process of elucidating and interpreting the unconscious through the skills of an objective, detached, and anonymous therapist, the feelings and responses of the therapist can be considered either artifacts or evidence of inadequate analysis and training. The early literature about psychoanalytic therapy was remarkable in the plethora of detail concerning the patient's unconscious, his libidinal development, and his attitudes toward the therapist, but striking in the absence of observations about the therapist's behavior.

The fact that the psychoanalytic process grew out of Freud's interest and utilization of hypnosis as a therapeutic tool determined the emphasis that was placed on the patient and his productions, and not on the interaction of the patient with the therapist. In spite of the changes produced by abandoning the hypnotic trance as a therapeutic tool, Freud retained and amplified the other elements in the hypnotic procedure, such as the recovery of lost memories. He eventually discarded the hypnotic technique, but never really relinquished the hypnotic goals. Certainly Freud and his students were aware of the effect of the therapist's personality on the therapeutic process, since it has always been a prime requisite that the therapist be analyzed to minimize these effects. Freud was aware that the therapist, being human, might have erotic and other feelings towards his patients—but naively and idealistically assumed that analysis would reduce them and leave only therapeutic attitudes. The therapist would resemble the surgeon who skillfully dissects the tumor out of the surrounding tissues without becoming too involved with the patient. One difficulty, however, was the troublesome element called transference. While it became clear very soon that it was more useful than otherwise, it played havoc with the programmed objectivity of the therapist. In this fascinating and crucial element in the therapeutic process, the patient regularly dealt with the therapist as if he were someone else— with flattering and derogatory characteristics. Not all these attitudes were irrational, although this was long considered to be the case. The patient's attitude did have some effect on the therapist, regardless of how well analyzed, detached, and competent he might be.

The mechanical, causal orientation and its object-subject duality was badly shaken in medicine as well as in the physical sciences by the Einsteinian revolution, when the concepts of interaction, transaction, field, and the significance of the effect of the observer on the observed were introduced into science. This was reflected in the growth of theories which developed the interpersonal aspects of behavior as emphasized by

Ferenczi, Lewin, Adler, Horney, and, finally, Sullivan, who called his approach an *interpersonal* theory of psychiatry. In therapy, this meant that not only the patient but also the therapist was the object of scrutiny, and particularly the relationship between them. This raised transference to a more dynamic and meaningful concept, and stimulated more interest and concern with what is called countertransference. Both these names are unfortunate historical accidents, and some theorists have preferred calling transference either "person perceptions or misconceptions." For Freud, transference referred to a special attitude every patient adopts toward his therapist, based on the infant–parent relationship. Nowadays, we are more inclined to think of transference as the broad spectrum of relationships the patient demonstrates to all people based on his particular attitudes and orientations to the world. In the therapeutic relationship, however, it may be exaggerated or highlighted, and be more available to examination. Thus, it could be called an acting out of the person's character structure.

In its classic meaning, countertransference refers to those responses of the therapist that are derived from the therapist's own unresolved parental attachments. It has been defined in a variety of ways, but mostly from the point of view of a phenomenon that implies some untoward response of the therapist toward his patient. D. W. Winnicott, for example, defines it as feelings that are under repression in the analyst. Fromm-Reichmann thought of it as distortions coming from the therapist, and tried to distinguish the private reactions from the professional ones. Ferenczi and Balint view it as the affectionate, positive, libidinous responses of the therapist to his patient. Mabel B. Cohen thinks of it as a development in response to anxiety in the therapist. Franz Alexander, on the other hand, uses the term in the way I think of it, as the totality of all the attitudes of therapist to patient.

The therapist's reactions are just as significant as the clues sought for in the patient—such as being late for interviews, being bored or preoccupied, or acting pleasant or unpleasant. The therapist must be attentive to such clues in order to bring his own feelings into awareness, where they can serve the purposes of the therapeutic enterprise. Such clues can relate to positive as well as negative feelings. For example, let us suppose that a therapist frequently feels belittled by his patients. He may notice this directly or indirectly in his subtle tendencies to feel annoyed or to be excessively critical toward the patient. Upon noticing this, he should determine if the patient has some subtle and pervasive techniques of depreciating others as well. If he does, then the therapist's response would be called rational, and we would expect him to draw the patient's attention to this tendency of which the patient may be unaware. Let us assume that after a careful search however, such tendencies on the patient's part are either not present, or only minimal, and should not produce an extreme response in the therapist. The response would then be considered irrational, and it would be the therapist's responsibility to search out his own difficulties or unresolved neuroticisms to account for his reactions.

In the light of the above formulation of therapy, any maneuver that serves to enlighten a patient about his patterns of behavior, their origins, and the sources of continued functioning should be an acceptable therapeutic tool. Countertransference phenomena in this framework constitute a veritable goldmine of information. For example, if we notice that the patient has a prevailing suspicious, compliant, or hostile attitude toward the therapist, we can safely direct the patient's attention to a feeling which manifests itself in the present, without any relevant provocation, and which must be involved with his preconceptions, distortions, or misconceptions derived from his past. We have identified it, and while we have some understanding of its role in the patient's life, we are still in the dark as to how it is currently provoked and sustained. We might notice when such feelings are more in evidence, and whether they occur in response to a patterned action on the therapist's part, or whether they result from some action or revelation in the therapeutic process. This would be helpful, yet it would lack the clarity and conviction of its irrational and destructive role in the personality structure of the patient.

However, if we discover that the patient's hostile attacks either annoy us or bore us, or that his compliance stimulates us to assertive, controlling behavior, or is simply flattering, we can then explore this tendency in a new dimension. Provided we are clear about our own responses, we now have *in camera* and in the clearest setting, unencumbered by reminiscences or distorted by some other defense, a picture of how this patient functions in the real world.

We can describe four categories of reaction of the therapist to his patient:

    (a) The tender reaction—which ranges from simply liking a patient, to becoming sexually interested or perhaps involved.

    (b) The hostile reaction—which includes all the responses from annoyance and irritation, to strong dislike, derogation, outright anger and resentment.

    (c) The bored reaction—which includes minor disinterest or inattentiveness to active discontent, unconcern, and detachment.

    (d) Anxiety responses—without the defense reactions described in the above categories. Here the therapist is aware of anxiety, uneasiness, and tension usually associated with psychosomatic manifestations.

The tender reaction can simply represent the benevolent aspect of any therapeutic relationship which some consider a necessity for successful therapy. In these instances there is a respectful, accepting attitude toward the patient as an individual, in spite of his behavior, and a genuine warmth and affectionate regard may be present. Knowing that he is liked and exploring the reasons for this is more rewarding, since all neurotics suffer from an inability to appraise truly what is likeable in themselves, and feel they are incapable of being liked. However, it is often equally fruitful to recognize, acknowledge, and explore with a patient why he cannot be liked just as he is. It may reveal crucial clues in his personality difficulty if we frankly express the negative feelings which he stimulates in others. It may open up areas of inquiry into his compulsive necessity to irritate and antagonize others in order to prevent them from liking him. This is a more widespread problem in the neuroses than a patient's tendency to be seductive. Another characteristic of the neurotic is his inability to deal with positive, tender feelings, and to use a variety of techniques to avoid closeness and intimacy. These problems can be explored only if the therapist can identify the tactics by noticing his own responses.

Other patients use the widespread technique of stimulating affection or sensual interest in others in order to evade or distract both themselves and others from their real difficulties. This occurs not only when patient and therapist are of opposite sex, but also when they are the same sex. This personality device has its beginnings in the baby's smile, and ultimately can become a formidable tool, both in a conscious and unconscious way, in interpersonal relations of a positive as well as a negative kind. For our present purposes we are interested in its capacity to distract the therapist through flattery or subtle admiration. This not only fulfills the therapist's need to be liked, but also allows him to like the patient. If this process goes too far, or is not noticed by the therapist, the situation may degenerate, as the therapist would become reluctant to expose and deal with the negative and unpleasant aspects of the patient's personality.

In more subtle ways, the patient may wince at the slightest criticisms, and thus ward off the more severe criticisms he anticipates. This not only divulges his low self esteem, but frequently gives us major clues about his need to control every event in his life. Or the patient may encourage criticism by proclaiming his ability to take it. The therapist must be careful to note that this is frequently a most effective way of preventing any tender or friendly gestures from the therapist.

When do we withhold statements about our positive feelings toward the patient? When do we express them? Should we ever indicate our erotic feelings? These questions can only be answered in the context of the clinical situation, but the same principles apply here as in all other therapeutic maneuvers. Any activity which furthers the patient's understanding and supports his esteem is useful, and vice versa. Obviously, many of the therapist's activities in the short run are deflating and derogating to the patient's false pride or neurotic esteem, but in the long run should be constructive. It may be very effective at times to indicate that a patient is attractive and interesting enough to stimulate sexual desires. This can be constructive insight, and can help overcome some doubts about the patient's charm. It can also function in a serious disintegrative way if it is clumsily done, or badly timed.

Should countertransference feelings ever be acted out? It must be evident that when this occurs therapy ends, and a personal rather than a therapeutic relationship takes over. There are times when withholding countertransference feelings serves the therapeutic situation best. This may be due to the extremely low or high opinion which the patient might have of himself. Holding back need not interfere with therapy if the therapist is fully aware of what he is doing. The decision rests on the value of the revelation to the clarification of the neurotic problem, and not simply on the moralistic notion of telling the whole truth, no matter how it hurts. There is a special problem which arises when the therapist finds himself interested in the homosexual patient. In these instances, if the therapist can deal with his feelings and not act them out, he can be of considerable use to his patient. Otherwise, it is essential that such patients be transferred, since it is obvious that such a relationship cannot have therapeutic possibilities.

The countertransference problems created by the immature, inexperienced therapist who covertly (or overtly) seduces all his patients to like, admire, or even love him are almost self-evident. He takes advantage of the special role that he is in and even develops a spurious rationale (based on a distortion of Freud's notions) that it is necessary and good for the patient to love him. Under such circumstances, therapy becomes converted to adulation, to the detriment of exploration, insight, and change.

The second category of countertransference reactions raises the paradoxical issue of how negative feelings of anger, irritation, etc., can be helpful to the patient. Strong negative feelings of hate, contempt, and disgust are inconsistent with therapy, and must be resolved by termination or transfer. However, the recognition of negative feelings stimulated by the patient as highlighted earlier can be most effective in illuminating covert patterns of behavior. Expressions of anger and irritation can stimulate and often provoke positive developments.

This issue was demonstrated in a paranoid patient who had regularly recurring depressive episodes, with marked grandiose fantasies.

I had been aware of a growing irritation towards his grandiosity, which frequently produced irritable responses from me. On the occasion of this incident, I was sharply annoyed, and spoke in an angry, derogating fashion. This patient was being supported by his wife because no job worthy of his status had been offered him. Besides, at any time, the call might come to acknowledge his "second coming," (he thought he was Christ) and he was holding himself ready for it. During the 7 months that I had been seeing him, he attempted to examine his living with respect to the major facets of his personality: his grandiosity, his contempt for the deficiencies and weaknesses of others, and, particularly, his special significance as a multigenius who would be acknowledged and given his true reward. At one interview, he described his ruminations about a device he had worked out to get larger rockets off the ground, which would beat the Russians and save the government millions of dollars. He would be awarded the medal of honor, and the Nobel Prize, as well as a fabulous reward. This device would use steam as a propellant, as is done on aircraft carriers to propel planes off the deck. I responded to this by saying very emphatically that his presumption had assumed fantastic proportions. I said that he was presuming to solve a problem which was currently being tackled by the most eminent scientists in the world who were experts in rocketry, who had probably devised steam propulsion for airplanes, and who were now spending all their time and energy and skill in trying to solve this problem. Yet, through a brilliant insight of 10 minutes spent in casual consideration, he, who knew nothing whatever about this subject, had devised a solution. I elaborated and emphasized his lack of humility. My tone was sharp, critical, and certainly angry. He attempted to defend his position by giving examples of other brilliant discoveries that had occurred in just this way, and finally said that he did not mean it seriously, anyway. At the next hour he arrived in excellent spirits, and described the hour-long ride home following his last session, and the intervening four days. He said that first he had been furious. Then he resolved to prove his point by developing the mechanism. Finally, he had to agree that I had been absolutely right. He recognized that all his living had been a succession of just such grandiose schemes, some of which he tried to actualize, with disastrous consequences. He further added that nobody had ever confronted him with the enormity of his distortions in the way that I had, but instead had tried to tone him down, argue with his scheme, or else say nothing, and just humor him. It was a real "come-uppance," but he recognized that he had had it coming for some time. He said now he understood why he thought he was Christ, since he assumed he was omniscient and omnipotent, and only Christ combined such virtues. He finally felt that *perhaps* he no longer needed to be Christ, and could go ahead with a project that he had organized recently with some friends. He was convinced that he had broken the hold which the delusions had on him, and for the first time in his life, he felt that the television cameras were not following him all the time, and that perhaps he "did not really need to be a bigshot."

The use of negative responses is also illustrated in the masochistic disorders in which the patient becomes self-defeating and self-destructive. This leads to a negative therapeutic reaction, arising from deeper unconscious needs of the person to suffer, fail, and negate all his experiencing. This is not an instinctual deformation, but rather a transference–countertransference situation, in which the patient's behavior is designed to annoy, irritate, and stimulate negative feelings in others. In therapy, defenses are utilized to thwart the analyst's efforts; consequently, an impasse is inevitable, no matter what the personality of the therapist is. The resolution depends upon the therapist's ability to engage the patient in a direct, frontal assault on the masochistic technique. This involves the ability to respond honestly and openly to the patient's provocation, so that the masochist can see precisely what effect he has on others. Nonintervention or passivity in these circumstances does not avoid the tug of war; it only alters its manifestation. The classic detachment of the analyst arouses intense anxiety and stimulates further masochistic or hostile defenses, which remain covert and unavailable to analysis. Under these circumstances, the patient may be cooperative, obsequious, catering and pleasant, but while peaceful relations obtain, therapy remains at a standstill. The patient may store up grievances regarding the therapist's inadequate, ineffective, and malevolent dealings.

As to the therapist's reaction of boredom, disinterest, and preoccupation with personal matters, we must clearly establish the reasons for such responses from the therapist. They are very revealing, and can effectively advance the analytic work. Most often they represent reasonable reactions to the patient's inadequate and dull existence, but often they are produced by the patient's pattern, which is designed to stir up just such a reaction to prove that no one can truly be interested in him. In such an instance, statements about the patient's emptiness and dullness must be withheld, since this would only confirm the already existing low esteem. It must be brought out in the open when it can serve the dynamic purpose of pursuing a neurotic pattern or illuminating a particular defense. The awareness of the therapist's reaction is, however, essential, since the patient is usually aware of the therapist's boredom, and may be reluctant to bring it out into the open. When faced with a direct question on this issue, particularly when the therapist is discovered to be dozing or dreaming, it is always essential to meet this challenge directly and honestly. Denial under these circumstances can only reinforce the patient's low esteem.

In the early years of my practice I pursued a rather active social life. This sometimes led me to doze, or at least to nod my head with a patient who, noticing this for the first time, reacted in a generous and self-effacing manner by suggesting that perhaps I had a fever and was drowsy. I snatched at this excuse, and readily agreed that this might be so, and that I was sorry to have been inattentive. My easy escape and limited physical capacity did not prevent recurrences, and although this patient did not comment on it again, I was surprised shortly afterwards to discover that she had experienced a miraculous cure and had decided to terminate her work with me. I have never again wittingly taken this way out. This type of reaction is largely eliminated when the patient faces the therapist. Such a response does occur in therapists who work long hours, or see too many patients.

It may also result from the reluctance to deal with the "ordinary neuroses" and to aspire to treat only the interesting and exotic cases. However, this reaction must be differentiated from the effect produced by those patients whose neurotic patterns are dedicated to boring and alienating people. In such instances, positive and interesting aspects of the patient's personality are buried in a morass of emptiness which superficially appears as dullness or stupidity. Because of the fear of closeness, warmth, or intimacy, these individuals advertise only their least attractive selves. The countertransference responses of the therapist can get behind this facade by responding to the charm which lies behind the boredom, or by noticing the undue emphasis on being unattractive.

The fourth category of countertransference reactions should include those whose response to anxiety has not yet produced the characteristic defenses of either exaggerated tenderness, hostility, or boredom. On these occasions, when the therapist feels anxious without the usual defensive reaction, he may be aware of physiologic changes, such as an increase in pulse rate, sweating, agitation, or he may manifest other evidences of anxiety in his verbal or nonverbal behavior. Such responses may be provoked by threatening, abusive, or overtly seductive behavior of the patient, and may occur most often in young, inexperienced therapists, although it is by no means limited to this group. The patient who threatens suicide, or the one who has been involved in homicidal activities in the past, or who threatens such activity in the present may stir up large measures of anxiety in all therapists.

When the therapist experiences such anxiety, he is immobilized and cannot engage in the required confrontation, exploration, or interpretation of the situation. If such situations recur and the therapist is unable to deal with his own responses of anxiety, it may be necessary to abandon the treatment and transfer the patient to another therapist.

REFERENCES

1. ALEXANDER, FRANZ: Fundamentals of Psychoanalysis. New York, W. W. Norton, 1948.
2. BINSWANGER, L. S.: Freud, Reminiscences of a Friendship. New York, Grune and Stratton, 1957.
3. COHEN, MABEL: Counter-transference and anxiety. Psychiat. J. Stud. Interpers. Proc. 15:231, 1952.
4. HEIMAN, PAULA: On counter-transference. Int. J. Psychoanal. 31:81-84. 1950.
5. FERENCZI, SANDOR: Further Contributions to the Theory and Techniques of Psychoanalysis. London, Hogarth Press, 1950.
6. FROMM-REICHMANN, F.: Principles of Intensive Psychotherapy. Chicago, U. of Chicago Press, 1950.
7. SALZMAN, L.: Masochism: A Review of Theory and Therapy. *In Masserman, J.* (ed.): Individual and Familial Dynamics. New York, Grune & Stratton, 1959.
8. WINNICOTT, D. W.: Hate in the counter-transference. Int. J. of Psychoanal. 30:67-74. 1949.
9. WOLSTIEN, B.: Transference. Historical Roots and Current Concepts in Psychoanalytic Practise. Psychiatry 23:159-172. 1960.

The Negative Therapeutic Reaction

by Claude H. Miller, M.D.

A KEEN AWARENESS of the process involved when a patient develops a negative therapeutic reaction during the course of intensive psychotherapy makes for more intelligent and expert handling of the episode, which, in turn, frequently determines the outcome. Such awareness also acts as a tranquillizer for the mutual anxiety of the participants.

Recently there has been a revival of interest in the negative therapeutic reaction; this is indeed fortunate because a great deal of confusion has arisen around this syndrome since it was originally described by Freud in "The Ego and the Id," in 1927. At that time he wrote:

> "There are certain people who behave in quite peculiar fashion during the work of analysis. When one speaks hopefully to them or expresses satisfaction with the progress of the treatment, they show signs of discontent and their condition invariably becomes worse. One begins by regarding this as defiance and as an attempt to prove their superiority to the physician, but one later comes to take a deeper and truer view. One becomes convinced, not only that such people cannot endure praise or appreciation, but that they react inversely to the progress of the treatment. Every partial solution that ought to result, and in other people does result, in an improvement or a temporary suspension of symptoms produces in them for the time being an exacerbation of their illness; they get worse during the treatment instead of getting better. They exhibit the so-called negative therapeutic reaction.
>
> "There is no doubt that there is something in these people that sets itself against their recovery and dreads its approach as though it were a danger. We are accustomed to say that the need for illness has got the upper hand in them over the desire for health. . . . This reveals itself as the most powerful of all obstacles to recovery. . . . In the end we come to see that we are dealing with what may be called a 'moral' factor, a sense of guilt, which is finding atonement in the illness and is refusing to give up the penalty of suffering. . . . This sense of guilt is dumb; it does not tell him he is guilty, he simply feels ill. This sense of guilt expresses itself only as resistance to recovery which is extremely difficult to overcome."

The above is a masterpiece of description distinguished by its clarity, accuracy and succinctness. Ten years later, however, Freud in "Analysis Terminable and Interminable," unfortunately confused and obfuscated the matter by tacitly equating the negative therapeutic reaction with therapeutic failure when he wrote:

"Nothing impresses us more strongly in connection with resistance encountered in analysis than the fact that there is a force which defends itself by all possible means against recovery and clings tenaciously to illness and suffering. We have recognized that part of this force is the consciousness of guilt and need for punishment and this undoubtedly is correct; we have localized it in the ego's relation to the super-ego. But this is only one element. . . . If we bear in mind the whole picture made up of the phenomena of masochism, of the negative therapeutic reaction and of the person's consciousness of guilt, we shall have to abandon the belief that psychic processes are governed exclusively by striving after pleasure. These phenomena are unmistakeable indications of the existence of a power in psychic life which, according to its aims, we call the instinct of aggression or destruction and which we derive from the primal death-instinct of animate matter. It is not a question of an optimistic as opposed to a pessimistic theory of life. Only by the interaction and counter-action of the two primal instincts— Eros and the death-instinct—never by one or the other alone, can the motley variety of vital phenomena be explained. How the elements of these two types of instincts combines to fulfill the various vital functions, under what conditions such coalitions tend to dissolve and finally to break up, what disturbances correspond to these changes . . . these are problems whose elucidation would be the most valuable achievement of psychological research. For the moment we must bow to these superior powers which foil our attempts."

It is imperative to distinguish between a therapeutic failure and a negative therapeutic reaction if we are to clarify our thinking in this regard. Actually these two entities are poles apart and perhaps it is the unfortunate labeling that seems to make them siblings. Certainly therapeutic failures occur frequently, but it is sloppy thinking to dignify them with the status of a negative therapeutic reaction. Let us attempt to establish some criteria that we can use to differentiate the negative therapeutic reaction from the therapeutic failure.

For purposes of exposition we have found it useful to distinguish between the acute and the chronic form of the negative therapeutic reaction. Clinically, the acute negative therapeutic reaction is an agitated depression; the chronic negative therapeutic reaction is a prolonged negative transference. These may occur singly or together in a given patient or they may alternate; likewise, a patient who has gone along in a positive transference for a prolonged period may blossom out with an acute negative therapeutic reaction as he gets closer to the core of his being.

DIFFERENTIAL DIAGNOSIS OF NEGATIVE THERAPEUTIC REACTION AND THERAPEUTIC FAILURE

Incidence

The negative therapeutic reaction is uncommon; we have seen five cases which satisfy our criteria for this condition in the past ten years. Unfortunately, therapeutic failure is very common; some writers place the incidence as high as 60 per cent while others report failures in 20 per cent of their patients who are adequately motivated at the outset.

Occurrence

The acute negative therapeutic reaction usually occurs midway to late in treatment, often after two or three years of profitable and rewarding reconstructive therapy. The chronic negative therapeutic reaction emerges after a more or less tranquil beginning when the patient begins to realize that the reality of the therapist does not coincide with his fantasy of what the therapist should be like. Therapeutic failures can occur at any time but are most frequently observed early in treatment; they can take the form of absence of change, flight into health or abrupt, unexpected termination.

Doctor-Patient Relationship

In the negative therapeutic reaction the patient's feelings toward the therapist, albeit negative, are deep and meaningful. His plight is similar to the boy away at camp for the summer, who wrote his parents, "I have only one friend and I hate him." In therapeutic failure, the patient's manner may be antagonistic, superficially positive or even glowing in praise of the therapist. Further probing will reveal, however, that the doctor-patient relationship is shallow and meaningless and actual involvement in treatment is minimal.

Feelings

In the negative therapeutic reaction there is a greater expression of feeling than ever before on the part of the patient. In the acute form this is evidenced by agitation and unrest associated with evidences of depression including anergia—a loss of interest in and capacity for work, anorexia, insomnia, anhedonia—the inability to enjoy any pleasure, suicidal ideation and frequently somatic complaints. In the chronic form there are intense, prolonged feelings of disgust, contempt and loathing of the therapist and consequently a loss of ability to communicate with him verbally. These developments are the result of mobilization of feelings that have previously been successfully avoided. The therapeutic failure often displays a facade of normality or emotional blandness consequent upon giving up certain vital aspects of personality functioning due to: (1) adoption of more rigid controls; (2) the gratification of certain neurotic drives; or (3) the repression of damaging conflicts.

Dreams

The dreams of the patient in the throes of a negative therapeutic reaction are alternately optimistic and terrifying, reflecting the conflict in which he is participating. In the therapeutic failure dreams are frequently completely disremembered, which reflects the generalized restriction of spontaneity and creativity.

Management

The management of these two conditions is markedly different. Once we decide that we are dealing with a negative therapeutic reaction it is imperative that we continue working with the patient to see him through this catastrophic experience that we have induced. Once we decide that we are dealing with a therapeutic failure we must think of securing consultation to validate our opinion and/or consider referring the patient to another therapist.

Prognosis

The prognosis of the negative therapeutic reaction in our experience is uniformly favorable provided that we recognize it as such, sustain the relationship and manage it constructively. Conversely, the prognosis in the therapeutic failure is poor but we must admit to the possibility that another therapist may succeed where we have not been able to influence the patient in a positive direction.

Dénouement

In our experience the patient who encounters a negative therapeutic reaction during the course of reconstructive therapy emerges more vibrant and alive by virtue of having had a deeply moving emotional experience in the company of another human being. The patient evincing a therapeutic failure becomes progressively more restricted and isolated unless he has a later life experience of a deeply moving nature or a successful therapeutic encounter at some future date. Essentially the negative therapeutic reaction is indicative of effective psychotherapeutic work while therapeutic failure bespeaks ineffective psychotherapeutic work.

THE ACUTE NEGATIVE THERAPEUTIC REACTION

Recognition

The acute negative therapeutic reaction may be defined as a paradoxical development occurring during the course of psychotherapy characterized by the patient's developing an agitated depression subsequent to a period of successful psychotherapeutic work. These patients display all of the classical signs of depression including anergia, anorexia, insomnia, anhedonia, suicidal ideation and somatic complaints.

There seem to be some similarities in the character structure of the individuals who develop an acute negative therapeutic reaction. We have found these individuals to be possessed of enormous energy and vitality, probably on a constitutional basis. We can speculate that it is this native power that enables them to react in such a dramatic manner during the acute negative therapeutic reaction. Also we have found these individuals to have been practitioners of a pattern of morbid independence or compulsive self reliance since an early age in response to an environment that did not permit them to enjoy the advantages of interdependence. Also the milieu in which they found themselves did not allow them to react with morbid dependency which is a much more common phenomenon that so many of our patients cling to.

Because of this pattern of being utterly self-sufficient, at least in their own inner estimation, they have avoided deep or meaningful sustained relations with others. They may have concealed this most effectively from their associates with what we call warm detachment which passes for genuine affection; they may be everyone's friend and no one's friend. In a way these individuals are caricatures of what we have come to view as the healthy person in our culture; they are apparently industrious, self-reliant, inner-directed, energetic, well liked, trustworthy and usually asymptomatic in the conventional sense.

In view of such an abundance of assets we might wonder why they seek psychiatric help to begin with. We must bear in mind that these pseudo-virtues are purchased at a very high price because of their driven, compulsive quality. The morbidly independent individual does not choose to behave in this way; he is obliged to do so because of stringent inner necessity. It is only when his neurotic solution begins to decompensate that he seeks psychotherapy to deal with anxiety that he is no longer able to deny. Even at this juncture he is not desirous of once again regaining the advantages of interdependence for he has given up on that a long time ago; what he does want is help in reestablishing his compulsive self sufficiency. It is understandable that he will be terrified and furious when it begins to dawn on him that he and the therapist are working toward different goals.

The acute negative therapeutic reaction seems to occur in certain morbidly independent individuals at a time when the therapist is succeeding in insinuating himself into the emotional life of the patient. The patient senses that he is reaching a point of no return in terms of interpersonal involvement and at this juncture he reacts with catastrophic anxiety for at some level he perceives that his overall solution of compulsive self-reliance, which means literally forsaking all others, is in jeopardy. In essence, he is going to be required once again to rely on others, or perhaps more accurately, once again to acknowledge his reliance on others, whom he thinks unreliable. Another unconscious factor which makes this all the more terrifying is the morbid dependency and feelings of impotence and helplessness that underlie the facade of total self-sufficiency; these feelings convince him that he will be completely at the mercy of the person upon whom he becomes dependent.

Management

The most important single requirement in the management of the acute negative therapeutic reaction is a clear understanding of what is going on; armed with this awareness the therapist will be able to function in a constructive and effective way. It is frequently a most unexpected occurrence when a patient who has been doing well develops an acute negative therapeutic reaction. It is also a most distressing experience for the therapist treating the patient; the suffering of the patient is an awful thing to behold particularly since the therapist must feel in some way responsible for this turn of events. Unless there is a clear notion of what is going on, as well as a thoroughgoing conviction that this is *the process* that must be experienced and resolved, it can be an alarming and discouraging development to see several years of effective therapeutic work disintegrate before one's eyes. Unless the therapist is conversant with the negative therapeutic reaction and its management, he may be sorely tempted to accede to the inner and outer pressures and abandon the patient when he is needed most. Under no condition should the therapist allow himself to be stampeded into terminating a patient in the midst of a negative therapeutic reaction.

In our experience a period of hospitalization has invariably been required in the management of the acute negative therapeutic reaction. Also a short course of electro-shock treatment, usually six or eight treatments, administered not by the therapist but by the hospital staff, has been of immense value in stabilizing the patient enough so that he can return to work and to psychotherapy. This has been experienced as supportive by the patient in every case.

Probably the most practical admonition that can be given on the management of the acute negative therapeutic reaction is this: "Sustain the relationship!" It is only within the framework of a sustained relationship that the problems, no matter how enormous, can be resolved. Consequently, the therapist who terminates a patient in the throes of an acute negative therapeutic reaction, whether acting from theoretical bias, rancor or guilt, may unwittingly and unwillingly convert a potential therapeutic success into a therapeutic failure.

During the dark days of gloom and despair the patient's dreams frequently prove to be a harbinger of optimism and better days. Also the therapist's dreams frequently can help to buoy up the relationship. Barring these or in addition to them, consultation with an experienced colleague may provide the needed illumination and support.

Invariably, in our experience, the patient who successfully resolves an acute negative therapeutic reaction comes to realize, by virtue of a deeply moving experience in the company of the therapist, that he can rely to some extent on persons other than himself and thus to recognize that his unconscious cherished expectations concerning the basic unreliability of others were based on irrational fears and not on fact. We can further suppose that if this acute negative therapeutic reaction is not successfully resolved, then the patient's unconsciously cherished expectations will be reinforced and the patient can only conclude that his fears of abandonment are rational and realistic for all other people, including the therapist, are basically unreliable when the going gets rough.

The Chronic Negative Therapeutic Reaction

Recognition

The chronic negative therapeutic reaction may be defined as a paradoxical development occurring during the course of psychotherapy characterized by the patient's experiencing strong conscious feelings of antagonism and contempt for the therapist over a prolonged period of time.

The chronic negative therapeutic reaction is similar to the negative transference in its manifestations but it is different in being of much longer duration. The negative transference is frequently a consequence of some interaction that has taken place recently between the therapist and the patient which has been alarming to the patient and to which he has reacted with bristling defenses. Usually this sequence can be interpreted and, as a consequence of the interpretation, the negative feelings of the patient are dispelled and the relationship again takes on a positive tone. The same is not true with the chronic negative therapeutic reaction which is a consequence of the character structure of the patient and not primarily due to any current interaction between the therapist and the patient. This is more evident as the history unfolds when it becomes apparent that the patient is either detached from and/or hostile toward all persons with whom he comes into contact.

It is very common for these individuals to have worked previously with many therapists and to harbor strong negative feelings toward all of them; so strong in each instance that it resulted in the termination of the therapeutic relationship. The previous therapists faltered because they failed to fathom the contempt and recognize it as the involuntary servitude of the inferior for the superior.

There may be one exception in the experience of the patient; e.g., he may have strong positive feelings for a dead sibling or even for a living sibling with whom he has no current dealings. This relationship gives evidence of having undergone retrospective glorification so that it is now recalled as grand, smooth, blissful and conflict-free.

These patients will stoutly maintain that the previous therapists did not understand them and that they received shabby treatment at their hands. Usually they have voiced these feelings to the therapist but sometimes not because they felt the therapist was so self-sacrificing that they could not bring themselves to punish him. In other words, the self-effacing manner of a therapist frequently has the effect of silencing the patient's feeling of contempt toward him.

In its most severe form, the patient in the throes of a chronic negative therapeutic reaction may be unable to speak spontaneously at all; he can only sit and loathe the therapist, viewing him as beneath contempt. The patient will spend the entire session in silence unless the therapist intervenes. Between sessions the patient may rehearse many things that he wants to say but when he enters the office, he is speechless.

Management

The management of the chronic negative therapeutic reaction will call for all the ingenuity and originality that the therapist can muster. A therapist should not undertake to have more than one, or at the most, two such individuals in his case load at a given time. In the first place, it is most helpful and illuminating to bear in mind that the patient's actions are far more eloquent and reliable than his words. It is in the actions and not in the words that the valid communications are to be found. For example, the patient will be prompt and regular in his attendance and may even ask for extra sessions even though all of his verbal productions are concerned with how rude, thoughtless, inconsiderate and incompetent the therapist is. Paying attention to the actions and discounting the words will make for a clearer understanding of the true state of affairs. Of course no therapist worthy of the name will ever make the gross error of asking, "If you feel that way, why do you keep coming?" Such a question indicates a complete unawareness of the process involved in the negative therapeutic reaction and validates the patient's suspicions that the therapist really does not understand him very well if he is so easily misled.

Also it must be borne in mind that the chronic negative therapeutic reaction is not resistance to treatment; it is rather one variant of the ongoing therapeutic process that some individuals display. Again, the fact that these patients pay their fees regularly and promptly is evidence of this and belies their continuing verbal tirades.

The patient with a chronic negative therapeutic reaction will repeatedly say that he does not feel that he is making any progress. This statement must be recognized for what it is , a test for the therapist to determine if he is dissatisfied with the patient. If the therapist falls into this trap, the patient is in effect told that he is not living up to the therapist's expectations for him. This complaint is usually best dealt with by silence for empty reassurance is worse than saying nothing; certainly under no circumstances should the therapist react defensively and blame the patient for the apparent lack of progress.

Patients with the chronic negative therapeutic reaction are exquisitely sensitive, so in the management of these individuals it is well to refrain from making any interpretations, even kindly ones, for they are almost always experienced by the patient as an assault and evoke more fear and defensiveness.

Conducting a session with a silent patient is hard work and requires a willingness to depart from routine. Some of the techniques that can be used are: playing checkers with the patient, letting the patient associate to the Rorschach cards, letting him make up stories about the Thematic Apperception Test cards in response to the therapist's questioning, doing jig-saw puzzles on the floor with the patient, turning the therapist's chair around so that the therapist is not facing the patient, etc. These procedures are not usually particularly effective per se but they do help to solidify the therapeutic relationship with the therapist as a potent, non-punitive individual and they have the constructive effect of showing the patient in actions that the therapist is imaginative, is interested and is trying to help. The demonstration that the therapist is favorably disposed toward the patient helps to undermine the patient's fears; also the fact that the therapist persists even though his efforts are not spectacularly successful is a good lesson for the patient and acts as an antidote to his hopelessness and despair. During this period, if the therapist does observe patterns and gathers significant data, he should keep these observations to himself for they only frighten the patient who is unable to deal with them.

After a time, frequently a long time, often measured in years, the patient will begin to talk a little. Again the therapist must listen and perhaps ask a few neutral questions but not make connections or insightful intrepretations which only have the effect of making the patient scurry back into silence. At this time it is possible and advisable to talk about the previous therapists and to let the patient project onto them, realizing all the while that the patient is also referring to the current therapy and the present therapist as well as to the qualities in himself that the patient has disavowed.

Another technique that is not offensive to these patients is to open the sessions with the question, "What did we talk about last time?" This has the effect of breaking the ice for the patient and, as time goes on, the information obtained thereby is most valuable and revealing because of the unconscious selection that takes place. The therapist will note that anything pleasant, positive or constructive has been disremembered and the negative, unpleasant and painful has been reinforced and accentuated.

The therapist should never tell the patient what has been omitted. The patient should be allowed to have the privilege and joy of re-establishing contact with what he has forgotten—even if he is unable to do so in a particular session. Often he will recall the repressed material as he closes the outside office door behind him after the session. This is the most personal demonstration for the patient of the existence and operation of unconscious forces as well as of the quality of the material that he habitually disremembers; it is also a confrontation with his own ability to recall things that were not immediately available.

Once this process is activated, it gradually becomes possible to inquire as to the origins of this need to dismiss the pleasant and to accentuate the unpleasant; this is really a major element in the character structure of the patient with a chronic negative therapeutic reaction. After this fear of pleasant, happy, joyful feelings is resolved, the treatment can proceed in the conventional manner and the patient can dare to admit that he is making progress.

Two Worlds: The Sighted and the Blind

by CHARLES MYRAN, M.D.

P SYCHOTHERAPY OF THE BLIND requires that one know the experiences of the person and the meaning of blindness to him. I have known blind people who talked of belonging to the blind world, referred to sighted people as members of the seeing world, and they expressed the feeling that there was social distance between them.

The Schilder[1] concept of body-image gives meaning to this alienation which exists between the sighted and the blind:

> "Our own beauty or ugliness will not only figure in the image we get about ourselves, but it will also figure in the image others build up about us and which will be taken back into ourselves. The body image is the result of social life. Beauty and ugliness are certainly not phenomena in the single individual, but are social phenomena of the utmost importance. They regulate and become the basis for our sexual and social activities."

Gordon[2] noted that in biblical times the blind were considered as the most degraded element in society and were kept outside of the city gates. *Oculus fascinus,* or the evil eye, was feared because it was full of hate, envy and destruction and could influence the minds of others. It was the alleged cause of ophthalmia neonatorum and blindness. The birth of evil spirits was attributed to the archangel Samuel who had cast lascivious glances on mother Eve; and the issue of this union was the tempter, Satan.

Gesell, Ilg and Bullis[3] describe the role of vision in the biosocial development of the infant and child and compare it with the maturation process in the blind infant and child. The cerebral cortex integrates the visual sensory function which consists of postural fixation and parasympathetic focusing of the eye on objects separated by space. The eye, the hand and the mouth form a complex in exploring the environment through locomotion, manual prehension, language and social response. The blind infant goes through the process of maturation in acquiring the same skills as the sighted child but uses auditory, tactile, and kinesthetic

115

cues in the place of visual ones; the mental life is, therefore, different.

Burlingham[5] analyzed a four year old girl and an eight year old boy at a residential school. Both children felt that they had been sent away by their mothers because they were blind, and much of their energy was invested in wishing for the miraculous acquisition of sight. The children had learned early in life that they were different from sighted people. The girl had slept with her parents and had the same reaction to the primal scene as a sighted child. Fear of silence in the blind boy had the same meaning as fear of darkness, because it left the child alone and he was frightened of instinctual temptations. Sighted people were invested with powers of omnipotence and were treated by the children with feelings of awe, envy, fear, resentment and subservience. The boy was passive, repressed aggressive feelings in an effort to become the love object of sighted people, and had unconscious homosexual strivings. Stimulation of the eyes, through rubbing, was a displacement of feeling from the genitals. The boy maintained that he was able to see and wished to be exhibited before the other blind children.

Deutsch[6] investigated the sense of reality in congenitally blind children. Of 28 individuals interviewed, only three verbally accepted that they were permanently blind; and five children who were born without eyes held the fantasy that an operation would miraculously give them sight. A common attitude expressed was: "I cannot see, but I shall certainly be able to see sometime. Something has robbed me of my sight. Somebody must be to blame." Another attitude was: "I cannot see; I once could see but I, myself, did something for which I lost my ability to see. I have done something wrong, this is the result." In some there was less fantasy life and a compulsive approach to appreciation of concrete experience by the depreciation of the value of vision: "I cannot see but that is not a great loss. I have no desire to see; and if I had been given the choice between losing my sense of hearing or of sight, I would not hesitate in giving up sight. I don't know what seeing is but it cannot be as splendid as they say." The majority of children did not accept their blindness and resorted to fantasy life or unreal thinking. They reacted very fearfully to any threats of loss of love objects and feared bodily injury.

Schlaegel[7] compared the dominant form of mental imagery in blind and sighted high school students. He confirmed the findings of Heerman, 1838, that if blindness occurred before the age of five years then the faculty of visual imagery was lost. The sighted person responded most frequently with visual imagery; and the totally blind responded primarily with auditory imagery on word association tests. Paradoxically, the partially-sighted blind person responded with a higher incidence of visual imagery than the normal controls. Even though he may have had light perception only, he would use the word "see" quite frequently, in an obvious attempt to deny blindness.

Cutsforth,[8] a blind psychologist, emphasized that neither the seeing nor the blind fully realized the difference that existed between their respective worlds of experience and reality. In the sighted, the process of education was primarily through the sense of vision, and vision itself was a form of reality-testing. The blind were educated to think and describe events in the same manner as the sighted person. The result was impoverishment of the personality and insincerity of character. The sense of reality in the blind was altered by blindness. His way of thinking was different from the sighted person. The sighted person visualized whole forms and then analyzed the components; whereas the blind person depended on tactile and other sensory cues to analyze details which had to be synthesized into total forms. Much concrete experience, of necessity, was beyond the reach of the finger-tips. The gestalt of form, color, space and movement could hardly be perceived realistically by the blind. Even congenitally blind children, on word-testing, tended to give visual verbal responses rather than their actual sensory impressions.

Diamond[10] interviewed 150 men at a rehabilitation hospital some one to three months after they had become blind in the services. Sixty per cent of the men seemed to accept their loss of sight stoically and were applying themselves well to rehabilitation. Twenty-two per cent showed minor behavioral problems; while the remainder showed pronounced behavioral difficulties with feelings of fear, anxiety, guilt, confusion and loss of self reliance. Displacement of feeling also manifested itself in somatic complaints. The patients with slight residual vision, particularly those who had had ocular disease prior to enlistment, had the greatest emotional upheavals and were overwhelmed by feelings of guilt and ideas of self neglect. And patients who had had neurotic problems before their illness generally had more difficulty in accepting their loss of vision.

Blank[11] analyzed the meaning of dreams in therapy with the blind; and used the same principles of interpretation as with sighted people. In patients blinded before the age of five years there was no visual imagery in dreams, but auditory imagery was reported. Newly blinded patients who were actively trying to adjust to blindness often had dreams in which seeing was a wishful fantasy. And the tensions of everyday living as a blind person showed themselves too in the wish-fulfilling dream of seeing. The blind patient who denied his blindness reported few dreams, found it painful even to talk about vision, and displaced his feelings into somatic complaints. Sexual desires manifested themselves in dreams in the wish to see and thereby gain social acceptance. In interpretation, the more manifest elements of the dream, dealing with reality experiences, were given preference over the deeply repressed feelings. Dreams were more fearful to the blind because it took them longer to orient themselves to their surroundings upon awakening, and to realize that what they had experienced was only a dream.

Hysterical Amaurosis. A 22-year-old man who sought vocational training related that he was of illegitimate birth and had never known his father. When he was 2 years old his mother married for the first time. His step-father was an alcoholic man who would beat up his mother and shout that the patient was a bastard. At the age of four years the patient contracted measles and was kept in a dark room during convalescence. When he complained that he had lost his vision he was placed in a residential school for blind children. He had little contact with his family. After graduation from the high school for the blind, he had difficulty in finding regular employment, and applied for vocational training as a blind person. An ophthalmologic examination revealed that he had normal visual acuity but was repressing vision. In his mannerisms and way of expressing himself he had the appearance of a blind person. He felt depreciated, castrated and suspicious. He was very passive and covertly hostile. He had normal intelligence and was in good health. He was raised with blind children and continued to associate with them after leaving school. In the blind world he had received recognition mainly for being an outstanding athlete. I diagnosed him as a person with hysterical blindness. He had no apparent conflicts and did not want psychiatric treatment.

Psychotherapy is strongly resisted by blind people. Therapy can proceed only slowly and with realistic goals of not changing all his beliefs. It does seem that the blind person lives in a world that is different but the degree of social comfort and acceptance can be modified by meaningful outside human resources.

The main aim of psychotherapy with the blind person is to help him function realistically within his limitations. If he can be helped to realize that he has worth as a person with feelings, thoughts and acts that can be shared with others, then he is more likely to accept his blindness as a limiting disability which narrows his range of movement but does not have to isolate him from the process of social life. Without the realistic acceptance of himself and his blindness he can live only in a world of fantasy and misunderstanding, and suffer the distress of not knowing the meaning of self fulfillment. Primitive feelings of anxiety are reactivated in the newly blinded, and the individual needs a meaningful relationship to effect a reconstruction of personality (taking into account the mechanisms by which he has handled stresses in the past, and has developed as a person). Re-education requires the learning of fundamental means of physically caring for himself, the acquisition of a useful means of verbal and written communication, such as the Braille touch system, and vocational training where desired. And the individual needs a system of social values that have meaning to him.

The individual who is unable to make use of primary educational and vocational services for the blind is often referred for therapy, and to the extent that he is dependent on social agencies for financial or other support he may feel that he is being forced to undergo psychiatric examination or treatment. It is important to point out the purpose and rules of therapy and put the onus of choice on him rather than hopefully accept him with no well-defined goals. It is important to examine his motivation and to avoid being manipulated by a patient who may use the relationship only as a means of passively fulfilling the demands being made on him that he do something about his problems.

The person who has just become blind goes through an initial phase of shock in which he appears almost catatonic and he is not really psychologically accessible for several days. His main requirement is nursing care and seclusion, so that he can gradually develop awareness of his feelings of loss of vision and associated feelings of helplessness. With the acceptance of being blind he will go through a period in which he will grieve for the loss of his eyes, and feel despondent about his future. He needs encouragement to master the acts of feeding himself and learning to walk again with the aid of a cane or a dog. His feelings of being depressed require insight therapy rather than repressive therapy; otherwise his fantasies of being punished for sinfulness which caused his blindness will give rise to a chronic masochistic depression. Persuasion and encouragement to master new skills is the first step in overcoming tendencies phobically to avoid the task of learning again by trial and error. Encouraging intellectual curiosity and the desire to be active may be associated with the development of compulsive traits. Aggressiveness and competitiveness in the process of learning produce anxiety in the blind person who is afraid of strong affective expression, and he needs sanction to be active.

The marginally adjusted person who becomes blind may be satisfied that he has no reason to become actively self-supporting, and may even demand that society take care of him. His motivation for therapy is poor and his attitude will be "You tell me what to do."

As the blind person has contact with fewer people, his dependency gratification may be more deeply invested in one or two significant persons. His transference reaction is intense and quickly developed in therapy. He needs help in knowing that he strongly desires—or even demands—approval from others, and that he often over-reacts to criticism as if he were being rejected. Loss of love objects is taken very hard, and depression occurs.

Countertransference tendencies require constant check on the part of the therapist; and realistic evaluation of the individual's function can be obtained through medical and social sources.

The parents of blind children require help in accepting blindness in a guilt-free manner in order to provide a healthy relationship with the child. They should be discouraged from placing their child in a residential school before he has gone through the oedipal period of development. Otherwise he is likely to become an affect-deprived individual with a poor sense of self-worth and no clear sexual identity, wandering around in what he calls the blind world, with the feeling that he is being ostracized by what he terms the sighted world. The degree of social acceptance which the blind person receives is a function of whether he relates to others in a socially understood and acceptable way. Only the individual who accepts his blindness can also realize himself as an adequate person who can participate socially with blind or sighted people, form love ties, and have a family and future of his own.

BIBLIOGRAPHY

1. SCHILDER, PAUL: The Image and Appearance of the Human Body. New York, International Universities Press, Inc., 1950.
2. GORDON, BENJAMIN L.: Oculus Fascinus. Arch. Ophthalmol. 17:290-319, 1937.
   Oculists and occultists. Arch. Ophthalmol. 22, 25-65, 1939.
3. GESELL, ARNOLD, ILG, FRANCES L., AND BULLIS, GLENNA E.: Vision: Its Development in the Infant and Child. Paul B. Hoeber, Inc., 1949.
4. GREEN, MAURICE R., AND SCHECTER, DAVID E.: Autistic and symbiotic disorders in three children, Psych. Quart. 31, 628-646, 1957.
5. BURLINGHAM, DOROTHY: Psychic problems of the blind. Am. Imago 2:43-85, 1941.
6. DEUTSCH, FELIX: The sense of reality in persons born blind. J. Psychol. 10:121-140, 1940.
7. SCHLAEGEL, T. F.: The dominant method of imagery in blind as compared to sighted adolescents. Pedagog. Semin. & J. Genet. Psychol. 83:265-277, 1953.
8. CUTSFORTH, THOMAS D.: The Blind in School and Society. The American New York Foundation for the Blind, 1951.
9. WEINSTEIN, E. A., AND KAHN, R. L.: Denial of Illness. Springfield, Charles C. Thomas, 1955.
10. DIAMOND, BERNARD L. AND ROSS, ALICE: Emotional adjustment of newly blinded soldiers. Am. J. Psychiat. 102:367-371, 1945.
11. BLANK, H. ROBERT: Dreams of the blind. Psychoanalyt. Quart. 27:158-174, 1958.

The Treatment of the Dying

by Thomas P. Hackett, M.D. and Avery D. Weisman, M.D.

A NY PROGRAM designed to help a patient face personal death must begin with careful consideration of whether or not the patient should be told he is about to die. Recent surveys[1] of physicians' opinions on this subject reveal that a majority favor withholding information. This opinion is often supported with the argument that offering truth to the dying can only lead to further discomfort, augmented fear, and deepened depression. The common underlying assumption is that the human being is unable to cope with the knowledge that he is about to die.

The reasons underlying this attitude on the part of the doctor seem to revolve around two primary issues. The first is that people in general tend to deny their mortality and that doctors, specifically, since they are in such close contact with death, tend to protect themselves with denial. Secondly, medical training offers little help to the doctor in the treatment of the process of death except familiarization with the use of drugs to alleviate pain and to blunt awareness of suffering. Because of the sweeping advances in medical science during the last century, death and dying have become symbols of defeat rather than conditions requiring a doctor's care and attention. However, despite our success in increasing longevity, death must still be dealt with on its own uncompromising terms.

Illness alters a patient's life and alienates him from the familiar world. When this illness is fatal, the patient's sense of alienation often mounts to profound loneliness—a state inaccessible to drugs. The physician, then, is left only with whatever resources he can bring to the situation. Like his patient, he finds himself alone. Because hope is what the patient seems to want, the doctor usually tries to supply it through veiled reassurance and a distant promise of health. In most cases the patient seems to respond favorably, feel better, or experience an elevation in mood. We believe that the hope and optimism often displayed by dying patients is an exterior maintained more for the sake of those about them than for themselves. Furthermore, we feel that by offering only false hope

121

and optimism, the physician reduces the possibility of true communication and thereby jeopardizes his chance to help the patient.

Our investigation of the dying patient began after we encountered six patients,[2] each of whom approached his death in a totally unique way. Each of the six viewed death more as resolution than as source of conflict. Not one was suicidal, depressed, or anxious. As a result of our experiences with this group, we began to wonder whether other dying patients, less favorably disposed toward death, might be able to assimilate and use the knowledge that they were about to die. We then examined the taped interviews of twelve patients with terminal cancer who had been in psychotherapy with one of the authors in connection with another project. In addition, eight dying patients were taken into psychotherapy. None of these twenty patients had been told he was terminal at the time he was first seen by the psychiatrist.

Early in our work with these twenty patients, two striking facts emerged. First, none of these patients ever alluded directly to his future or to dying. The second fact was less obvious and revealed itself only after the doctor–patient relationship had been well established. Each of these patients knew, to some extent, that he was dying and that facts were being withheld. The theme of death, revealed through associations, dreams, slips-of-the-tongue, subtle queries and silences, was a constant, ever-intrusive partner. That these patients were not direct in expressing apprehension was no proof of ignorance. The form of inquiry forced on the physician the choice between truth and deception. If a middle-of-the-road course was attempted, the doctor soon found himself unable to reply to questions without altogether avoiding the topic of death or being forced to truth.

An example of this dilemma and of one solution is evident in the case of a woman with a terminal breast cancer who asked why her headache persisted. When the doctor said it was probably nerves, she asked why she was nervous. He returned the question. She replied, "I am nervous because I have lost 60 pounds in a year. The Priest comes to see me twice a week, which he never did before, and my mother-in-law is nicer to me even though I am meaner to her. Wouldn't this make you nervous?" There was a pause. Then the doctor said, "You mean, you think you're dying." She said, "I do." He said, "You are." Then she smiled and said, 'Well, I've finally broken the sound barrier; someone's finally told me the truth."

Another patient, a retired minister, beleaguered his physician daily with a host of questions about minor symptoms. The doctor patiently reassured him by explaining away each symptom. It became a boring litany, hollow and meaningless to both patient and doctor. One day the patient asked whether the soul could catch measles. The doctor did not know what to do, so he smiled and uttered the comfortable cliché, "You have to get worse before you get better." The patient smiled and said, "I begin to get worried when the doctors begin to sound like young clergymen. When you put a straight question to them they start talking wind."

This type of questioning took place only after the doctor had known his patient for some time and had shown himself to be open for discussion. If the contact had been brief, as on rounds, it is more than likely that these patients would have appeared content in their ignorance, avoidance, or acceptance of their fate. Left to themselves, they would probably not have asked the question of paramount personal importance.

Patients may know they are dying, but, at the same time, be unable to accept the fact that they will be dead. This paradox has been described elsewhere[2] and is by no means confined to the dying. All of us recognize that death is a property of life, but still find it impossible to imagine ourselves dead. The terminal patient cannot avoid facing this paradox. It presents a conflict—a state of mind wherein the patient can repudiate death while realizing that he dies. Because he is between what he knows and what he cannot know, we call this state of mind Middle Knowledge. The patient vacillates between hope and despair. Pulled, on the one hand, by the optimism of physician and relatives, he is quickly reminded of dying by pain and the persistence of symptoms on the other.

Middle Knowledge is neither static nor standard and varies from patient to patient as well as within the same patient at different times. At its simplest, it can be regarded as the knowledge that one is dying without the ability to know fully or anticipate the fact of death.

Middle Knowledge bears an inverse relationship to denial. The more a patient is able to deny that he is dying, the less Middle Knowledge he possesses. Denial can result from displacement, rationalization, avoidance and other defensive measures. Middle Knowledge can be gained from learning about one's disease, from an inability to deny the facts of one's condition, or from a disbelief in reassurance.

The processes of denial are notoriously active in the dying patient. It is not unusual to hear a moribund patient speak of going on a vacation. Taken at face value, this optimism would be a tremendous asset in easing the anguish of the dying. Some patients are excellent deniers and appear to use this defense effectively to the very end. With such patients open and honest confrontation by the doctor with the facts of their condition is not assimilated. The facts do not seem to register. This type of global or massive denial seems to be more common among patients facing sudden death than among those dying slowly. For example, 16 out of 23 patients on the cardiac pacemaker for heart block flatly denied fear or concern with death in spite of the fact that they had been fully informed of the danger. In such patients Middle Knowledge is at a minimum. With patients who die slowly, on the other hand, denial tends to become less sturdy and Middle Knowledge, revealed in the form of subtle questions about persistent symptoms, dreams about dying, or reversal of affect, comes through. We are left then with the fact that a few people can deny splendidly, others very little. The effective use of denial depends on a variety of factors, all special to the individual.

It is a mistake for doctors to assume that all dying patients believe what they are told and accept proferred hope because they desperately need to. There are many patients who value truth in communication and who will lose confidence as soon as trust is violated. The dying patient needs communication and exchange with those around him more desperately than do other types of patients. Dying is lonely, and closeness and warmth are the only remedies. This is our principal reason for advocating truth. We do not mean that the physician must bluntly tell the patient that he has a fatal, incurable condition and will be done in within the month. Truth has many faces, each of which can be employed as it is needed. Nor does truth, under these circumstances, altogether cut off a source for hope. Hope for improvement is never lost, even when a cure is impossible.

That truth and hope are not mutually exclusive is illustrated in the case of a middle-aged widow with a metastatic breast lesion. Her family had been told the prognosis, but only one brother fully understood its implication. The rest of her relatives treated her as though she would recover soon, and chided her for not gaining enough strength to do housework. She felt guilty about her weakness, suspicious of her brother's unaccustomed kindness, and angry at the evasiveness of her doctors. Her apprehension was evident to the psychiatrist as was the extent of her Middle Knowledge, revealed in questions. He told her that she must know the answer to her questions. There was a silence and she cried. She was then told what could be expected and her internist repeated the explanation. She was told that her doctors would stand by her and do everything in their power to prolong life. As months went by, symptoms accumulated and, had truth been strictly adherred to, the physician would have been no more than a morbid commentator on her state of decline. Instead, talk of symptoms could often be avoided, and, when reassurance was offered, it was accepted as intended. When she became despondent, she was returned to the hospital and given nitrogen mustards. Although the word "cure" was never mentioned, she was always aware that she was being cared for. The hope that a new drug would make her more comfortable for a few days was enough to lighten her spirits.

Shortly before her death she wrote a note saying, "Thank you for putting up with me and listening to what I said."

The easiest course for the physician to follow in treating the dying is to withhold the truth and to support the patient's use of denial. There probably are cases where this policy must be used, but we have not as yet uncovered one valid contraindication to the use of truth. The doctor sometimes misinterprets a patient's silence on matters of mortality as evidence that denial is operating effectively. A case in point was that of a charming and worldly man dying of tongue cancer. Throughout our long contact with him, he always managed to avoid talking about the future and behaved as though his illness were a transient thing. He was considered an excellent denier. A few days before he died, the tumor suddenly enlarged and swelled his tongue to such an extent that he could not speak. On the night of his death, his psychiatrist visited him, but could think of nothing to say. So he sat on the bed and put his arm around the patient's shoulder. The patient reached for a pencil and pad and wrote, "Don't take it so hard, Doc." He had known the prognosis throughout those many months of conversation, but had not spoken of it. As one can see from this case, the physician must have a constant awareness of his own tendency to avoid talking about painful issues.

The physician's attitude determines the policy for the patient's family and friends. When he advises them not to disclose the grim truth, a lie is born. To act out a lie requires acting ability which the physician may or may not possess. Even if he does, the other characters may not play their roles convincingly. How, for example, can a wife "be herself" with a husband who is dying, but supposedly does not not know it? One wife told her husband the truth the very day she learned he would be dead in a few weeks. Neither of them informed the doctor, who continued to behave as though his patient would improve until his patient died. The wife apologized for the deception, saying she could never have acted the part. Most relatives are not as willing to realize their limitations as was this wife and enter the plot without questioning the practicality of it. Unprepared to meet the constant questions of the dying patient, they tend either to avoid him or to adopt an unfamiliar manner. The distance between them and the dying can quickly become enormous. Deception cannot flourish where openness and honesty have been the rule. One of the saddest dramas enacted is the silent conspiracy between doctor and relatives to keep the patient happily uninformed, when, all the while, the patient has been playing his assigned role and protecting the feelings of the other actors.

Even when the relationship between doctor and dying patient has been established in truth and when a climate of open discussion prevails, it is a taxing and trying job to treat those about to die. The physician should be prepared to cope with an initial anger when the prognosis is disclosed, an anger directed toward him and toward medical science as well. He will have to adjust to a constant feeling of helplessness, unable to do anything but sit and listen and talk when there is something he can say. The physician must contend with the guilt evoked by the questioning glance of the dying, with the unspoken question, "Why should I die while you live?" The term deathwatch can only be appreciated after one has watched at the bedside until the patient has died. The nearer the patient approaches death, the more he reaches out toward life. Touch is often important, sitting close to him, holding his hand, staying near him even without words. All of these things make the chasm between the living and the dead less terrifying and lonely.

In summary, we believe that it is a mistake to assume that everyone feels the same unutterable fear of death. Furthermore, we believe that it is almost impossible to withhold the knowledge of death from a dying person, and that to attempt to do so blindly imposes an unintended exile on someone facing ultimate loneliness. In order to treat the dying patient, the physician must be familiar with the concepts of Middle Knowledge and denial and must act with this knowledge to insure closeness, confidence, and care between the living and those about to die.

REFERENCES

1. OKEN, DONALD: What to tell cancer patients, J.A.M.A. 175:1120-1128 (April 1), 1961.
2. WEISMAN, A. D., AND HACKETT, T. P.: Predilection to death: Death and dying as a psychiatric problem. Psychosom. Med. 23:232-256 (May-June), 1961.

The Physician's Management of the Dying Patient

by CHARLES WILLIAM WAHL, M.D.

T HE FEAR OF DEATH is in many ways unique in psychic life, for unlike other fears and anxieties which owe their frightening import to the possibility only of a foreboding and dreaded circumstance, death is certain and unavoidable for all mankind. Uniquely, it is the one known fear whose referent is based on an absolutely unavoidable circumstance. In strict objectivity, it is the one inescapable fear with which we deal, based on the reality, which we often tend to ignore, that life is finite and we are finite with it. Aeschylus expressed man's plight in a very graphic way 2300 years ago:

> Alone of gods Death loves not gifts; with him
> Nor sacrifice nor incense aught avails;
> He hath no altar and no hymns of gladness;
> Prayer stands aloof from him, Persuasion fails.

While it is with awe and with pride that we survey man's fantastic progress since Aeschylus wrote these lines, with the phenomenon of Death it remains exactly as he has described it. We can postpone death, we can assuage its physical pain, but escape it we cannot.

Since the inescapable hallmark of the human estate is its finitude, then on one level the fear of death is the deliberate and rational apprehension that one day we shall cease to be. One might expect that under this condition all of us would be in a state of chronic apathy and depression; yet it is a noteworthy and remarkable paradox that while we all must die, we do not all fear death to the same degree nor in the same way.

Now this should prompt us as psychiatrists to ask several germane questions. First, does the fear of death, or thanatophobia, as it is designated in its maximal form, because of the inescapability of its referent

EDITOR'S NOTE: With reference to the preceding chapter, the policy of this series is to present contrasting views when these are held by authorities in important fields of psychiatric therapy.

127

evoke or necessitate unique methods of defensive reduction in the psychic economy? We know that the fearful concept, object or circumstance in a phobia is comparable to the manifest content of dreams, i.e., its ostensible concern only conceals another one which is more unacceptable to the self, which is latent and repressed. Is thanatophobia an exception to this rule? Can there be anything more fearful to the organism than the cessation of its being?

It is a matter not without its dynamic import that these questions, germane as they are, have never been properly addressed by psychiatry— a profession that prides itself on investigating things which others wish to shun. An entire bibliography on the subject makes very scant reading indeed. For the sad truth is that we do not have very satisfactory answers for these questions. The massive psychological defenses against death that are more fulsomely applied by mankind in the handling of this fear than in any other area of human experience have not exempted psychiatrists from their employment. The elucidation of this whole area remains one of the great tasks of our generation.

The scope of these defenses may not be immediately apparent to us without reflection. Until quite recently the very word death was taboo. Cumbersome and elaborate euphemisms were employed instead, such as "passed away" or "passed on," and the dead were referred to as the "departed." The persistence with which man has believed in an immortal state without the slightest shred of evidence that he chooses to collect in the establishment of other beliefs is noteworthy. The very word "perish" is from the Latin "perire," meaning "to pass through," an insistence that death is a transition rather than a cessation. There are those who maintain that religion can be explained as a gigantic defense against death by the guarantee of an immortal state which it is purported can be obtained by adherence to its system of belief. In addition, at gigantic cost and expressly against the tenets of the prevailing Judeo-Christian ethics, there is maintained a multibillion dollar industry, "the undertakers," to shield us from ever looking at an untreated dead person. They purvey to us an illusion, an illusion of sleep and incorruptibility. These cultural defenses are so effective that the vast majority of persons live their entire lives without ever viewing death in its pristine form.

These complex social taboos against death protect from involvement with it all segments of the population except for two groups only—the medical and the nursing professions. The physician and the nurse cannot isolate themselves from death. They see it not in its prettified form, but before the intervention of the artful hand of the embalmer. They see the deceased with his rigor mortis, agape mouth, staring eyes, and with the slack expression of the newly dead. It is the rare physician who does not remember his first such contact. It is a powerful and compelling experience.

It is significant, however, that this experience rarely provokes in a physician or a nurse the fear that such an experience might presume to produce in other groups, and this seemingly has not just to do with the physician's habituation to these sights. It is appropriate for us to consider how this may be.

The usual defense against death is a precipitate of the infantile omnipotence, and this reflects itself as a complete inability to unconsciously credit or believe that the immutable self can ever cease to be. This precipitate is stronger in previously loved and cherished persons in childhood, for reasons discussed elsewhere.* And so it may be that persons who become physicians can forego the usual defenses which require separation from "memento mori" and choose a profession that brings them into contact with the dead and dying because of exceptional ego strength and feelings of magical invulnerability resultant from such childhood experiences. I am sure that oftentimes this must be so. An opposite pattern, however, also could result in the choice of medicine as a profession. I have been struck, in the physicians whom I have treated in psychotherapy for other matters, how frequently one encounters a strong antecedent fear of death of considerable proportions in their history. It would appear that the later choice of medicine as a profession sometimes may represent a counterphobic defense against death, a reaction formation to an earlier fear of it mastered by the doing of the very thing that was previously frightening. It seems sometimes to represent a kind of identification with the aggressor, a wish to be on the winning team. Just as the guilty little boy may end up as a lawyer and be comforted by being the judge rather than the judged, so the physician may handle the fear of death by identification with the profession of medicine, for by paleologic definition it is always the patient who gets sick and dies, not the doctor. In the unconscious, the M.D. degree confers immunity to all the ills and vicissitudes that beset our patients. Perhaps another indication of this is the oft-noted tendency of doctors to give sage advice that they never follow themselves. Most of us smoke and are overweight, we work too hard, we tend to ignore the rules of simple hygiene, we fail to get sufficient exercise and rest. These are of course dangerous things to do, and we would get quite angry with a patient if he did these things. It is significant that they do not evoke in us, however, the same sense of self-preservative horror. Doctors, too,

---

*Wahl, Charles W.: The Fear of Death: *In* The Meaning of Death, edited by Herman Feifel, Ph.D. New York, McGraw-Hill Book Company, 1959.

as any nurse will confirm, are notoriously bad patients when they themselves are ill. It is as if they are shocked and outraged at the wholly unbelievable fact that they themselves can be ill. In addition to this another defense for the handling of this or any fear is to learn all about it. Knowledge gives an illusion of control, and one is rarely so frightened of a thing well known to one.

These patterns of behavior have particular relevance to the physician's management of the dying or the terminally ill patient. For this antimony in the physician's character, his earlier fear of death handled by denial, reaction formation and identification with the aggressor, and his subsequent counterphobic feelings of magical omnipotence and invulnerability may result in a failure to perceive the fear of death and illness in his patients and particularly leads to mismanagement of the dying or terminally ill patient. The price of his comfort may be to remain oblivious and consequently uninvolved at a time when the patient badly needs his care.

The unconscious attitudes towards the dying which exist covertly and implicitly in our culture are often overt and explicit in more primitive cultures. Anthropologic scrutiny of these cultures helps us better to see our own subtle practices.

In many cultures the moment the process of dying begins the dying ones become an object of fear and uncanny dread. The onlookers, even the close family, respond as though contact with them may cause themselves to die. In some cultures, the dying are removed from the community to die neglected alone in the "death hut" outside the village. We do not have to look far in our hospitals to see that our dying too are often in a sense abandoned. It is not a rare sight on a ward to see a terminally ill patient alone in a room at the end of the hall with an IV rigged, the oxygen hissing, and the staff far away comforted by the feeling that they have done all they can.

In other cultures the dying person is presumed to commit a hostile act by so doing, and in one instance it is the custom to "beat him to it," so to speak, by hitting him over the head with a club. Do we ever, as physicians, feel that the patient, by perversely dying, has turned traitor, so to speak, by challenging our omnipotence, and is our detachment from him an expression of unconscious anger which the savage experiences more directly? Apropos of this, the arguments adduced in favor of euthanasia often appear to be in the service of relieving the doctor of his hostility, care and guilt rather than being such a service to the recipient. Moreover, when a patient begins to die, he is hard to love. There is a natural, though primitive, wish to free libidinal cathexis from him. It is also a common experience for the terminally ill patient to regress and to become more selfish and infantile, narcissistic and demanding. We are often not prepared to face these character traits which are unpleasant, and we may respond with a vague, guilty anger. Also when a patient knows he is going to die, unconsciously he wants to punish the ones who will survive, particularly the doctor who does not save him. This may serve too to provoke the physician or the nurse to view the patient as alien, separate and frightening and justify a gradual detachment from him. These primitive practices, "anläge" of which are residual in our own unconscious, may give us clues as to how we may better help the dying patient.

Hence the most important and necessary precondition in the management of the terminally ill is that the physician have the willingness and capacity to look deeply within himself not only in scrutiny of his attitudes towards living and dying and some of the unconscious equivalences of the latter, but also an addressment to what might be called the eternal questions—"Whence came I? Whither go I?"—and have derived in terms of his own needs and understanding answers that are meaningful and significant for himself.

With this as a preludium, it is then possible to consider objectively what are the goals in managing the care of a terminally ill patient and how may this best be done. The primary goal is to assuage the terror of death and of the process of dying in the patient, not only to prevent these from adversely affecting the course of the disease, since it is quite possible to be "frightened to death," but to enable the patient, if needs be, to die with dignity and serenity in the fullest possession of his human faculties that his state permits. To this end, it is important that the patient not be deprived of hope. It is a surprising thing that the possibility of personal surcease is not resident in the unconscious. Even though the rational probabilities of survival may be slight, the individual is obdurately immune to reality testing in this area. The defense of denial in the face of death is absolute and inveterate and is persisted in even in those patients who assert that they recognize and accept this fact, and even in patients who had been categorically told so by their physicians.

The extent to which this is operative has to be seen to be believed. I recall a physician who suffered from a neoplastic disease of great malignancy. He was deeply depressed until on looking up the literature he discovered that there was a five-year survival rate of 4 per cent. He became immediately much more cheerful, convinced against logic and probability that he would be of the 4 per cent, not of the 96 per cent, and this overweening optimism persisted until his death. Las Vegas should convince us that we all, in the depths of our selves, feel immune to the laws of chance that govern others. Unconsciously, we all agree with the psalmist David who said, "A thousand shall fall at thy right hand and ten thousand at thy left, but it shall not come nigh thee." The task of the physician is to strengthen and buttress the natural and ever present defenses of denial. This small area of paleologic unreality is permitted to exist, so that the rest of the personality may be preserved reachable and intact. It must be remembered that the peculiar torture of capital punishment is not death itself (for we all must die and the death of execution itself is not a painful one), but in the fact of knowing exactly when death will occur.

The physician then, for humanitarian reasons as well as scientific ones, must never give a sentence of death and the patient is never permitted to be bereft of hope. It is my conviction that no patient should ever be told he is going to die, even if he assures his physician that he wants the "naked truth." He should be told, "You have a serious problem, but no illness is without hope and you should remember that." The patient is helped to utilize his best defenses, namely, those of denial and infantile omnipotence. To make the hope more believable it is also important not to overassure the patient or to be unduly cheerful out of context.

It is important that the patient also not be permitted to be isolated, either from friends and relatives or from the staff. The Greeks said that the most horrible of ills was not to die but to die alone. Regularity and predictability of contact with the physician implies continuity to the patient, continuity of care to the conscious, but the probability of continuity of life to the unconscious. It implies a promise, "I will see you again tomorrow at the same time and you have nothing to fear in the interim." And this dependable certainty alone has great efficacy in making the patient more comfortable. For just this reason, however, great care must be taken not to omit a promised visitation. Relatives should also be encouraged not to isolate the patient, though constant and unduly prolonged visitation should not be permitted. This implies to the patient the "death watch."

The patient is helped to make a symbolic displacement from his concern about his incurable illness to ones which are curable. He should be encouraged to be somewhat hypochondriacal and the physician should listen with interest and attention to all his complaints, particularly the physical ones and ones related to intercurrent infections, colds, skin rashes, etc. which can be treated and cured. These should be vigorously treated. The patient, by "trading up" illnesses, receives an intense reassurance and a magical relief, as though he were exchanging his fatal illness for others less lethal.

To the same end one should deliberately focus attention on the patient's "immortal physiology," such as the processes of digestion and elimination.

He should be questioned at length about these functions, and it is remarkable to see how often the obsessive–compulsive narcissistic regression of the terminally ill manifests itself in an extreme overconcern and interest in bowel movements. It represents a regressive return to infantile logic and the infantile conception of disease—"If I just avoid drafts and have a good bowel movement I can never be ill."

One should listen attentively to the patient's complaints and to the key words with which he voices them and pay particular attention to those which express a symbolic fear of death. Terminally ill patients may have a recurrence of fear of the dark, or of closed doors, or of lying recumbent or of numbness or coldness, and the wording of such phrases as "I'm deathly afraid of the dark," "I feel boxed in when the door is closed," show the primary anxiety. Recumbency may be equated with "laying down to die." All of these demands, and many of them are quite idiosyncratic, should be unobtrusively complied with. For the same reason it is not a service to the patient to utterly ablate any pain he may be experiencing. To feel nothing is to be dead, and the terror complete analgesia may produce far outweighs the advantage. The same considerations apply in the use of ataraxic or sedative drugs. These are, in my experience, rarely efficacious, particularly since the isolation and detachment from reality which they may produce cause terror in its own right. Admittedly there is a need for further experience with their use.

The patient should be touched. Not only because this assuages the fear of being "untouchable," the dying thing, a feared object, but because the touch, the caress, is the most archaic pre-verbal way we possess of communication, solace and comfort. The mother uses it long before words can solace, and to lightly pat or touch the patient who is disturbed or frightened communicates a comfort that words can never convey. Frequent backrubs and massages, therefore, not only engender physical well being, but psychic as well. Also cosmetic care of the patient should not be neglected. This is particularly important for a woman.

The patient should not be treated as if he had no future. All patients should be encouraged to plan for the future for themselves and for their relatives and children. Children are, in the unconscious, "the fruit of our loins," immortal extensions of ourselves, living defenses against the fear of being blotted out. Terminally ill patients derive comfort and satisfaction from visitation with relatives and children and in planning for them. No hospital should be organized in such a way as to prevent this contact with family members. And it is a service not only to the patient but to his survivors. Their own guilt and sadness is assuaged by opportunities to make such a service to their loved one.

Lastly, if the patient is a member of a religion that makes mandatory that he be told of any possibility of his death, this should not be done "in extremis," but should rather be done while the patient is well enough to make what plans may seem to him to be important and while he still has time to re-employ the usual denial defenses.

While the physician does not bludgeon the patient with the full and exact truth about his status, it is important that one or preferably two of his close family be informed. This is necessary for legal reasons and to enable them to have time to adjust also to the possible death of the patient.

It is remarkable to note that these simple measures, when practiced by a warm and empathetic physician, acting in concert as they do with the powerful defenses of denial, reaction formation and undoing which the seriously ill person can call upon, usually suffice in themselves to enable the terminally ill patient to cope successfully with his situation.

In a small minority of patients, however, these measures are insufficient to produce relief. In these patients the prospect of their imminent death may provoke a terror, depression or apathy that can progress to a psychotic decompensation if unchecked. The treatment of choice for these patients is intensive psychotherapy and it should begin as soon as possible after consultation.

The following is a brief enumeration of some of the factors which appear to inhere in psychotherapeutic work with the terminally ill. In the treatment of these patients it is remarkable to note, considering the seriousness and inexorability of the reality situation, how quickly the terror and depression which they have experienced is moderated and how greatly they appear to be benefited. This appears to be explained by two factors. Firstly the psychiatrist attempts to supply the patient with a unique experience in that he, in contradistinction to the other persons who surround the patient, is better able to tolerate the discussion of material frightening to him without utilizing the defensive isolation, detachment and fearful projection which others may have employed. The psychiatrist takes particular care to see the patient faithfully at the stated intervals and makes himself available to the patient at any other time he may urgently require it. Secondly, a significant difference between psychotherapy with the terminally ill and other psychoneurotic conditions is that with extraordinary rapidity a strongly positive and dependent transference to the therapist is established and very archaic aspects of ego function and interpersonal relationship are evidenced. The speed with which this archaic, regressive transference is established is not paralleled by any other treatment situation known to me. The therapist becomes in rapid order the omnipotent, primordial parent imago, and as

*Eissler, K. R.: The Psychiatrist and the Dying Patient. New York International Universities Press, Inc., 1955.

soon as this kind of transference is established the patient appears to have an almost complete assuagement of the terror, anxiety, depression and reality alienation that preceded treatment. The healthy usual denial defenses and the feelings of infantile omnipotence and invulnerability are then reconstituted in their pristine strength and the patient, even though consciously aware of the seriousness of his illness, and often experiencing considerable physical pain, acts as though he had "a new lease on life."

In psychotherapy with any other kind of neurosis this "transference neurosis" would be explored, studied and analyzed. In psychotherapy of the terminally ill, scrutiny of it is deliberately avoided. In addition, everything which will further reality contact and serve to limit regression to this single area of exaggerated magical relationship is done. The patient is seen, if he is ambulatory, *vis-à-vis,* and never should be worked with on the couch. The face and person of the therapist should be constantly available for testing scrutiny.

The therapist is often in a dilemma when material relating to a concomitant or antecedent neurotic problem is produced. To work with this material dynamically may in some patients produce a serious depression, since the patient unconsciously knows that he is preparing himself for better function for a future which he will not possess. And yet perhaps even more frightening to him is the thought that the therapist by so doing employs denial defenses more patently magical than his own. It is necessary to be very individualistic in the approach to the patient. Just as some persons facing certain death may be solaced by engrossing themselves in a chess game, so occasionally, after the denial defenses are re-established, the patient, with serene detachment, studies himself as though he were another. Other patients deal with quotidian experiences only or experience a second childhood which often seems to subserve the same purpose the second childhood does in the old, namely, a counterphobic reaction formation against age, death and dying, and a return to that period in life in which one was most alien and distant from the concept of death. They experience a most pleasurable revivification of early days and memories when death was far off, and this identity with one's former youthful self may persist unabated until the final moment.

It is clear, too, that another avenue of relief for the patient is based on the unconscious conception of cure—one which is described and utilized by all primitive tribes, that is, that of transference in the concrete sense— a *transfer* of the patient's ills to the therapist, as does the witch doctor who, for a fee, takes upon himself the illnesses of his clients. The dreams of the patient show decided evidence of the hope, the expectation even, that "the therapist will die instead of myself." Needless to say, this is left uninterpreted to the patient. He is instead allowed the magical lift in his spirits which it produces and it is presumed that the therapist has worked through his own feelings about death and dying so that it may not be necessary for himself to feel the need to empathetically detach himself from the patient when he perceives these wishes on his part.

Finally we come to a question that perhaps you have perceived I have not dealt with previously, namely, the countertransference of the therapist and how he is affected by developing an intimate identification and relationship with a person who will soon die. I must candidly acknowledge that doing psychotherapy with the few such patients I have treated has been the most difficult and challenging professional experience of my life. Martin Grotjahn* has said that a therapist must be like the harp player in that like him he develops a callus on the tip of each finger so that he may pluck the strings without bleeding. And yet, despite this, he must have a sure and delicate touch and a consummate sensitivity to all the nuances of the strings. This is harder to achieve in psychotherapy with the dying than with any other patient; and short of one's personal psychoanalysis, I know of no experience which gives one deeper insights into oneself or others.

Perhaps this shows us that what one really does for and with a patient in this most inescapable of all life situations is to say covertly to him, "Time and Space have no representation in the unconscious. Be solaced by the knowledge that but an eyeblink of time separates my death and the death of all mankind from your own." The willingness to do this without horror or abandonment of the patient gives him a solace that one day we shall have a right to expect from another for ourselves. It will enable him and later ourselves to follow Bryant's advice in *Thanatopsis:*

> So live that when thy summons comes to join
> The innumerable caravan which moves
> To that mysterious realm where each shall take
> His chamber in the silent halls of death,
> Thou go not like the quarry slave at night,
> Scourged to his dungeon, but, sustained and soothed
> By an unfaltering trust, approach thy grave
> Like one that wraps the drapery of his couch
> About him and lies down to pleasant dreams.

*Personal communication.

REFERENCES

Shapley, Harlow, Rapport, Samuel, and Wright, Helen: A Treasury of Science. New York, Harper and Bros., 3rd ed., revised, 1954.
Wahl, Charles W.: The Fear of Death. Bull. Menninger Clin. 22:214-223, 1958.

PART IV

Treatment of the Psychoses

Dynamics and Psychotherapy
of Depression

by WALTER BONIME, M.D.

A BASIC, unifying formulation for understanding the psychological
forces that generate and constitute depression is that *depression is a practice*. The view that depression is not a passive, intrapsychic
response to external or endogenous circumstances, but an active way of
relating interpersonally, may also serve well as a guiding concept for
dealing with the condition psychotherapeutically.

The dynamics of depression are obscured by attempts to define a
*pre*morbid character. The illness is not a supervening emotional response
which inhibits tendencies to 'normal' functioning. On the contrary,
depressive symptomatology, varying in intensity from sulk to psychosis, is
a consistent reflection of the basic pathological functioning of the personality. Anger, in part a response to the frustration of the functioning and in
part and implementation of it, is a central element of depression.

Descriptively, in the wide range of clinical pictures, the outstanding
common features are the aspect of gloom and a major recession from an
achieved level of productive activity. There is not merely a reduction of
motion, but a decline of useful activity. There is often monotonous,
repetitive, slow or agitated, indecisive, impulsive, unconsummated pre-
paratory behavior. Although anorexia is characteristic, compulsive eating
may also occur, and this latter feature may sometimes lead to an obesity
which is confused with pyknic habitus. Cases of psychotic severity tend to
be characterized by feelings of unworthiness, persecutory, preoccupations,
hypochondriasis, 'guilt,' and self recrimination. These features appear also
in the milder depressive disturbances and probably underlie some forms of
insomnia—it is difficult to sleep in anger. While its association with the
age of involution is generally recognized, depression—characterologically

and symptomatically—is frequently amalgamated with homosexuality, alcoholism, migraine or lesser headaches, and gastrointestinal ulcer. Finally, in duration, the outstanding features of lowered mood and decline in productiveness may involve anywhere from a few hours or a weekend of moping to years of institutionalized inertness. Since its brief or less severe expressions are often neither discerned by the observer nor acknowledged by the subject, depression tends to be recognized only in its more dramatic forms and then regarded as a clinical entity divorced from the afflicted individual's pre-existing ways of living. In order to see the relationship between the individual's personality and the depressive exacerbation, it is necessary first to examine the chief pathological features of his way of relating.

Manipulation of others is a cardinal element of the patient's behavior. Control over the activity, feelings and attitudes of others is the chief goal of manipulativeness. Gratification comes from the success of the controlling effort, rather than from the specific response. Making someone do something is more important than what he does.

Dependency, for example, is a common covert form of managing the activities of others. Sexual seductiveness may be covert and unaware, but even when it is overt and conscious the individual may not recognize that the manipulative gratification greatly outweighs the sensual. The 'hypomanic' quality of personality often associated with the depressive may itself represent the interpersonal technique of sweeping people along, bending them to one's will in numerous activities, especially social activities. What appears to be exclusively friendliness and enthusiasm for people in the hypomanic can be primarily an enjoyment of their influencibility. The seemingly physiologic ups and downs of the manic-depressive may be alternations of bouts of controlling people by enthusiasm and infectious energy, followed by gloomy, angry, 'depressive' retardation in response to manipulative failure. In the excessively religious or moralistic individual, manipulativeness may appear as righteous tyranny. Manipulativeness may involve no more than implicit threats or bribes, or be accomplished by the enslaving devices of self effacement and self sacrifice, or by an insidious showering with excessive service in order to impose dependency.

A long history of minor depressions—sulks, moping, and sudden inertias—probably exists in most patients, and will often be found to be related to failures of manipulation. These types of minor depression are not always clinically correlated with the patient's practices or even fully elicited in the anamnesis. The high incidence of intense depressions in the involutional period can be understood in relation to the diminution of various forms of manipulative effectiveness: the decrease of parental authority, loss of occupational status, and loss of sexual allure, to suggest a few. A frequent basis for a common form of depression—'feeling rejected'—a depressive reaction charged with angry vindictiveness that at times reaches homicidal intensity, is the inability manipulatively to elicit love.

A corollary of manipulativeness is a *pathologic aversion to being influenced* by others. The individual makes little discrimination between healthy, cooperative, reciprocal influence and the undue manipulation of him. Frequently the sense of coercion comes from a distorted interpretation of the intent of another person.* Almost any interpersonal influence produces a sense of being subtly coerced or used, a sense of weakness and helplessness. This is intolerable because it nullifies the individual's own basic operational effectiveness, his own manipulating.

Since this manipulating is the basis of the patient's sense of self, the interference with and the threat to this sense of self would ordinarily produce profound anxiety. However, the anxiety usually does not occur, probably because the depressive exacerbation, the sulking and withdrawing or more serious manifestations, themselves secure gratifications through effectively fulfilling his manipulative goals. Anxiety, when it is nevertheless present, is likely to occur during a period of anticipation of a failure of manipulative effectiveness; if success ensues, the anxiety gives way to relief, an excessive pleasure, or even elation.

The personality of the depression-prone individual is characterized, then, by both manipulativeness and hypersensitive aversion to influence. The combination of these elements, as will be indicated later, is fundamentally implicated in the punishing, demanding, thwarting and inaccessible withdrawing behavior in both manic and depressive exacerbations.

The genetic matrix of such emotional and functional distortions may be found in the highly competitive interpersonal currents of our Western culture. Children are raised in a milieu of both open and covert striving for dominance between man and woman, particularly their parents; between younger and older, stronger and weaker, brighter or slower, the arrogant and the meek. Competing as such is not a distorting activity, it is the absolute necessity of winning that creates difficulties. Competing is usually thought of as applying to striving for greater material power or privilege, greater skills, higher status of any kind; however, in the form of

---

*This kind of distortion is traditionally explained by the somewhat mechanistic concept of *projection,* the displacement of one's own impulses onto another. More accurate, I believe, is the consideration that a great deal of what the individual understands about others comes through his subjective experience of himself; he does not displace his motives, but interprets the motivation of others, much of the time unawarely, by the subjective criteria of his own patterns of motivation.

undeviating interpersonal struggle to effect and oppose influence it becomes a distortion of the personality. The tenacity of resistance and the frequency of negative therapeutic reactions in the therapeutic interpersonal relationship with the depressive type of individual are, in part, often expressions of the patient's excessive competitiveness.

The common feature of *guilt*, of self recrimination and sometimes psychotic delusions of destructiveness must be dynamically and clinically re-evaluated. The patient's sense of evil is usually regarded as a distortion. However, every individual with the sulking and other depressive personality practices including, in some, alcoholism, hypochondriasis, headaches and dependency, has dampened or more seriously corrupted the lives of those about him. Usually he has been unaware of his own anger and intent to frustrate, restrict, disappoint, exploit and punish. But a vaguely sensed record of inflicted pain constitutes a reality base for whatever guilt the patient experiences; behind whatever forms of exaggeration or grotesqueness of distortion he may clinically present, the destructive course of his depressive practice can be identified.

The not uncommon depressive exacerbation occuring as a reaction to success is another dramatic manifestation of this. The patient, refusing to yield to the demands of his new responsibilities, competitively outwits those who expected the fulfillment of his promise, or the consummation of his potentialities. In these and comparable situations, such as achievement of marriage, becoming a parent or perhaps entering college, the depressive disengagement from responsibility disappoints, thwarts, hurts others and also, moreover, simultaneously exacts forebearance and attention.

The guilt of the depressive patient is then quite appropriate to his infliction of real injuries and does not issue just from fantasies of evil and destructiveness toward others. The fantasies themselves merely reflect more vividly, or sometimes symbolically, the intensity of the existing anger, the desire to hurt even more, to dominate, to punish. Preoccupation with guilt, especially that associated with *illusory* injury to others, serves to divest him of responsibility for changing his *actual* behavior toward these others. The seemingly remorseful destructiveness toward oneself, including self maiming (and even suicide) is not an effort to punish any "incorporated object." Punishment is directed, rather, contemporaneously at real people in the environment, who become morally, economically or otherwise penalized by the self-destructive act. The "guilt" which appears to be an exaggerated, overly moral and severe self blame also serves to protect the depressive from retribution, and to exact consolatory service, thereby achieving another victory in his unceasing, unawarely competitive, interpersonal struggle.

The commonly observed paranoid tinge or sometimes strong persecutory element may also, in this context, be seen as a reaction consistent with the dynamics of the depressive personality. The individual may simply feel rejected; this has a mild paranoid coloration. Even, however, if the persecutory element shows severe or bizarre emotional and conceptual distortion, the same dynamics are present. The irrational fears of ostracism and victimization must be considered hypothetically as rooted in a subjective sense of the possibilities of retaliation from others for his own angry, thwarting, anarchic and often sadistically punitive practices, both in and out of his periods of symptomatic exacerbation.*

The occasional suicidal termination of the depressive way of life may to some extent be motivated by a desire for an absolute source of release from suffering and insularity and from a pathetic enslavement within what is subjectively sensed as an inescapable vicious cycle of depressive living. It may in part be an escape from fear of utter nullification of the capacity to influence others, fear of bankruptcy of the manipulative functioning which has been the source of a sense of self. It may often, however, also be an ultimate punitive blow, a final frustration of the efforts of others to help. It may be an extravagant, anarchic rebellion against all forces leading toward mutuality and responsible, reciprocal human effort, against all influences upon him from other people, against all that the depressive person experiences as control.

Psychotherapy

On the principle that one finds the basic dynamics of depression in the nonexacerbative ordinary functioning of the personality, one may often detect and deal with the problem clinically without even a presenting complaint of depression. Such experiences can prove instructive for understanding and handling the more intense, frank expressions of depressive illness. For example, often in the course of working clinically with a "neurotic" one finds the patient experiencing depression of which he is not aware. In the midst of protestations of good relationships and favorable prospects, a shade of dullness in his tone of voice, a faintly discernible slowness and heaviness of speech, may gradually impinge upon the clinical ear. "There seems to be a discrepancy between what you're saying and how you seem to be feeling—is there something bothering you?" Such a query may bring a quick denial. Leading the patient to focus concentratedly upon the immediate emotion, however, will often lead to his

---

*There is, in addition, the paranoid distortion described in: Bonime, W.: Paranoid Psychodynamics. *Psychotherapy I*: 1955. The individual attempting to manipulate, but being thwarted, feels attacked because a crucial mode of functioning has been impeded.

recognition of dissatisfaction. A pursuit of the dissatisfaction is likely, then, to grow associatively into complaints about the behavior of others. As this area is invaded, always with attention intensively focussed by the patient upon his feelings, it will often be found that memory fragments of competitive struggles with spouse, parents, children or others closely related begin to appear. Flashes of "annoyance," "upset," resentment over being coerced or thwarted in attempts to get one's way, come to light. As the patient becomes more honestly self-observant and communicative, these "annoyances" and "upsets" come to be indentified as something more intense—anger or rage. Then the barely perceptible depression, first detected by the therapist, turns out, in its context, to correspond directly to the sulks and moping, the dejections and crankiness (often accompanied by headache, insomnia, lassitude or other psychosomatic manifestations), which the patient eventually discovers to be common constellations of experience. The *sulk pattern* emerges and becomes an invaluable indicator of the dynamic settings of the practice of depression. In the discovery of such a pattern it often develops that the patient originally appearing to be a neurotic has a personality with distinctly depressive features. With him as a clinical reference, we can learn about much to look for in the more obviously, more traditionally depressive subject.

Engaging the depressed patient in the psychotherapeutic process by which insight is achieved and gradually applied in breaking up the vicious self-defeating cycle, is a profoundly difficult problem. All the psychoanalytic skill and dynamic understanding at the therapist's command must be marshalled for long, continuous effort. It is in this pursuit that therapeutic compassion demands the firmest pressure upon the patient to mobilize his own healthy resources. It is only seemingly a paradox that compassion dictates more strenuous demands upon such unhappy, apparently helpless people. No other patient seeks more desperately to manipulate the therapist into therapeutic bankruptcy, into the abandonment of demands upon the patient, into fruitless commiseration, coaxing, guidance and ultimately the substitution of pharmacological and physiological methods. Those methods even if they temporarily alleviate, leave the patient to resume the practices which again lead to his being the agonized victim of his own behavior. Persistent and firm effort to engage even severely depressed patients in an examination of their emotions and practices may succeed. Firm, explicit confrontation, as well as clearly focussed query are necessary. As in any dynamic interpersonal therapy, with the depressive the delineation of the personality in operation in the therapeutic relationship itself is a primary approach. It is essential to explore his denial of anger and his manipulative and counter-influential maneuvers toward the therapist; and it is essential to work out correlations between his negative therapeutic reactions and his withdrawal from favorable developments outside therapy. These correlations serve to define the patient's problem in terms of his personality and its consistent reflection in interpersonal practice. Slowly, by learning to recognize his precise role in a seemingly hopeless continuum of hurt, rejection and failure, the patient begins to find at least new choices of behavior, the possibility of using his personal resources in such a way as to bring about new, more gratifying consequences.

It is essential not to waste time and energy to *convince* the patient of one's sympathy; no amount of it can ever fill the void he has created in his life. Furthermore, such activity conforms with his pathological demands, and, most important of all, it clutters, vitiates and postpones genuine therapeutic activity.

Patients often seek sympathetic bolstering by saying, "It just can't go on like this." It must be made clear that it *will* go on, unless the patient changes what he is doing. But it is necessary also to let the patient know that your therapeutic goal is not alleviation of the misery he is causing others. Such a goal is too often contrary to the (unaware) objective of the patient. Sometimes it must even be stated explicitly that the alleviation of the misery of a resented husband or parent, for example, is a calculated risk! The patient simply cannot achieve a healthier, more enjoyable existence without benefitting this or the other hated target of his depressive tactics. Realistic sympathy is adequately expressed by some such statement as I once made to a depressed woman: "Whenever you are prevented by reality from fulfilling unrealistic plans, you go into a vindictive depression. Through your depressed tactics you punish everyone around you. My concern is what this does to *you*."

The greatest therapeutic compassion is expressed not by the comforting word but in practice, in addressing oneself to the patient's genuine needs. One may be firm without being unkind. An example is that of a forty-five year old father of three who, after hinting suicide to his wife, was persuaded to seek analysis rather than undergo a second series of electro-convulsive therapy for recurrent depression. He initiated the first interview pacing rapidly back and forth and then saying with agitated, polite and gloomy intensity: "I hope you don't object if I pace—I can talk better if I pace." I answered at once that I found it distracting and did object, and that I thought if he paced he would ramble instead of concentrating —we had serious work to do. As therapy progressed his life revealed a frequent pattern in which friends and family sought to help him and were thwarted in their efforts by his constant shifting, back and forth, in hopeless, depressive indecision. Symbolized in a sense by his initial office behavior (the parallel was pointed out to him), his vacillation had for years embroiled his friends and this had provided him a cheap substitute for greater, more meaningful gratifications. Both in treatment and in his professional work—he was a gifted journalist—he gradually became more productive by staying in one place, facing the problem or the job. He began to experience a subjective harmony and strength more rewarding than the sense of power from enlisting the concern of friends and family, and then thwarting them. The parallel activity and feeling in relation to his analyst was also kept in view.

When the threat of suicide comes up during psychotherapy, it is important to make clear compassionately that the threat of suicide can not in any way change the nature of the activity in which the patient and analyst are engaged. It can be helpful to state that a premise upon which therapeutic activity is based is interest in the patient, and that the analyst or other psychotherapist uses every force and skill at his command to help the patient identify and deal with his difficulties. *The threat of suicide, whether in the spirit of painful desperation or implied blackmail, cannot increase therapeutic ability nor artificially muster for the situation any beneficial approach that has not already been brought to bear on the solution of the patient's problems.* The sharp, and at the same time adequately kind definition of this basic reality of the therapeutic enterprise tends to reorient the patient away from his impossible demand for rescue, and toward his positive personal resources and the possibilities offered by intensified collaborative therapeutic activity.

There is no quick or magic *entrée* to psychotherapy of the depressive. It is a long, slow process, but a cardinal consideration is the earliest possible and most persistent engagement of the patient in understanding and changing his way of living. He has spent his life seeking alleviation from others, and seeks it from the therapist, too. Sometimes insight offers the depressed individual an innervating release from the sense of being paralyzed in the grip of external circumstances. It must be borne in mind, however, that the imperative to change that accompanies insight may also produce a recalcitrant intensification of depression. Both responses may occur—this being a succession which is frequently the dynamic basis of *negative therapeutic reaction.* When the achievement of insight after long and painful struggle leads to an exacerbation of depression, the elucidation to the patient of this dynamic of recoil is often the most effective therapeutic approach.

The pursuit of this therapeutic policy was most fruitful in treatment with a recently married depressive young man. He at first felt relief when he reached the insight that, again in his new life situation, he was seeking to institute the sulk as an instrument of punishment and tyranny. However, after a few days of achieving deeper intimacy and harmony with his wife, he rebelled (experienced a negative therapeutic reaction). But he communicated in treatment more searchingly and precisely than ever before. He began: "You can't make me change even if it costs me my life. My parents never tried to get close to me—all this is retribution. I'm just going to drain everybody till there's nothing left—and go on to somebody else." Then he proceeded to describe the suddenly deteriorated relationship with his wife: "There was nothing she could do—and that's what I wanted. I watched her, and I thought to myself, 'It's too bad—there's nothing I can say that can make you feel better. It's too bad, you're just going to have to go on like this.' There were several moments there where I sat and couldn't say a single thing to her. It was like I was dead. I think I felt: 'You can't get at me (and referring without interruption to the analyst, he appended) like *you* can't get at me.' " When he was helped to grasp the relationship between his sudden retrogression and his withdrawal from the influence of analyst and wife consequent to his insight, he was able to resume constructively and use the newly acquired insight.

Depressive patients—often those with a singular record of poise—frequently may be helped to find in dreams evidence of otherwise even subjectively undetected fury. There is a fairly high correlation between depressive reactions and dreams of nuclear destruction. But the variety of explosiveness is great. One very calm scientist smashed with a sledgehammer the head of the symbolized analyst who refused to die. Another man—a most stable physician who suffered from migraine and depressions—dreamed of having a bit of car trouble. As he calmly inspected he "suddenly saw that the metal of the engine was glowing. The heat was terrific. The entire car was white hot. I got out and *walked* (!) about to the front. From there I could see that there was a roaring blaze like a molten iron furnace."

The depressive patient can find in working with his dreams a rich source of data about his personal role in hampering the use of his potential. One woman, for example, found an exquisite symbol of her destructiveness in a dream in which she deliberately lopped off the top of a young "slow-growing" tree she had been cultivating in her much-loved garden. In another of her dreams depression was symbolized by the "sensation of leaden feet," as she hurried to catch a train. By this time in therapy she was becoming aware of her own role in missing what she wanted in life. Spontaneously she interpreted this dream episode with the remark, "I felt *I was really struggling hard to 'miss the boat,'* that I was holding back." She was, however, beginning to deal with her self-defeating activities: in the same dream she put on a spurt and caught that train, and in interpreting she said, "The fact that I made it, made me feel very good."

There remains the question of how much the pharmacological and convulsive therapies are justified or welcome in these pursuits. When these methods are used today, I feel they should be employed as far as possible only as ancillary to psychotherapy, as a means to achieve more ready accessibility to the patient. If the psychiatrist feels insufficiently prepared to undertake psychotherapy in the depressions, he has no choice but to resort to other methods. When clinical approaches other than psychotherapy are used, however, either to achieve psychotherapeutic accessibility or to relieve suffering, difficult questions always arise: To what degree does the use of drugs achieve accessibility, and to what degree does their use relieve the depressive individual of responsibility for seeking solutions of life problems on a more integrative rather than a palliative basis? By the use of pharmaceuticals, are we depriving the patient of incentive for cultivating his own personality resources, and are we to some extent subsidizing the depressive process itself?

In summary, the recognition of the personality pathology of the depression-prone individual directs therapeutic attention and efforts (certainly in the younger and more accessible) upon alteration of the underlying personality deviations rather than upon the symptoms of the depressive exacerbation. This focussing upon disease process instead of upon symptoms is consistent with progressive therapeutic trends in psychiatry as well as in other fields of medicine. With this approach the patients who now feel themselves caught by a dismal and agonizing disorder may eventually find their way to understanding their depression as a practice which they have the resources to change, and from the painful effects of which they can therefore free themselves.

First Stage Techniques in the Experiential Psychotherapy of Chronic Schizophrenic Patients

by Carl A. Whitaker, M.D., Richard E. Felder, M.D., Thomas P. Malone, Ph.D., M.D. and John Warkentin, PhD., M.D.

THE MOST FREQUENT failures occur in the early stage of psychotherapy with difficult schizophrenic patients. The authors have found some empirical techniques useful in dealing with these problems. There is little doubt about the diagnosis of schizophrenia on the basis either of the presenting symptoms or the patient's history. Excluded from the group are the pseudo-neurotic schizophrenic patients and the schizoid characterological problems. The patients described here do not readily relate to a therapist in any meaningful way. Their transferences are primarily internalized, i.e. are not operative interpersonally. The distortion of their interpersonal relatedness and communication is so gross that the ordinary ways of responding on the part of the therapist are both inappropriate and ineffective.

The difficulties in the early stages of treatment of these patients arise out of their interpersonal poverty and the therapist's consequent dilemma. Effective psychotherapy requires a personally meaningful relationship between the two.[1] It is not enough that the therapist becomes meaningful to the patient in terms of the latter's delusional system. The therapist finds himself in a vacuum at the onset. Schizophrenic patients are then meaningful only in terms of stereotyped feelings about "the schizophrenic." These are on a similar feeling level with the delusional system of the patient. The therapist somehow has to relate to the patient in a way that the patient becomes personally meaningful. To say it negatively, the patient must reach the point where he is unable to ignore the person of the therapist, either by including him in his delusional system or by withdrawal. In the same vein the therapist must reach a point where he is unable to ignore the patient either by becoming administrative in his relationship to the patient or becoming lost in a labyrinth of concern over psychopathology. Intense reciprocal involvements are usually momentary. A problem in the early stage of treatment is to preserve and extend these periods of involvement in order to assure a solid interpersonal matrix for treatment.

Confronted with such patients, we recently have begun to strive for certain limited objectives. The early phase of treatment takes shape around the achievement of these objectives. They in no way cover the complete treatment program, but are rather limited objectives which we see as necessary in the early phase of treatment in order to provide the kind of therapeutic relationship within which the long range therapeutic objectives can be attained.

These immediate and limited objectives[2] are, first, *the provocation of affect in the patient.* The stimulation of any affect within the relationship is constructive and a necessary forerunner to a transference relationship. Our second objective is *the reduction of terror in the patient and, to some extent in the therapist.* We think of this as the core affective experience of the schizophrenic. Therapists exposed intimately to this terror frequently experience anxiety allied to unreality feelings. These at times come close to terror. Our third immediate objective is to *establish some sort of relationship with the patient outside of his delusional system.* We consciously and persistently resist any effort by the patient to neutralize his relationship to us by including it in his delusional system. Our fourth immediate objective is *the neutralization of critically pathogenic relationships.* By this we *do not mean* the resolution of pathogenic introject relationships within the patient. This we consider a long range treatment objective. We do feel that it is essential in the early phase of treatment to neutralize real relationships in which the patient is involved since they currently either bind, immobilize or terrify the patient.[3]

OBJECTIVE No. I: PROVOCATION OF INTERPERSONAL AFFECT.

Technique A: Intensification and reinforcement of affect.

As in other techniques, the patient is kept "off balance" in his perception of the therapist. He is shown that the ordinary social restraints are inoperative, and is likely to get the feeling that "This is the damnedest thing I ever ran into."[4]

Example:

P:* (Simple schizophrenic†) I can't trust you—I can't trust anybody.

T: You hadn't better—I never fight fair.

---

*P is abbreviation for "patient", T for "therapist."
†Abbreviated to "simple" hereafter.

Technique B: Direct Confrontation.

In our experience, confrontation with factual or logical inconsistencies is ineffective. Forcing the patient to acknowledge his psychosis is useful.

> Example:
> P: (Paranoid) (Looking stealthily at the window)
> T: You hear voices outside the window.
> P: (Nods slightly)
> T: You're really crazy, aren't you?

Technique C: Deliberate Affect Flip.

Schizophrenic patients often elude a relationship with the therapist by sudden unexpected flip or reversal of affect. In this technique, the therapist pulls the same trick on the patient. The therapist does it by being aware of his own affect and deliberately switching to the opposite, then amplifying it as far as possible.

> Example:
> P: (Catatonic) (Time for the interview to be over) I appreciate your interest in me.
> T: (Flippantly) Time's up.

In this technique, as well as in the others, the therapist refuses to make any effort to explain his behavior, or to be consistent.

Technique D: Contrived Double Binds.[5]

The use of a deliberate double bind may be effective in stimulating anxiety and transference.

> Example:
> (This is probably the prototype of all double binds).
> T: (Provokes the patient to anger by flipping cigarette ashes in patient's hair.)
> P: (Simple) (Looking very angry, clenching his fists, saying nothing)
> T: If you feel angry, why don't you express it?
> P: (Expresses his anger verbally)
> T: (Plaintively) What are you mad at me for? All I'm trying to do is help you.

Technique E: Calling the Patient's Bluff.

The purpose is to make fun of delusional systems, inappropriate responses, pseudo-affect, and seductiveness. It presupposes that the therapist can be more cynical than the patient.

> Example:
> P: (Paranoid) (Smiling) I'm sure you know what you're doing.
> T: Wipe that shit-eatin' grin off your face.

Technique F: Negation of the Sacredness of the Interview. (The Home).

The ritualistic quality of the relationship is negated in order to make room for the human encounter.

> Example: (Multiple therapy)
>
> P: (Simple) Do you think I'll ever get better?
>
> T1: (Speaking to the other therapist and completely ignoring the patient) Did you get your steps made in the back yard over the weekend?
>
> T2: Yes, let me tell you about it.
>
> P: Do you think I'll ever get better?
>
> T1: Don't interrupt; we're talking about something important.

Technique G: Silence.

Silence is for us an encounter between patient and therapist with no speaking, no smiling, no movement at all. It may be eye to eye, or staring at a fixed point or into space. This may be empty, useless and futile and when it is we suspect the ineffectiveness to be due to the self-consciousness of the therapist. Such a silence may include any feelings; for example love, hate, togetherness, isolation. When it intensifies the isolation of the patient it may provoke overt psychotic responses. Presumably, it produces a vacuum of initiative which the patient may fill. Silence may be continued in spite of the patient's effort to get into conversation. Each time the patient speaks he may be told to shut up, with increasing aggressiveness at each repetition. If the patient speaks with feeling we respect his communication.

Technique H: Threats.

The effort to produce affect in the patient by forcing him to take some initiative and some responsibility for himself.

> Example:
>
> P: (Simple) I'm not getting anywhere.
>
> T: You're going to get in the back ward of the State Hospital for the rest of your life if you don't get something out of this.

Technique I. Use of Primitive Language.

Various types of primitive language may be provocative as well as effective in communicating with schizophrenic patients. Vulgar language or dirty jokes, for example, are not perceived by the schizophrenic as offensive or humorous—nonetheless his response indicates its significance.

> Example:
>
> (Any dirty story may be told that comes to mind, assuming the therapist to be sensitive to the situation and using good judgment. They are not told as jokes, but presented as parables).

It conveys to the patient our willingness to go beyond customary social expression. It is a method of inviting the patient into the psychotherapist's fantasy life. We use this technique intuitively, and on a trial and error basis.

Technique J: Destructuring.

We consciously endeavor to devalue the magical quality of the interview situation, so that the patient loses his faith in what the therapist will do for him and to him. The natural tendency to retreat to stereotypes is broken. This helps resist the patient's effort to subsume the therapeutic program under his psychosis. Destructuring disrupts psychopathy as a defensive avoidance system and provokes anxiety or confusion.

> Example:
> P: (Paranoid) Have you had any insights about me since my last interview?
> T: Yes, many, I've been staying here every evening for three hours praying for you.

OBJECTIVE II, REDUCTION OF TERROR

Technique K: Professionally Acceptable Acting-Out in Interview.

Schizophrenic patients do concrete thinking. They must have some opportunity to express their thoughts in behavior. If this is forbidden in the presence of the therapist, then the patient is likely to get in trouble socially. The involvement of motor and proprioceptive systems in the therapist and the patient tends to modify the awesome fantasies and to provide a kind of interpersonal contact. Provision of symbolic activities which suffice to express intense and terrifying feelings of the patient, for example murderous feelings, reduces the patient's terror.

> Example:
> P: (Simple) What's wrong with me?
> T: Let's play checkers and I'll show you. (The patient sacrifices himself endlessly on the checker board and this activity becomes symbolically cathected.)

Technique L: Counteraction of Wedging Effort on the Part of the Patient[6]

Terror is intensified by any feeling in the patient that he can separate the parents. We have referred to this as "wedging". In individual therapy we have noted that the terror of the patient is increased when he is able to split the maternal and paternal functions of the therapist. He may also try to wedge the therapist and the patient's family. This splitting has been more obvious in multiple therapy. Techniques which reaffirm the primacy of the relationship between the multiple therapists over the relationship of either of the therapists to the patient seem markedly to reduce the anxiety and terror of the patient. In our preliminary contact with the patient, we verbally affirm the primacy of the relationship of therapist to therapist. For example, one patient was told, "We two therapists have been married for years, and we do not believe you can do a thing about it." Other safeguards against wedging include any refusal to accept administrative restructuring, which would separate the therapists. For example, one therapist refuses to see the patient during the absence of the other therapist, where wedging has been a problem. Another example is the refusal on the part of one therapist to accept criticism of the other therapist during his absence from the interview, and his insistence that the patient bring this directly to the other therapist. Another common example is the willingness of the multiple therapist to reinforce the other's decision in the interview situation, even when he has verbally disagreed with him. Sometimes however, despite these measures, the patient is successful in splitting the therapists and his terror is intensified. Techniques for repairing these splits are many. One technique is to place the responsibility on the patient, by saying, "You have succeeded in splitting us, now what are you going to do about it?" Another is to exclude the patient from participating until the therapists can work out the repair themselves. For example, "You have managed to split us, now you shut up while we work this out in your presence."

Technique M: Physical Contact.[7]

The rationale of the initiation of bodily contact by the therapist, or by the patient, has to do with the infantile functioning of the regressed schizophrenic. In some respects, the therapist accepts the patient as a real child, where words make relatively little difference, and it is important to the patient to have some sense of physical nearness and contact with the therapist. Sometimes a brief touch of the hand can change the course of the interview, or even of the therapy. It is important to remain clear about the fact that the behavior of the patient is motivated by his need, while the behavior of the therapist is motivated by professional awareness of the clinical situation.

Example: Touching of Hands
P: (Catatonic) I don't know what to do with my hands. (As he moves restlessly)
T: Your hands seem lost.
P: (Sits silently, looking confused, questioning, but unable to speak)
T: (Holds out his left hand, palm down and says) "Could you lay your hand on mine?"
P: (Stares uncertainly for a few moments, then slowly and laboriously lays his hand lightly on the therapist's. Both the thera-

pist's and the patient's hands tremble and seem tense and awkward).

T: I like the warmth of your hand.

(At this point the patient relaxed, rested his hand comfortably on the therapist's, and seemed ready to continue on a new basis in the interview relationship.)

Technique N: Sleeping.

On occasion we find ourselves going to sleep for varying periods of time during the interview. While going to sleep is involuntary, we tend not to resist it. This may be a powerful technique in reducing the terror of the schizophrenic patient.

Example:

T: (Just waking up from a short nap)

P: (Paranoid) Aren't you afraid I'll kill you?

Although in some instances the therapist probably goes to sleep out of anxiety, it is still obvious that he is not afraid of the patient's aggressiveness toward him.

Another reason for going to sleep may be that the therapist is feeling no response to his patient and goes to sleep in an unconscious effort to locate his relationship to the patient. Sometimes as the therapist begins to go to sleep, the patient is stimulated affectively. On other occasions, the therapist may dream of the patient and report his dreams in the interview.

Another effect of the therapist's sleeping is to state in an emphatic way that his responsibility for the patient and for the therapeutic movement has a limit. Finally sleep seems to be a powerful form of postural kinesis; with the relaxation of the therapist, the patient himself may become more relaxed and this may be a way of helping to reduce his terror. Our sleeping occurs more frequently when the therapeutic situation is in the form of multiple therapy. If the patient begins to go to sleep in the interview, the therapist may or may not interfere with this, according to his feeling about it at that moment.

Technique O: Waiting It Out

The therapist assumes that his just being there is therapeutic. This technique is attitudinal rather than behavioral. The attitude of the therapist includes a casual approach to the interview, no sense of urgency about relating, and no thought of termination.

Example: (Comfortable participation in small talk with expansion ad absurdum.)

P: (Simple) It looks like rain.

T: I expected it would rain yesterday, but maybe it won't rain until tomorrow—etc.—etc.

Technique P: The Periodic Assumption of Omnipotence.

This reduces terror in the patient by providing a strong and directive parental image. The therapist communicates his sense of being able to help the patient, his sureness of the relationship, and conviction that the patient is susceptible to interpersonal contact.

Example:

(A hebephrenic patient who couldn't get to the interview on time because he was having fecal incontinence and vomiting, when it was time to come to the interview).

T: You are to come here an hour early and if you have to shit or vomit, do it in the waiting room and bring it into the interview in a bag.

Example:

(A catatonic patient beginning the interview, snaps his fingers three times.)

T: Trying to destroy us, eh? (Snaps his fingers three times and the patient jumps.)

T: You'd better be careful or I'll do it the fourth time.

Technique Q: The Periodic Admission of Impotence.

The patient needs an opportunity to identify with the therapist. This is not possible if the therapist maintains an omnipotent role. Identification is fundamental in reducing anxiety and terror in patients. Much of the terror in the schizophrenic patient seems to be a byproduct of his dependent feelings.

By placing as much responsibility for getting well on the patient as the patient's ego strength will allow, we reduce his terror. This has to be delicately judged. It is better to leave the responsibility with the patient than assume it for yourself. Choice itself reduces terror, particularly in terms of double-bind dynamics. There is no choice if the therapist is God. His admission of his impotence may take many forms.

Examples:

1. T: You have defeated me.
2. T: Perhaps continued psychotherapy would be a mistake.
3. T: If we're lucky we may be able to keep you out of a hospital.
4. T: (Paranoid patient who has seen several therapists over period of years) I'm no better than the other doctors you've seen.

OBJECTIVE NO. III: ESTABLISHMENT OF RELATIONSHIP WITH THE
PATIENT OUTSIDE HIS DELUSIONAL SYSTEM

Technique R: Change of Technique.

The therapist must be able to keep the patient off balance. For this purpose, the changing of techniques unexpectedly, may in itself be effective. This change may involve a reversal from one technique to another directly opposite. Schizophrenia involves opposites; such reversals recognize this. An example is the use of the technique for the assumption of omnipotence on one occasion, followed by the use of the technique which involves the admission of impotence.

Technique S: Shared Fantasies of the Therapist.

The therapist relates to the patient's initial limited participation with his own fantasies. These fantasies emerge spontaneously and free associatively to the patient's limited behavior and speech. They are shared by the therapist without any interpretation. They appear indirectly to present the patient with some underlying dynamic of his delusional system in such a way that the patient has to continue to struggle with the problem within himself. This prevents him from avoiding the problem by the interpersonal extension of it into delusional thoughts about the therapist.

> Example: A paranoid patient, apparently relaxed, closed his eyes. The therapist shared a fantasy which he spontaneously had that the patient had slits in his eyelids, through which he was peeking at the outside. The patient remarked "I feel ashamed, suddenly. I have never known what a feeling was before. Now after two minutes of this feeling, I am completely exhausted." (The therapist was conveying to the patient 'You are the one who peeks at people—it is not other people who peek at you').

Technique T: Denial of Secondary Symptoms.

The patient may present symptoms as an endeavor to avoid relationship with the therapist. The therapist denies these symptoms frontally by calling them fakes, or by pressing for something more real.

> Example:
> P: (Mixed) (Giving a long story of imagined interplanetary travel).
> T: (After repeatedly interrupting) Are you interested in getting help from me?
> P: I've been needing some help.

Technique U: Mirroring.

This is a type of psychiatric judo. The therapist responds to the patient by expanding the patient's delusional presentation.

Example:

P: (Paranoid) "Is that desk lamp a microphone?"

T: Of course. The phone is also recording, and the recordings are published in invisible ink in the daily Atlanta Journal.

Technique V: Reification and Anthropomorphizing.

Many times the schizophrenic has distorted people by making them into things. He desperately defends this delusional system until the therapist breaks into it. This may be done by fragmenting his experience in the interview, or by making the therapist's experience identical with the patient's delusional system.

Example:

T: (With no preliminary comments from the patient). You are a marble statue standing in the middle of a Greek square.

Technique W: Upside-down Language.

The patient's defenses include a kind of denial which takes the form of saying the exact opposite of what he feels. He may verbalize complete hopelessness, particularly on the day that the psychotherapy shows some evidence of getting into motion. Since the therapist cannot directly counteract this dynamic, one technique is to join the patient in talking upside down. Sometimes, this resembles sarcasm on the part of the therapist, although it may not be at all hostile. This is a technique which de-values words, and emphasizes that there needs to be some sort of exchange between patient and therapist.

Example:

P: (Simple) I want you to know that my Mama had nothing to do with my being sick.

T: I'm sure you're right, your mother is a wonderful person who could help you a great deal now. She has already done everything she possibly could.

Technique X: Reversal of the Double Bind.

The double-bind is the outward presentation of acceptance with the meta feeling of cold rejection. In this technique, the reverse is true. An outwardly hostile presentation is made with the meta feeling of warm acceptance. This technique may help break the "spell" of the original double-binding.

Example:

T: What do you want me to do that for?

P: (Hebephrenic) It might help me.

T: I'm not interested in helping you.

OBJECTIVE NO. IV: THE NEUTRALIZATION OF CRITICALLY PATHOGENIC RELATIONSHIPS

Over the years in our treatment of schizophrenics, the most difficult problem in the early phases of treatment has been the administrative relationship of the therapist to the patient's family. We have utilized a multitude of techniques for neutralizing the family in such a way as to allow psychotherapy of the patient to proceed. By and large, all of these techniques have been inadequate. We have attempted to remove the patient from his family by a variety of isolating techniques. We have attempted to put members of the family into collaborative therapy. We have had the family members as visitors in interviews with the primary schizophrenic patient. In all instances, however, there were serious difficulties. We increasingly were made aware that an essential problem of the schizophrenic person is his assumption of a saviour-like responsibility for members of his family, particularly his parents. All of our techniques have been aimed at negating this self dedication. It appears now that the most effective way to neutralize critically pathogenic relationships is to treat the whole family of the schizophrenic as a unit.[8]

SUMMARY

We have outlined and briefly described some techniques which we have found useful in the psychotherapy of schizophrenic patients in the early phases of treatment. These techniques reflect some general attitudes. First is a willingness to accept the limits of what is possible, with these patients, at this point in psychotherapy. Second is a willingness to take more responsibility for and with these patients than we do with other patients. Part of this responsibility involves relating more directly to the "child" in the patient and the sickness of the patient.[9] This contrasts with psychotherapy with neurotics where we relate primarily to the "adult", the wellness of the patient. The primary dynamic of psychotherapy is the human encounter.

REFERENCES

1. MALONE, T. P., WHITAKER, C. A., WARKENTIN, J., AND FELDER, R. E.: Rational and nonrational psychotherapy. Am. J. Psychother. 15:212-220, (Apr.), 1961.

2. ——: Operational definition of schizophrenia. In: Psychotherapy with Schizophrenics: Dawson, J. G., Stone, H. K., and Dellis, N. P., eds. Baton Rouge, Louisiana State Univ. Press, 1961, pp. 123-135.

3. WHITAKER, C. A., WARKENTIN, J., AND MALONE, T. P.: The Involvement

of the Professional Therapist. In: Case Studies in Counseling and Psychotherapy: Burton, A., ed. Englewood Cliffs, N. J., Prentice-Hall, 1959, pp. 218-256.

4. WARKINTIN, J., FELDER, R. E., MALONE, T. P. AND WHITAKER, C. A.: The Usefulness of Craziness. M. Times 89: 587-590 (June), 1961.

5. BATESON, G.: *In*: Psychotherapy of Chronic Schizophrenic Patients: Whitaker, C. A., ed. Boston, Little-Brown & Co., 1958.

6. WHITAKER, C. A., MALONE, T. P., AND WARKENTIN, J.: Multiple Therapy and Psychotherapy. *In*: Progress in Psychotherapy: Fromm-Reichmann, F., and Moreno, J. L., eds. New York, Grune & Stratton, 1956, pp. 210-216.

7. WARKENTIN, J., AND TAYLOR, J. E.: Case Fragments: The Experimental Physical Contact in Multiple Therapy with Schizophrenic Patients. Vol. III of Report to 2d International Congress for Psychiatrists, Zürich, 1957.

8. MALONE, T. P.: Experimental Encounters in Family Therapy of Schizophrenia. Read at the American Psychological Association Meeting, Sept., 1961 (to be published).

9. WHITAKER, C. A., AND MALONE, T. P.: The Roots of Psychotherapy. New York, The Blakiston Co., 1953.

Family Concept of Hospital Treatment of Schizophrenia

by Ivan Boszormenyi-Nagy, M.D. and James L. Framo, Ph.D.

THOSE WHO HAVE RECOMMENDED changes in the contemporary practices of mental hospitals have proposed coordinated multilevel
programs for the treatment and resocialization of psychotic patients(e.g.
changes in the mental hospital per se, day hospitals, halfway houses,
ex-patient groups, etc.)[15] The socio-psychotherapeutic philosophy of
these programs can mainly focus either on the fostering of independence
in the chronic mental patient or on the cultivation of personal relationships during hospitalization. The first focus has logically led to "therapeutic community" programs[16] and patient government, which encourage patient responsibility, whereas the second emphasis suggests hospital
organizational designs which would promote a variety of relationship
models and their emotional elaboration by the participants. Excellent
studies of the psychologic climate and sociologic implications of mental
hospital living have appeared in recent years.[1, 7, 12, 21] Almost all of
these writings about the mental hospital have emphasized its undesirable
"total institution," or dehumanizing character.[11] Yet, while we do not
question the demoralizing effect on the patient of being an outcast, it is
the thesis of this paper that hospital living comes to have a deeper, more
personal meaning to the patient which can be put to therapeutic
advantage.

The observations serving as the basis for the present report originate
from a research project of the Eastern Pennsylvania Psychiatric Institute,
organized in 1957 for the purpose of gaining a better understanding of the
relationship characteristics of schizophrenia and for learning more effective methods of treatment. The patient population on this 20-bed unit
consists of young adult female schizophrenic patients ranging from acute
to "hard core" chronic cases. The therapeutic staff consists of two full time
and three half time psychiatrists, two psychologists and a social worker,

as well as nurses, aides, and student nurses. The small size of the unit allows sufficient time for a wide range of psychotherapeutic endeavors. From the inception of the project, further, family members as well as ward personnel have been involved in the treatment process.

While the personal relationship dimensions of hospitalization have long been recognized, their systematic utilization for treatment has not been exploited, perhaps due to the lack of a comprehensive model. We were already aware of the need for implementing these dynamic, interpersonal principles in the early stages of the organization of our hospital treatment program for schizophrenia. However, it was not until we actually had conducted treatment of schizophrenic families for several years that we were able to formulate a unitary framework for our milieu approach. This approach integrates the concepts of the human relations aspects of hospitalization with the family-based viewpoint of schizophrenic pathology.

The conventional medicopsychiatric view about schizophrenia states that the psychotic symptoms constitute an illness which, ideally, should be removed so that the patient can return to a comparatively healthy family and function productively afterwards. Those who have come to know patients and their families in conjoint therapy have developed an entirely different nosologic perspective about schizophrenia, departing from the usual concept of a disease as etiologically confined within a single individual.[6, 14, 17, 23] The seemingly bizarre and meaningless symptoms of the patient gain an interpersonal meaning when seen in the gestalt of family living, where they "make sense" and are perhaps the only appropriate responses to the interlocking pathologic system. Even the symptomatic picture of the schizophrenic as a lonely, withdrawn person on the ward is regularly seen to change to that of an overinvolved participant in the presence of the family in conjoint therapy sessions.

We propose, in particular, that the study of the psychopathology of schizophrenic family interaction can provide one of the basic sciences for hospital psychiatry, inasmuch as these family interaction patterns are "transferred" to and elicited from the hospital staff. Family transference is a term we have coined to connote a multitude of phenomena. The symbolic interpersonal meaning of the patient's behavior can frequently be decoded as a set of "transference" messages patterned after family models. The documentation of these transplanted competitive, succorant, protective, exploitive, hostile, proprietary, manipulative or loving attitudes as they occur on the ward is contained in our previous publications.[4, 5] It should be emphasized that family transference manifestations occur not only in one-to-one relationships but in more global responses of one person to interactions between others, to an entire network of group interactions, and even to the physical, non-human environment of the hospital.[20]

The psychological atmosphere of the hospital, which of course is overtly very different from that of the family, nonetheless corresponds to family living, most significantly at its deepest instinctual level—viz., they are both uniquely conducive toward the stimulation of relatively unrestrained expressions of hostility and of infantile forms of sexuality (physical handling, bodily exposure, sharing of physical intimacies, etc.) with a minimum of social consequences. Intensive temptations and taboos pervade both family and hospital living. What patients feel free to do in the privacy of their own homes they expect the hospital to tolerate.

Another theoretical consideration of our treatment approach derives from the characterological understanding of the pre- and postpsychotic personality structure of the patient herself. Therapists who have conducted long term, intensive, individual psychotherapy of the schizophrenic, beyond the removal of overt psychotic symptoms, have to contend with enduring, schizoid personality deficiencies which manifest themselves in typical anomalies of social functioning.[8, 10, 13, 18, 19, 22] The relationships formed by the post-psychotic schizophrenic are fragile and so painfully ambivalent that only two alternative solutions seem to be available: a solitary existence or extreme dependence. Those patients who seek outpatient psychotherapy establish a dependence on the therapist which threatens to develop into a lifetime proposition.[13]

Our family treatment experience, however, has revealed that what seems like the patient's exclusive need for symbiotic attachments turns out to be one component part of an amorphous sticking together of the family as a whole, or of several members of the family. Therapists of families with a schizophrenic member have used different phrases to emphasize aspects of the mutually dependent cohesiveness of these families. Bowen writes of "undifferentiated family ego mass," [6] Wynne of "pseudomutuality," [23] and Boszormenyi-Nagy of "pathologic need complementarity." [3]

A corollary of these "sticky" family interaction patterns is the relative absence of a variety of differentiated relationships within and outside of the family. This observation led to a rationale of therapeutic organizational planning for our unit. Just as the normally growing child widens his realtionships from mother to father, to siblings, to friends, and to marriage partners, we hoped to provide the opportunities for patients and their families to differentiate themselves as individuals via exposure to new relationships. This is in line with a principle of psychoanalytic psychology which specifies that it is essential for healthy functioning to have a multiplicity of relationships of varying intensity of emotional investment. In like manner, Sullivan has stressed the lack of "chum" relationships during the pre-adolescent period of the schizophrenic.[22] Recognizing, then, the enormous pull of symbiotic styles of relating in these families, we developed a spectrum of programs with varying parameters of relatedness in order to provide therapeutic leverage for breaking up their rigid patterns.

Every patient is seen in intensive individual psychotherapy at least three times a week. Group sessions are held daily with all of the patients, the ward administrator, and most of the nursing personnel. The family character of the meetings is reinforced when, once a week, most of the therapists join this group. In this meeting the patients hear reports read by the nurses on their behavior of the previous week. The patients frequently dispute their reports, and this usually stimulates strong feelings on all sides; we have found very complex counter-transference reactions taking place in this meeting (e.g., who is regarded as a "good parent".) Another activity consists of weekly meetings of all patients, some therapists, nursing personnel, and as many of the parents as can attend. The simultaneous presence of original and transference family figures provides a setting for growth-promoting diversification of meaningful relational opportunities. The most specialized therapeutic activity for the exploration of relationships is the formal conjoint family therapy which has been conducted with twelve selected families over the past three years. These therapy sessions,[2, 3, 9] have furnished a wealth of understanding about repetitive patterns of mutually sustained conflicts, alliances, and pathological forms of need gratifications. Family treatment has intrinsic value as a basic treatment method of schizophrenia but it does not necessarily have to constitute part of the hospital treatment approach outlined here.

In addition to these regular programs, other relationship-centered activities are initiated as the occasion comes up. We have found ad hoc psychodrama sessions constructive; in these sessions the patient assigns roles to the participating members of the staff, and the ensuing family context is acted out. Occasionally it has been productive to have the patient's mother spend all day in the hospital, ministering to her autistically regressed daughter. This measure has been beneficial in cases where the mother's relationship to the patient appeared distant rather than overinvolved.

The over-all effect of the program was that many patients and their families found increasingly important relationships which helped to replace or dilute the intensity of the family unions. This therapeutic effect could be conceived as being analogous to a stage of normal child development and therefore another family dimension of the program is implied. The milieu of our unit helped to cultivate peer level, "chum-like" relationships, even between very disorganized patients. For many of the patients it was the first time in their lives that they had a friend. These friendships typically occurred as a rebellious alliance between patients against the authority of nurses, replicating a phenomenon which normally occurs during latency with peers. We found that, like parents, the nursing staff needed help in overcoming their resentful feelings about patients withdrawing from them in this fashion. They have sometimes pointedly reported to the doctors that some patients "are getting much too close." Another instance of the emergence of friendship has been seen when our patients shifted their attachment from the head nurse to the student nurses, who had relatively peripheral authority roles in the unit. This shift was frequently associated with a marked decrease in the patient's need for severely regressed behavior.

All the observations from the various approaches of the unit are fed back into regular meetings between therapists and nursing personnel, where the elusive family interaction patterns can be discussed, and the staff can recognize the deeper meaning of the roles they have wittingly or unwittingly come to adopt in these "family dramas." We have observed repeatedly that the nursing staff were considerably supported in their difficult dealings with hostile, regressively demanding patients if these behaviors could be unmasked as attempts to transform professional attitudes into those of an involved, angry, impatient, or nurturant parent. Members of the staff needed to be alerted to the patients' gambits at creating staff divergencies, much in the manner of the child manipulating the parents so as to gain the possession of each separately. Latent interprofessional rivalries, based on possessive needs for a patient, were frequently capitalized upon by patients and their families. On other occasions the staff needed support when parents and patients collaborated in projecting all badness on them as a way of displacing intrafamilial negative feelings. It was necessary for personnel to recognize that the abuse hurled at them for being cruel and authoritarian frequently stemmed from the patient's view of the hospital as the family's punishment agency, especially in those cases where the patient regarded hospitalization as libidinal rejection on the part of the family. On the other hand, since projections are usually based on a germ of truth, ward personnel needed to examine their own overprotective, jealous, retaliatory behaviors as they dovetailed with the roles assigned to them by the patients. The deep seated, unconscious need of the parents to keep their daughter available to them, even if this requires that she remain psychotic in the hospital,[3, 9] can find its counterpart in the unconscious reluctance of the staff to lose the patient. We have interpreted the bitterness which a patient and staff member may feel toward each other when the patient is ready to leave the hospital as an indication of unadmitted mutual attachment.

At times delayed stages of development, impossible to achieve in the patient's family, can be embarked upon in the hospital. What appears as grossly destructive, aggressive behavior on the patient's part, upon closer examination is often revealed as an exaggerated, inappropriate adolescent rebellion. The impersonal, authoritarian structure of the hospital reestablishes a child-parent complementarity inasmuch as the regressed behavior of the patient finds its needed control by a parental substitute. At the same time, this implicit parental authority role of the hospital renders it eminently suitable as a target for rebelliousness. The need of some patients to have enemies, or to be the rejecting one, should be recognized; even this negative form of relating should be temporarily accepted for ultimate therapeutic gain. Patients' chief complaints are consciously oriented toward the all-encompassing regimentation of their life with its consequent loss of personal dignity and rights.[11] The mobilization of meaningful relationships within the family context of the ward, on the other hand, is instrumental in counteracting the pull of antitherapeutic forces which exist in every institutional setting. The home-like meaning of the ward helps explain, at least in part, the inner reluctance of patients to leave the hospital; patients who meet crises after discharge frequently turn for security to the hospital as a second home.

In evaluating the patient's response to a therapeutic program of this sort, the removal of overt psychotic symptoms is not of primary relevance. Indeed, it is not incompatible with our therapeutic approach that symptoms frequently become accelerated or exacerbated as interpersonal involvement intensifies and massive defenses come under therapeutic review. We have been concerned with criteria of improvement which are more far reaching than those set conventionally. Our approach was directed at the long range perspective of the individual's life functioning, which necessitated dealing with deep psychological problems of an interpersonal as well as intrapsychic nature. Furthermore, customary standards of evaluation of treatment effects would not comprehend changes in the attitudes of relatives and staff. It has been our persistent finding that members of the families we have worked with repeatedly exchange the role of who is the sick one. As the primary patient improved another member of the family would transitorily develop near-psychotic or psychosomatic symptoms. We defer judgment, then, on the whole question of what constitutes genuine improvement, but we can give our clinical impressions. One of the striking results we have witnessed is the improvement in the marriages of the parents of our patients. A number of parents who for years had been hopelessly deadlocked were able to reexamine constructively their partnership and free the patient thereby to relate to extra-familial figures. Young schizophrenic patients probably have the greatest opportunity to grow when they no longer have to feel responsible for the marriage or psychological equilibrium of their parents.

The very special conditions of our research ward (small number of patients, their youthful age, and intensive therapeutic coverage) does raise the question of the applicability of our findings to other institutions, particularly the large state hospital. The phenomena we have described, however, are perhaps more sharply etched versions of what we are sure occur in every mental hospital. While the occurrence of "transference" to the hospital climate is obviously a spontaneous product of the patient's relationship to the ward milieu, certain of its conditions can be provided by administrative design—e.g. constancy of nursing personnel, reinterpretation of role relationships among staff members, inclusion of relatives, etc. Subsequently, the principles learned in programs similar to the one described can then be translated into training and operational practices in larger mental institutions.

REFERENCES

1. BELKNAP, I.: Human Problems of a State Mental Hospital. New York. McGraw-Hill, 1956.
2. BOSZORMENYI-NAGY, I.: Goals and methods in individual and in family therapy of schizophrenia. Paper delivered at symposium on "Clinical and Research Aspects of Family Treatment of Schizophrenia," American Psychological Association Meetings, New York, 1961.
3. ——: The concept of schizophrenia from the perspective of family treatment. Family Process, Vol. 1, No. 1, March, 1962.
4. ——, AND FRAMO, J. L.: Hospital organization and family oriented psychotherapy of schizophrenia. Proceedings of the Third World Congress of Psychiatry, Montreal, 1961.
5. ——, FRAMO, J. L., ROBINSON, L. AND HOLDEN, E.: Family concept of schizophrenia and treatment organization of the psychiatric hospital. Paper read at the 117th annual meeting of the Amer. Psychiatric Assn., Chicago, May 1961. (To be published.)
6. BOWEN, M.: A family concept of schizophrenia. In Jackson, D.: The Etiology of Schizophrenia. New York, Basic Books, 1960.
7. CAUDILL, W. A.: The Psychiatric Hospital as a Small Society. Cambridge, Harvard University Press, 1958.
8. EISSLER, K. R.: Limitations to the psychotherapy of schizophrenia. Psychiat. 6, 381, 1943.
9. FRAMO, J. L.: The theory of the technique of family treatment of schizophrenia. Family Process, Vol. 1, No. 1, March, 1962.
10. FROMM-REICHMAN, F.: Principles of Intensive Psychotherapy. Chicago, University of Chicago Press, 1950.
11. GOFFMAN, E.: Asylums, Essays on the Social Situation of Mental Patients and Other Inmates. Garden City, New York, Doubleday & Co., Inc., 1961.
12. GREENBLATT, M., et al.: From Custodial to Therapeutic Patient Care in Mental Hospitals. New York, Russell Sage Foundation, 1955.

13. HILL, L. B.: Psychotherapeutic Intervention in Schizophrenia. Chicago, University of Chicago Press, 1955.
14. JACKSON, D.: Family interaction, family homeostasis, and some implications for conjoint family psychotherapy. *In* Masserman, J. H. (Ed.): Science and Psychoanalysis, vol. 2, Individual and Familial Dynamics. New York, Grune and Stratton, 1958-61.
15. Joint Commission on Mental Illness and Health, Action for Mental Health: Final Report, 1960. New York, Basic Books, 1961.
16. JONES, M.: The Therapeutic Community, New York, Basic Books, 1953.
17. LIDZ, T., AND FLECK, S.: Schizophrenia, human integration, and the role of the family. In Jackson, D.: The Etiology of Schizophrenia. New York, Basic Books, 1960.
18. SEARLES, H. F.: Dependency processes in the psychotherapy of schizophrenia. J. Am. Psychoanal. Ass. 3:19, 1955.
19. ——: Positive feelings in the relationship between the schizophrenic and his mother. Int. J. Psychoanal. 39:569, 1958.
20: ——: The Non-Human Environment, In Normal Development and in Schizophrenia. New York, Internat. Univ. Press, 1960.
21. STANTON, A. H., AND SCHWARTZ, M. S.: The Mental Hospital. New York, Basic Books, 1954.
22. SULLIVAN, H. S.: Conceptions of Modern Psychiatry. Wash., D. C., William Alanson White Psychiatric Foundation, 1947.
23. WYNNE, L. C., RYCKOFF, I. M., DAY, JULIANA, AND HIRSCH, S. I.: Pseudo-mutuality in the family relations of schizophrenics. Psychiat. 21:205, 1958.

ACKNOWLEDGEMENTS

We are indebted to Leon R. Robinson, M.D. and Miss Eddis Holden, M.S.S. for their part in executing the therapy programs and for contributions made during numerous discussions.

Adult Diagnostic Court Clinics

by JOHN A. ORDWAY, M.D.

T HROUGH ADULT misdemeanor courts passes a daily stream of alcoholics, shoplifters, wife beaters, child deserters, husband-haters, exhibitionists, and homosexuals. Because the evident psychopathology of such a group has been lost on neither judge nor psychiatrist, psychiatric diagnostic teams are provided in the courts of many American cities. Although some court clinics carry out a considerable amount of therapy, this chapter will deal with administration, treatment, and referral by clinics that are mainly diagnostic.

Court-referred patients run the entire range of diagnostic nomenclature; and their treatment includes traditional psychiatric techniques and parameters of therapy. But quite as important as this therapy are the agency relationships that enable diagnosis, treatment, and follow-up by court-oriented professionals to take place. "Administrative psychiatry" not only provides a balanced team for the diagnosis of the patient, but also maintains optimal liaison with cooperating agencies. Because they are relatively new and their purpose not generally understood in the community, court clinics find it essential to add to the usual psychiatric report statements of the mechanism by which the referral is to be carried out. If the mechanism is not spelled out in detail, an agency may pursue an independent, unintegrated course of action adverse to the original plan of rehabilitation.

For example, a court clinic referred a 20 year old exhibitionist to a mental hygiene clinic for psychotherapy as a condition of probation. The court clinic report stressed the *need* but did not spell out in detail a *method* for the probation department to keep track of the patient's attendance at the clinic. It was necessary for the probation officer to know whether this young man was following instruction to go for psychotherapy because the patient was markedly rebellious toward authority and in the initial transference reaction would probably view the psychotherapist as a rather weak edition of authority, and one easily flouted. Since the patient had responded favorably several times to firm neighborhood verbal limits on fast driving, it was felt that these limits would again be useful in the hands of the probation officer. As predicted, the patient breached his probation by failing several appointments with his psychotherapist, who properly interpreted the patient's rebelliousness but did not inform the probation officer of this patient's failures. The officer, in his ignorance of the broken probation, then set no limits. The patient's anxiety over his success at flouting authority mounted; and seeking relief from this anxiety, he exhibited himself once more in such a way as to be absolutely certain of identification and arrest. He thus set limits on himself which poor liaison had made impossible.

While it is quite possible that the dynamic formulation of the court clinic in this case is incorrect and the patient untreatable, reports from court clinics treating sex offenders indicate very real therapeutic possibilities for a man of this age and character structure. Closer liaison and clear understanding between clinic and therapist of the latter's exact responsibility to the probation department might lead to the successful results reported by Maas and Mills[1] and Lamers and Bradman,[2] who have had patients in psychotherapy as a condition of the patients' probation.

In addition to interagency contacts formalized by reports and conferences, a court clinic may be further linked to four or five treatment facilities by interlocking personnel. For example, psychiatrists in court clinics supervise, teach, or do psychotherapy in their community's mental hygiene clinics. When a patient is referred from court to a mental hygiene clinic, a psychiatrist who has taken part in the diagnostic workup of the offender in court conveys the court's wishes—not only by a formal letter of referral, but also by his presence and discussion of the case in this second clinic. By his continuing interest in the patient and the type of problem, he directs his colleagues' attention to court referrals. This stimulation of interest is of the deepest importance and is perhaps a sine qua non for successful referrals from a court clinic to other treatment facilities. It also helps dispel the aura of fear and mystery about the workings of the judiciary that may otherwise lead psychiatrists, psychologists, and psychiatric social workers to avoid working with court cases.

Additionally, of course, psychiatric social workers and psychologists from court clinics often work for family guidance organizations, alcoholism clinics, and mental hygiene clinics. They take part in hospital teaching seminars and, of course, share their experiences through papers or informally at professional meetings. The growing number of professional contacts between formally trained court clinic personnel and their opposite numbers in non-court agencies has helped ease the strained situation that has existed between these agencies and the non-professionals in court who in the past have handled referrals from court to agency. Improved therapy seems to go hand in hand with improved court–agency relations.

Beyond considerations of liaison and coordination of efforts, an important parameter of treatment is a type of combined or tandem therapy carried out in concert with the probation department. In this co-operative enterprise, the court clinic first works out a defendant's clinical diagnosis and psychodynamics. It then conveys this information to the judge. If the clinic and judge decide that in addition to psychiatric therapy probation is indicated, their thinking is further shared with the probation department. After this consultation, responsibility for limit setting and reality planning in the case is assumed by the probation department while psychiatric therapy is carried out elsewhere.

For example, a 32 year old, single waitress was charged with "drunkenness" and "common prostitution." Referred after conviction and before sentence to the court clinic, she was found to be a narcissistic, dependent woman, angry and lost in the Big City away from her Appalachian home. By identification with an alcoholic father, she had made an uneasy adjustment to her bargirl life, in which she found some satisfaction in closeness to her patrons and to a succession of "friends." Because her heavy drinking seemed ego-alien at least in part, it was felt that she should be offered therapy at the local alcoholism clinic. But because of her anger at the world, it was also felt that she would disobey a mere clinic recommendation to go for treatment. Furthermore, she needed guidance with day-to-day planning in the confusing and complicated city. She was, therefore, placed on probation and weekly attendance at the alcoholism clinic made a condition of probation. Although this "enforced therapy" was not a success for some of her psychotherapy group, this patient gradually integrated herself first into group psychotherapy, and later into her neighborhood life. Her heavy use of alcohol disappeared; and, interestingly, she married.

In cases where, for example, reinforcement of a wavering superego or stepwise provision of a particular executive function for a maladaptive ego can be carried out only by identification with the probation department, the clinic outlines the goal and the specific steps by which this goal may be attained, and makes the referral only to the probation department. In this sense, of course, the probation department has been the only therapeutic arm of many courts since the days of John Augustus, the shoemaker and "first probation officer" who befriended the friendless of a mid-nineteenth century Boston court.

As foundation stones beneath these parameters of therapy and "liaison psychiatry" always lie the traditional and basic psychiatric techniques with in- and outpatients. It is only the *use* of these basic techniques rather than of jail with "criminals" that is relatively new. There is no need to labor their usefulness with the considerable number of psychotics and psychoneurotics that are so obviously ill as to demand immediate suspension of a patient's trial and his referral for medical help. But the promise of these techniques with particular types of ostensibly "healthy" offenders is of interest and will now be considered.

Between 1957 and 1960, the Cincinnati Municipal Court Psychiatric Clinic[3] noted among shoplifters an apparently low rate of recidivism, a high incidence of pre-crime depression, and a frequency of recent object losses. Investigation revealed that the shoplifters as a group had a lower (38 per cent) rate of recidivism than the over-all group of Municipal Court defendants (66 per cent). Furthermore, shoplifters who had been referred to the Clinic had such a low rate of recidivism (1 per cent) as to suggest that they had profited by referral for various combinations of psychotherapy, casework support, drug therapy, hospitalization, electroshock therapy, or whatever combination of help seemed appropriate to a particular case.

Tabulation of the depressions from a shoplifter group indicated that these shoplifters were four times (43 per cent) as likely to be depressed as the non-shoplifters (10 per cent). Most were acute psychoneurotic depressions, traceable to recent object losses.

The importance of these object losses were difficult to evaluate; but throughout this group divorces, separations, deaths, etc. were numerous (61 per cent) and apparently of greater frequency than amongst the non-shoplifter clinic population (15 per cent). The following case reflects a not uncommon shoplifting situation.

A 21 year old secretary from a well-to-do family was arrested and convicted of stealing sweaters, a girdle, and makeup from a department store. She had no explanation or understanding of this act. She carried money sufficient to pay for the articles. She remembered only that she felt "real empty, lonely, and blue" on the day of the theft. For five days before the shoplifting she had additionally suffered from insomnia and anorexia. On the weekend preceding the misdemeanor her fiancé had broken the engagement, her brother had told her to "get out and stay out" of the family home, and her mother had returned from the hospital "a stranger with a changed personality" after electroconvulsive therapy. On direct examination the patient was described as "mildly depressed." The diagnosis was psychoneurotic depressive reaction, acute, mild. The clinic recommended to the judge that the patient not be jailed or placed on probation, but be given a small fine to help alleviate her guilt and then be referred for limit-setting, supportive psychotherapy. The court fined the patient $10.00 and costs and referred her to the psychiatry resident in the court clinic for psychotherapy. A detailed description of this particular psychotherapy would reveal a course little different from many another similar case of mild reactive depression following the loss of important love objects—with the *exception* of the special meaning of the theft which symbolized an act of love, a gift to her by the lost love object (mother). In other words, she carried out a gift to herself that she wished that her mother had given her. She was discharged after only two and one-half months of psychotherapy, her depression having completely left her. Like so many other patients charged with shoplifting, she has not been brought back to court for a theft or any other type of misdemeanor.

Other more severely depressed shoplifters need hospitalization, drug and/or physical therapy, and agency help to bring order to their lives. But these judge-selected patients do respond in such a way as to suggest that jail is not the appropriate way to return them to happy and law-abiding lives.

And so it may be with sex offenders. Following in the footsteps of Samuel Hadden's work with homosexuals[4] in group psychotherapy, other workers (Maas and Mills,[1] Bradman and Lamers[2]), are reporting success in treating sex offenders with either combined (group and individual) psychotherapy or only group psychotherapy. Over a four and one-half year existence the Cincinnati Municipal Court Psychiatric Clinic has observed *no* reappearance in court of sex offenders *actively* participating in group psychotherapy. The only known repeater repeated his offense immediately after the termination of his group psychotherapy.

Other types of offenders, such as those who "abuse" their families and who are not candidates for psychotherapy, drug therapy, or any other type of medical care, may be placed on a combination of family service guidance and probation. The psychiatric clinic stands by as a consultant, ready to guide the probation department in an understanding of the psychodynamics of their probationers. In this situation Family Service Organization or another similar agency teaches the technique of living, and probation applies appropriate limits and insists upon standards of conduct that the community expects of the probationer.

Each morning in the United States tens of thousands persons appear before the bar of justice. There is no promise that the United States with its huge prison population is approaching the situation reported by Baan[5] of Holland (population: 12,000,000), where less than 2,000 languish in prison; but more and more often the modern judge and psychiatrist combine talents to return defendants to a healthy, lawful existence. And with shoplifters and sex offenders this combination shows some real promise.

REFERENCES

1. MAAS, JAMES W. AND MILLS, ROBERT B.: Group Psychotherapy with Sex
   Deviates on Probation. In press.
2. BRADMAN, B., AND LAMERS, W.: Group psychotherapy with sexual offenders.
   Read at the Tri-State Group Psychotherapy Society meeting, October 21,
   1961, Toledo, Ohio.
3. ORDWAY, JOHN A.: "Successful" Court Treatment of Shoplifters. Read at
   the 117th annual meeting of The American Psychiatric Association, Chicago,
   Illinois, May 8-12, 1961.
4. HADDEN, SAMUEL B.: Group Psychotherapy with Homosexuals. Read at the
   Tri-State Group Psychotherapy Society meeting, April 19, 1958, Cincinnati,
   Ohio.
5. BAAN, P. A. H.: The Treatment of Criminal Psychopathy Canadian Journal
   of Corrections, January, 1960.

Psychiatric Treatment of the Sex Offender

by Asher R. Pacht, Ph.D.; Seymour L. Halleck, M.D.; and John C. Ehrmann, Ph.D.

D URING THE LAST DECADE, increasing public attention has been focused on the sexual criminal. In an effort to cope with this perplexing problem, many states have developed special legislation for dealing with this group. For the most part, this legislation has been wholly inadequate. Public concern tends to emphasize the responsibility of psychiatry for developing effective treatment programs. To date, the psychiatric treatment of these offenders has been considered unrewarding and only a limited body of knowledge has come from the profession. This paper offers information in this area by detailing some of the unique experiences involved in the effective treatment of a large group of sex offenders.

Based on nine years experience with an operative Sex Crimes Law, the authors have developed a cautiously optimistic outlook toward the psychiatric treatment of this disorder. Favorable therapeutic results are, however, dependent upon the incorporation of specific factors in the program. Briefly stated, these are:

A. The necessary administrative machinery for differential handling which stresses indeterminate sentencing for those who need psychological treatment.

B. Over-all support from progressive judicial and correctional administrators as well as appropriate institution facilities and adequate staff.

C. A diagnostic appraisal which insures intensive study of the psychodynamics of the individual offender.

D. A flexible program which includes all modalities of psychiatric treatment.

While the emphasis in this paper is directed toward treatment, brief attention must be given to the first three factors which are considered necessary prerequisites.

The administrative and legal structure of our program is based on the Wisconsin Sex Crimes Law which was instituted in July, 1951. This law specifically recognizes the psychological nature of many sex offenses and establishes the machinery both to identify and provide specialized treatment for the "deviated" sex offender. Under this program any person convicted of rape, attempted rape or indecent sexual behavior with a child, *must* be committed to the State Department of Public Welfare for a pre-sentence social, physical and mental examination. Any other offense prompted by a desire for sexual gratification may be examined at the discretion of the Department. During a sixty day examination period, the Department attempts to determine if the individual is in need of specialized treatment for "mental or physical aberrations." If the individual is found in need of such treatment, the court *must* either recommit him indeterminately to the Sex Deviate Facility at the State Prison, or place him on probation with mandatory outpatient psychotherapy. Unlike most sex crimes laws, this program fulfills two needs. It provides treatment for those who can benefit from it and maximum custody for life, if necessary, for those who cannot utilize treatment and who remain a danger to society.

No law, regardless of how well it has been written, can be effective unless it has the wholehearted support of all those concerned with its operation. The Wisconsin Sex Crimes Law was developed by a large committee which included judges, lawyers, correctional administrators, mental health personnel, and representatives of civic and religious groups. These groups have maintained an active interest in the operation of the program and continue to lend their support. Equally vital has been the cooperation received from all levels of personnel at the State Prison where the program is conducted. Despite the limits imposed by a maximum security setting, modalities of rehabilitation comparable to adjunctive therapies in mental hospitals are available. Where specific treatment needs cannot be met at the Prison, the facilities of mental hospitals and other correctional institutions can be used. In addition, after-care services are provided by a large, well trained state parole service. Most important, it has been possible to maintain (although with considerable difficulty) an adequate staff of qualified psychotherapists and consultants.

Adequate diagnostic facilities are available during the pre-sentence observation period. Social history material is obtained from two sources. Trained social workers in the field submit a report based on direct contacts with the individual's family, acquaintances, and appropriate agencies. In addition, an intensive psychiatric social history is obtained from the individual at the prison. Each offender receives a battery of psychological tests and has a series of interviews with a psychiatrist. When the different disciplines have completed their examinations, the offender is discussed at a staff conference and a group decision is made with respect to his diagnosis and his proper committability under the Sex Crimes Law. A report of the staff decision is then submitted to the Department of Public Welfare and from there to the committing court.

The law is worded in a manner that makes it unnecessary to conform to a rigid rule of responsibility or committability in recommending a person for treatment. The staff is free to develop their own criteria for selecting the most suitable candidates for recommitment into the treatment program. In practice, we recommend commitment under the Sex Crimes Law for those people who present two basic qualities in their personality and behavior. First, we look for an immaturity in the development of sexual functions, which also encompasses other areas of the individual's personality and social behavior. Second, we look for a deviation of the individual's normal sexual aim or object which he has little ability to control by conscious rational thought. We then speak of this individual as having a compulsive need to live out his sexual immaturities.

Although our population presents a wide variety of social backgrounds, intellectual abilities, and previous levels of achievement, it is rare that we see an offender with a relatively intact personality. The majority of our patients demonstrate few ego strengths and few conflict-free areas in their lives. Histories of severe trauma and emotional deprivation during early childhood are commonplace. Approximately 40 per cent of our population has had previous correctional experience and many others have been wards of the State. Our experience indicates that sex deviates as a group function in the world as inadequate individuals.

Sexual behavior, for most of our patients, is associated with tremendous needs to satisfy passive wishes, bolster self esteem, find identity and, in a figurative sense, be fed. Many of these individuals would fall into the category of ambulatory schizophrenic or borderline states.

The treatment begins when the individual has been recommitted to the prison under the law. At this institution, he immediately becomes involved in a program which includes orientation, classification and job assignment. The scope as well as limitations of our treatment may be clarified by examining the personality patterns of our offenders, particularly as related to the impact of the prison milieu. Given the inadequate ego skills and passivity of our patients, we are faced with problems created by placing these individuals in a prison environment. Their overwhelming passivity is accentuated by arrest and commitment. The impact of arrest on a sex offender leads to feelings of shame and humiliation. When the passive, inadequate individual encounters these emotions, he becomes even more helpless. He seeks easily grasped concepts or structures that will afford him an explanation for his behavior. Many sex offenders dismiss their behavior as being entirely the product of overindulgence in alcohol. Sometimes the offense is denied in its entirety both to the authorities and to themselves. More often attempts are made to rationalize deviant behavior by claims that the patient was seduced by sexually aggressive, precocious young boys or girls. Given the personality limitations of our patients and the impact of the prison milieu, there is a need for immediately creating a climate of acceptance which at the same time discourages rationalization, denial, and projection.

Each new inmate is placed in an orientation group led by two members of the psychiatric staff. These groups contain between ten and twenty patients and meet for a total of ten sessions. Basic principles of mental health as well as the mechanics of normal sexual behavior are explained and discussed. Wherever possible, relevant films are used and free discussion is encouraged. These meetings attempt to create a climate devoid of blame or punitiveness toward the sex offender. The orientation group also serves the purpose of giving our staff a second chance for evaluating the patient's potential for psychotherapy, and it is not until the end of this period that a specific treatment program is outlined.

A majority of offenders are offered psychotherapy. We currently provide both individual and group psychotherapies ranging from insight therapies to supportive and even didactic approaches. For those individuals who we feel are able to make personality changes, the major goal of treatment is to provide a degree of self understanding sufficient to help them resolve their impulsive sexual motivations. For those who do not demonstrate a potential for personality change, treatment may consist of strengthening useful defenses, education, and emotional support.

Based on their needs, many individuals are recommended for expressive individual or group psychotherapy. While all members of our staff accept the role of unconscious processes in determining behavior, the backgrounds and training of different individuals leads to a variety of approaches. Thus, free association is frequently supplemented by a variety of techniques based on client-centered and learning theory. Success in therapy seems to depend more upon the offender's motivation and the therapist's skill than on specific theoretical investment. In general, therapists tend to use techniques directed at uncovering unconscious material when working with patients who are appropriately motivated and can tolerate anxiety. Group therapy was originally inaugurated to provide for a maximum number of contacts with a limited professional staff. It has, however, proved so markedly effective in helping establish positive self-identification quickly, and in bringing about the development of social and interpersonal insights that we now regard it as a treatment of choice for many.

Psychotherapy is less frequent than we feel to be optimal, and runs the gamut from a few who receive therapy twice a week to a greater number who are seen weekly or biweekly. The average length of treatment time for both group and individual therapy is approximately fourteen months.

The process of our reeducative therapy with sex offenders may be broken down into three phases. The initial phase is devoted to creating a climate which allows the establishment of a therapeutic relationship. This period may encompass several months to a year. Only after the development of such a relationship can the individual begin to examine his behavior without resorting to defensiveness or intra-punitive mechanisms. The second phase is the period of working through nuclear conflicts. During this period, therapy focuses upon those factors in the background of the individual that have contributed to the development of deviant trends. Considerable attention is also directed toward the day to day interactions in the prison setting emphasizing those vignettes of behavior that are similar to self destructive actions that have led to incarceration. The last phase of therapy is devoted to problems of separation and planning for the future. This is often a very complicated process. Returning to the free world from a closed institution presents an additional burden to the stresses of community attitude, vocational problems, family attitudes, and separation from the therapist.

Termination of therapy does not necessarily mean automatic release from the institution. The final responsibility for release rests with a Special Review Board which is independent of the treatment service and consists of a social worker, a lawyer, and a psychiatrist. The majority of offenders released are assigned to an after-care program which includes supervision and counselling by trained social workers.

The combination of a correctional setting, an indeterminate sentence, and the inadequate personality structure of the sexual deviate tends to produce specific problems in psychotherapy which may not be encountered elsewhere, The most outstanding of these is the type of resistance in which the patient eagerly grasps onto a psychological or moralistic formula which provides him a rationalization for his behavior. This serves as a superficial explanation for his difficulties which may also lead him to the conviction that he will not repeat the offense. If he merely promises to stop his aberrant behavior, and holds to his belief on the basis of an alleged change in his morals or an alleged understanding of his difficulties, he sets up a tremendous road-block to treatment. The patient who clings to such a position effectively removes the need for a therapist or any further therapeutic change. The most satisfactory way to avoid this resistance is for the therapist to be constantly aware of any tendencies in himself toward adopting a psychiatric "partyline" which the inmate can learn and parrot back to him. The inmate must be constantly questioned as to what he actually does understand about himself and both he and the therapist must realize that the areas involved are so complex that they can never be treated with certainty.

It is essential that the offender take responsibility for his actions. Rationalizing behavior through invoking alcoholism, unfortunate circumstances, or even psychoanalytic formulations, does not lead to therapeutic progress. The offender must recognize that it is he who has committed the crime. It is neither the alcohol, nor the environment, nor the neuroses. Optimally therapy should be conducted in a situation where the offender is moderately anxious and both uncertain and concerned about his propensity to repeat the offense. The inmate who leaves the institution with doubt and apprehension is perhaps a better risk than the one who leaves with an ultimate assurance of being cured.

A sizeable number of offenders are not selected for expressive therapy primarily because they either show little motivation or do not have sufficient ego strength to cooperate in this type of treatment. For this group we have been experimenting with a wide variety of other techniques including supportive educational sessions, environmental manipulations, and even exhortative approaches. Many of these offenders have been unable to tolerate close contact with another person without feeling aroused by all sorts of infantile sexual and aggressive feelings. Few are able to appreciate that a close benevolent relationship with another individual is a possibility. These men are provided therapeutic contacts ranging from "friendly chats" to specific didactic sessions on sexual problems. Through such techniques many offenders are able to discover a new type of interpersonal relationship and to markedly strengthen their internal controls. Adjunctive services such as religious, occupational, and educational counseling are used.

There are a few offenders who are neither interested in nor able to cooperate in any type of psychotherapeutic venture, but who will respond to the basic correctional program of the institution. For those who do not, our program functions primarily to protect society. Some of these individuals will be committed far longer than they would have been under ordinary sentencing. We feel that the failure of ordinary psychological treatment techniques with this group represents an inadequacy of psychiatric knowledge, and that until techniques are more refined, treatment must consist of indeterminate custodial care. This is analogous to the case of the chronically psychotic patient in the mental hospital who often must be institutionalized even though there is little definitive treatment available.

All in all, our experience in working therapeutically with this group has taught us to be flexible in our thinking, daring in our experimentation with new techniques, and realistic with respect to the establishment of meaningful goals. Only by modifying orthodox concepts have we been able to produce positive results.

The parole experience and discharge record of individuals who have received treatment under the law is encouraging. Only a few of the more relevant statistical results will be presented. Of 1,605 male offenders examined under this law over a nine year period, only 783 were found to be in need of specialized treatment. Parole experience with this group has been excellent. Of the 475 individuals granted parole through May 31, 1960, only 81 have violated that parole—a rate (17 per cent) considerably lower than that found with parole granted to the general prison population. It is particularly noteworthy that only 43, or 9 per cent of the total paroled, violated their parole by commission of a further sex offense. For individuals who have been discharged following a period of institutional treatment and parole supervision, the results are even more outstanding. Through May 31, 1960, 414 individuals were discharged from Departmental control; only 29, or 7 per cent of this group, committed a new offense following discharge. We feel that this law has been most effective, not only in providing protection to the public, but also in demonstrating that most sex offenders are capable of responding to treatment.

The Treatment of Psychopaths

by MELITTA SCHMIEDEBERG, M.D.

PSYCHOPATHY and criminality overlap, but are not synonomous. Some ordinary persons break the law under pressure or temptation; habitual criminals however are abnormal or abnormalised and usually psychopathic. On the other hand, many well-to-do psychopaths manage to remain within the law. Psychopathy is not an entity, nor a rarity. With three million serious felony offenders in the USA the number of psychopaths must run into millions, yet they have hardly been studied, even diagnostically. They range from the borderline psychotics, such as those committing horrible types of murder or bizarre acts, to the borderline neurotics, who often still have some social or family ties, suffer from depressions if they fail, and may commit suicide if the game is up. Even the ordinary person may, under the pressure of certain situations, as in wartime, develop psychopathic reactions and even become psychopathic. The neurotic, again, does not always correspond to the textbook version of overconscientiousness, and even obsessionals may show psychopathic reactions and act antisocially. This is still more true of borderline psychotics, schizoid and paranoid personalities. Some psychiatrists tend to minimize antisocial traits in their patients and call them "character cases" or "passive aggressive dependents." The line between the "bad boy" in adolescence and the psychopath is not easily drawn, and it is hard to distinguish the product of the slums, devoid of moral and other training, from the "true" psychopath. Many alcoholics and other "acting out" patients are actually psychopathic; most drug addicts many of whom are former gang boys.

The psychopath behaves antisocially and has antisocial ideals and fantasies; he both "wants to be a villain" and is forced to be one, since he is unable to succeed socially. Often there is deep underlying hopelessness. Psychopaths are not altogether devoid of anxiety and guilt, but they manage effectively to cut off these levers of socialisation, the temporary awareness of which frightens them excessively. While anxiety and guilt

180

help to make the neurotic and normal person more social, they incite the psychopath to antisocial acts in his attempts to prove himself master of these emotions which he fears and despises.

A patient felt guilty towards his wife whom he mistreated; to punish her for having made him feel bad, he beat her and when she cried he beat her harder.

The cliché that psychopaths "fail to learn from experience" is only partially true. Time teaches them to become a more skillful criminal, but not to socialize, though some give up their fight against society as they get older. Their failure to learn from social experience is based on their ability to take their behavior out of its social context, to break the continuity of cause and effect and the continuity of time. Punishment to them is not consequence, but merely ill luck or injustice. They continue to believe that they will go scot-free, irrespective of how often they have been caught, and are almost delusionally convinced of their superior intelligence. Their excessive narcissism makes them immune to social pressures and rational thinking. The problem for therapy is that they want no treatment, because they have no wish to change and find no fault with themselves, but only blame others and society. Their denial mechanisms and narcissism make them, as a rule, immune both to severity and kindness. The only time they are somewhat amenable to influence is when their narcissistic bubble of grandeur has been burst, when they have been caught and await trial. Incidentally, the anxiety they then experience and the desperate efforts they make to avoid punishment is proof that they desire punishment neither consciously nor unconsciously. Although I have examined thousands, I have not yet seen a single serious offender who was motivated by an unconscious wish for punishment. The fact that antisocial personalities and psychopaths have been mistaken for "neurotic offenders" and been treated as such has had disastrous consequences, likely to bring psychiatry into disrepute in legal circles.

Probation which developed empirically, has hit intuitively on the one avenue by which many offenders can be influenced, namely a combination and delicate balance of fear and kindness, by approaching the offender when the apprehension of punishment and the experiences of trial have stirred him and he is relieved because he has not been sent to prison.

Though the patient usually can be reached when the harsh reality has pierced his narcissistic defences, such influence is as a rule only short-lived, owing to the psychopath's remarkable ability to reestablish his antisocial mental balance with the help of his ideas of grandeur and denial. Hence we need a situation of continuing pressure. The attempt of some psychiatrist to win an antisocial patient over by siding with him against authority and removing external pressure, usually results in the patient feeling relieved and staying away. The patient comes for treatment unwillingly, and his good resolutions are attempts to manipulate the therapist. He must be allowed such hope for manipulating or he would not try, but the therapist must be careful how far he allows himself to be manipulated; rather, he must manipulate the patient to socialize him. The enforced attendance must be used to establish a more genuine relation; this can only be done by showing understanding and by giving help in teaching the patient to solve his problems and to gain satisfaction in a social manner. We must constantly fight the patient's tendency to denial and to insensitizing himself by evoking two opposite emotions almost simultaneously, i.e., giving him sympathy for having been wronged, yet highlighting the wrong he has done and warning him of the consequences of his behavior, thus evoking guilt and building on whatever rudiments of social feelings he possesses. This must be done so that he feels the doctor is on his side, e.g., would regret it if he went to prison. Unbearable anxiety or guilt stimulate his antisocial mechanisms, yet no influence is gained unless sufficiently strong emotions are evoked.

These patients have tremendous energy, probably because so little of it is inhibited and sublimated and are able to wear out their environment and the therapist. Effective therapy should turn the tables on the patient and wear him out: create situations for him to which he must conform rather than allow him to control the situations. The more persons are involved in the treatment situation, provided they are well co-ordinated, the better. In the Association for the Psychiatric Treatment of Offenders in New York City we utilize many persons, each playing his own role. The clinical director sees the patient on intake, trying to motivate him, thus making the task of the therapist easier. She remains a figure of authority to whom the therapist can refer. The probation officer, with the judge behind him, plays his legal role and represents final authority. The therapist is more on the patient's side. Then there may be a reading instructor, medical doctor, members of family or friends, with all of whom the therapist seeks contact and whom he tries to co-ordinate.

I had, as Clinical Director of APTO, succeeded in getting a young recidivist out of detention, after he had been arrested for new offenses during treatment. He needed a letter from APTO for the court hearing and I insisted that he see me. When he phoned for an appointment I discovered that he had no job. "Look here Billy, what can I write in this letter? The judge knows that you have been in trouble before, that you stole cars again while on probation. If I write that you have no job, what will he think? I give you a piece of advice. Do not see me till you have a job." But there were only three days left to the hearing. Next day Billy had a job, the first one in his life.

Treatment of the psychopath, then, is the opposite of the passive, detached, nonjudgmental therapy currently used for neurotics, since this type of patient contrasts in all essentials with the neurotic. The latter is too inhibited, overconscientious, worries too much, acts too little and too slowly, is afraid of change; the former is consumed by restlessness, is in constant motion, acts on the spur of the moment, is underconscientious, and asocial. The task of therapy is to build inhibitions, social feeling and conscience, to teach him to delay action, to think within the context of reality, to establish a sense of continuity, to solve his problems and gain satisfaction in a social manner. To do this we must be active and alert, manipulate him and his environment; not only be judgmental, but teach the patient values and judgment.

Cooperation with the courts is essential. For this it is necessary to know and respect the prerogative of the courts, have some knowledge of law, institutions, criminal mentality, know what, can and, cannot be condoned, what recommendations to make to the Court and how reports should be written, what information should be given or withheld, etc.

Since this highly specialised knowledge and approach is essential for the treatment of offenders, and even for evaluating them diagnostically, criminal psychiatry should be developed and taught as a specialty. Psychiatrists lacking such experience should not advise courts, educators, parents, etc. on the handling of delinquents as analogies drawn from private practice with neurotics are misleading.

Captive Outpatients: A Psychotherapy Program for Parolees

by Virginia Patterson, M.A.; M. Robert Harris, M.D.; and
William Bewley, M.D.*

T HE OUT-PATIENT psychiatric treatment of adult offenders has generally been regarded as a difficult, if not fruitless, psychotherapeutic task. It has been the experience of many who have attempted to work psychotherapeutically with criminal offenders, that they lack motivation for treatment, that they discharge anxiety through impulsive action, and that these actions frequently bring about a disruption of the treatment relationship through the necessary reinvolvement of law enforcement agencies. These cases generally show a high drop-out rate after an initial contact or a brief series of interviews. The pressure from courts, probation or parole officers has been regarded as intensifying the individual's rebellious, resistive feelings toward treatment even though it may insure the individual's physical presence at the interview. The hope to escape a prison sentence has often appeared to be the primary motivation for a request for treatment and this alternative has been sanctioned by legal authorities. Often the motivation has disappeared when the case has been adjudicated. All of these factors have led to a reluctance on the part of voluntary agencies and private practitioners to offer or enter into a psychotherapeutic relationship with individuals in conflict with the law.

*The Langley Porter Neuropsychiatric Institute and the Department of Psychiatry, University of California School of Medicine, San Francisco 22, California. Also participating in a major way in this project were Dr. Marietta Houston, former psychiatric director of Langley Porter Neuropsychiatric Institute Outpatient Department, and Mr. Herbert Wadler, former senior psychiatric social worker in the Department. Psychiatrists participating for a portion of the project were Dr. Peter Ostwald, Dr. James Stubblebine, and Dr. Jean Hayward Malerstein. Parole officers and officials from the State of California, Department of Corrections, Division of Paroles were: Mr. Walter Stone, Director, Division of Paroles; Mr. Patrick Smythe; Mr. Joseph d'Angelo; and Mr. Eugene Luttrell.

These considerations led us to develop a program which could meet the formidable treatment problems presented by patients of this type. At the outset, the critical questions seemed to be (1) how to engage a unmotivated patient in psychotherapy; (2) how to hold these individuals in treatment despite stresses both in the treatment relationship and their life situations; and (3) how to limit acting-out with its disruptive consequences.

The referring correctional authority provided the clinic with an initial answer to these questions by offering to make participation in psychotherapy a condition of the parole contract. The concept and the conditions of mandatory treatment were central to the project and will therefore be discussed in more detail.

It has been an implicit assumption that therapy cannot take place under conditions of coercion. Attendance may be commanded, but the process of therapy has seemed to require a willingness to engage with a therapist in self exploration and effort toward personality change. Yet we know that there are many individuals with varying behavior disorders who have little inclination toward introspection and whose dynamics are such that an adaptive balance is maintained with difficulty. Careful therapeutic work with the "unmotivated" patient utilizes whatever conflict-free ego functions are available for self examination and problem solving may sometimes prove effective. With neurotic patients, those aspects of psychotherapy which parallel the parent–child relationship are analyzed for the purpose of freeing the individual from transference distortions. The function of therapy with patients who show less adequate ego development is in large part to provide a safe, predictable, non punitive relationship in which experimentation and learning can take place.

It was our hypothesis in the project that if the prospective parolee patients expressed at least an initial willingness to engage in the therapeutic effort and, if they could be held to the task for a sufficient period of time, some useful characterologic changes might result. The reluctances, the anger, the lack of motivation, and the externalization could gradually be worked with in the context of an ongoing therapeutic relationship in which the individual is not permitted to run away either through conscious intent, indifference, hostility, involvement in extratherapeutic pursuits, or other reasons.

Mandatory therapy found many of the therapists in serious conflict. Some therapists considered this approach as punitive and too aggressively intervening in the life of the patient. It was seen as a process akin to "brainwashing." Some therapists felt that they would be simply sitting

out the parole with the parolee. Considerable staff discussion was necessary to reach a consistent therapeutic attitude toward these patients. The
project staff met weekly to discuss the treatment and the many issues
involved. Changes in staff required repeated reexamination and working
through of the attitudes toward mandatory therapy and toward the
general problem of treatment of the criminal offender.

In considering the therapeutic approach, the aspect of control of
impulse appears critical in the dynamics of the criminal offender. These
men in their early experience, often in identification with parents with
similar problems, failed to learn socially integrated ways of handling
impulses. Their efforts toward impulse gratification were characteristically
met in punitive ways, so that what was learned was that the only way to
get anything was to disregard the consequences. A profound pessimism
regarding the possibilities for satisfaction in socially approved channels
resulted.

Society has generally taken the responsibility for control of individuals
who do not control themselves. The controls offered by imprisonment,
while essentially restrictive, serve a function in relation to the impulsive
acting-out features of the behavior of offenders. However, the prison
experience may also shape later behavior in the direction of increased
dependency and a reliance on external controls. The parole period continues many of the controls which have been provided by the institution.

In our design of the project, we felt that it would be important for a
time to maintain this type of situation, that is, to perpetuate the system
of external controls until the individual could be helped to develop his
own. For this reason we collaborated closely with the parole officers.

One of our initial conditions in setting up the project was that the
parolees should be assigned to a limited number of parole officers who
had time to work closely with the project staff. The twenty-two parolees
who were included in the project were assigned to two parole officers,
although there were later shifts in assignment due to personnel changes
in the parole office. The parole officers assisted the men in finding living
quarters and employment. They talked with employers with the aim of
facilitating the work adjustment. They helped the men to keep their
appointments, sometimes in practical ways such as giving them rides to
the clinic. We reported missed appointments as violations of the parole
contract. Meetings with the parole officers were scheduled biweekly, and
later, monthly. In addition, there was informal contact by phone, and
special visits during emergencies.

Rather than emphasizing the confidential and exclusive nature of the
therapeutic relationship, we obtained the permission of the men to share

information with the parole officers. The shared communication had to do less with the content of the therapy than with mutual decision-making on how to handle various aspects of the men's behavior.

The problems of the parole officers in relation to the men and their own self image became apparent in such meetings. They showed uneasiness at times with a perception of themselves as either too lenient or as punitive and authoritarian. They possessed considerable authority in relation to the parolees and were required to make decisions of major importance. Their recommendations to the parole board were crucial in determining whether individual parolees might marry, move from the county, be returned to prison, etc. The behavior of the parolee was of such a kind as to present many dilemmas to both the treatment staff and the parole officers. For example, there was the question of what action should be taken regarding a homosexual relationship which was a violation of the parole conditions and yet which seemed to offer a stabilizing influence and some gratification to a man who had few relationships with others. Again, how should petty thievery be handled? It was clearly illegal, but was it of the proportions that a formal parole violation with its complicated legal consequences should be recorded? Too many violations reflected upon the work of the parole officers. On the other hand, the parole officer was not fulfilling his function in overlooking an illegal activity.

A doctrine of permissiveness in child rearing practices and in therapeutic procedures has been prevalent in the past decade. The dilemma of reconciling permissiveness with law enforcement was frequently encountered in staff discussions although in many ways it appeared to be a spurious issue. We believed that it was important for both the treatment staff and the parole officers to acknowledge any activity on the part of the parolee which was illegal and to help the man to take corrective action. In work with the parolees, we attempted to clarify the choices as well as the consequences of their behavior. We did not attempt to protect them or intervene in their behalf if legal action was forthcoming.

It was our experience in the project that when, as a result of changes in the men's living situations, parole officers were assigned in addition to the two with whom we usually worked, problems resulted. The issues on which some resolution had been achieved again became confused. Negative attitudes on the part of the new parole officers toward a therapeutic program often became apparent. They raised questions as to whether therapy was necessary. The hardships on the men in terms of time off from work, treatment fees, and transportation costs were stressed. In effect the resistances of the parolees were reinforced.

Another way in which we attempted to modify the social situation of the parolee patients was to work with relatives or persons of importance in their life situations.

The staff of the project consisted of the director of the out-patient department, one or more psychiatric residents, a clinical psychologist and a psychiatric social worker. These individuals set aside a regular weekly time to discuss the project. In addition, a series of evening seminars was arranged for the staff of the project which provided background material in criminology, sociology, psychoanalytic theory of criminal behavior, and forensic psychiatry. There were also periodic joint meetings with the staff of a local child guidance clinic who were working psychotherapeutically with juvenile delinquents and their families for whom therapy was a condition of probation.

DESCRIPTION OF THE PROJECT

Twenty-two paroled criminal offenders from a prison medical facility were accepted for study and treatment by the adult outpatient department of the Langley Porter Neuropsychiatric Institute. The board which grants paroles in the state selected two men during each month of the year and, with the agreement of these men, attached a special condition to their parole contract which required that they come to the Institute for psychotherapy. The basis for selection of the men was unknown to the outpatient department staff although subsequent perusal of the prison records permitted speculation about the factors which determined the choice. Some of the men were regarded as "good" psychotherapy candidates on the basis of their participation in therapy while in prison; some were labeled as "dangerous;" a number were sex offenders at a time when sex offenses had aroused considerable public indignation; and, for some men, no rationale for selection could be determined. The range of offenses included robbery, burglary, forgery, homicide, drug addiction, and sexual offenses.

The project continued for three years.

TREATMENT

Initially, each parolee was seen for a series of diagnostic studies and interviews. Because of staff limitations, not all of the men could be seen in individual treatment although this might have been desirable in an exploratory project of this type. Certain of the men were therefore chosen for group psychotherapy and a group composed of parolees was formed.

As had been anticipated, resistance was the primary feature of both the individual and group therapies. The men complained constantly about the fact that they were required to come for treatment and about the assessment of a fee. They felt that they were being used in various ways, for example, by the prison authorities to justify the funding of an out-patient clinic for parolees. They talked about innocuous subjects. The main affectively toned topic of discussion, particularly in the group, was reminiscence about life in prison.

These men were in continuous search for external sources of blame. For example, one man told with considerable feeling of having taken his wife to a public lecture on crime and prisons by a well known psychiatrist. He described the psychiatrist pointing his finger at the audience and saying, ". . . . but the biggest difficulty of all is the attitude of society."

To the extent that life problems and decisions were involved, both parole officers and therapists attempted to help in whatever ways were available to them. As soon as it was feasible, we began to interpret the defensive nature of their complaints, their resistances, distrust and hostility. Their manipulations at the clinic, efforts to get the fee revised, to have appointment times changed, to make clinic attendance impossible, to enlist the sympathy of parole officer versus therapist or vice versa, were used to elucidate patterns of behavior and underlying motivations.

Attitudes toward the therapist were particularly difficult to deal with. Transference aspects had an all or nothing quality. The therapist was seen as a sinister and all-powerful representative of a hostile social system or as a helpless tool of the prison authorities, unable to wield enough influence to free the man from his parole condition regarding therapy. Therapists were generally perceived as cold and distant. The men began to relate to their therapists only very gradually.

Five of the parolee patients got into difficulties almost immediately after release from prison. One patient was frightened by the responsibility of life outside prison, several committed crimes similar to the ones that had brought about the recent prison term, one sex offender with an unstable, borderline psychotic and perhaps organic pattern repeated alcoholic excesses which necessitated his return to prison. Psychological testing indicated that the individuals who got into difficulties immediately upon release were more disturbed than the group as a whole, in particular showing more evidences of anxiety. It appeared that the more "hardened" and resistive men were better able to make the transition to life outside of prison.

TREATMENT OF RELATIVES

A therapeutic contact with relatives was seen as a possible means by which the interpersonal milieu might be positively altered. It became apparent, however, once the men were interviewed, that many of them were without family or had made long term separations from their relatives, or had very tenuous relationships with family members. Where possible, we did interview parents, wives or fiancées and, in some instances, we were able to engage them in a continuing therapeutic relationship. For many of the men, the work of therapy appeared to be to help them build emotional relationships of some substance. An unusual proportion of the men married during the time that they were in therapy. For the most part, the prospective spouses appeared to share the distrustful attitudes of the parolees toward the therapeutic program. In some instances, it appeared that the relatives wished to avoid the official linkage with the paroled family member as if there were an implication of being an accomplice in a crime. Parolees avoided involving their relatives as though they were concerned about being informed upon. The general impression was that the relatives, both parents and spouses, were as resistive to therapy as the parolees themselves.

EVALUATION OF THE TREATMENT PROGRAM

The results of this pilot project did not indicate that the treatment techniques could be considered critical in reducing the social problem. Five of the twenty-two men in the project got into trouble during the period of the initial study and were returned to prison. Another six had been re-arrested or disappeared during the first year following their release. The remaining 50 per cent completed their paroles successfully. This percentage is not significantly different from the rate of parole success reported by the Department of Corrections for the parole population as a whole.

An evaluation of the program by the parolees themselves was obtained through a follow-up questionnaire administered six months after termination of the project. For the most part, the questionnaires revealed the same ambivalence which the men displayed in the treatment situation. The prevailing attitude expressed in the questionnaire was one of contempt for the program, denial of its usefulness, and negation of any need for it. Interspersed were contradictory statements of agreement that psychotherapy should have been a condition of the parole, and recommendations that it be provided for *other* parolees. Paradoxically, the questionnaires returned by the reincarcerated parolees were generally more favorable in their retrospective evaluations than those who "made" parole and are currently in the community.

For the most part, this project did achieve one of its primary goals, namely the definition of those conditions under which treatment could be offered to paroled criminal offenders in the setting of an out-patient clinic. Our own conditions in setting up the study were not always met, e.g., not all the men were released as planned to the environs of the clinic, additional and sometimes unsympathetic parole officers were assigned, etc. But the project enhanced the staff's knowledge about, interest in, and comfort in dealing with these patients. The aspect of mandatory therapy prompted many of the therapists to study carefully the whole area of motivation, and to give serious considerations to possible techniques and treatment modifications which may be developed to approach this and other resistant, unmotivated but obviously needful patient groups.

RECOMMENDATIONS

In designing a future treatment program for criminal offenders, we would incorporate certain changes based upon our experience with the present project. It seems of primary importance that the contract regarding psychotherapy be made between the parolee and the clinic staff rather than between the parolee and the parole board. Members of the clinic treatment staff and the parole officers should personally describe the therapeutic program and obtain acceptance from the prospective patient (criteria for selection did not emerge clearly) before the condition regarding treatment is attached to the parole contract. At the same time, permission should be requested to interview significant relatives with whom the man will be involved while on parole. Prior to the man's release from prison, these relatives *should be* contacted with the hope of involving them, too, in concurrent therapy. The therapeutic media may include both individual as well as group psychotherapy in a socio-recreational setting for each patient, with the parolees being included in groups which are not composed entirely of parolees; however, the individual psychotherapeutic setting may be the treatment of choice. It would also be desirable to have an administrative arrangement whereby the men could be either temporarily returned to the correctional facility or hospitalized briefly at the point of a significant threat of acting out.

Occupational Psychiatric Therapy

by RALPH T. COLLINS, A.B., M.D., MED. SC. D.

T HE WORK THAT MEN DO is an essential part of their lives, not mainly because by it they earn their bread, but because a man's job gives him stature and binds him to society. The worker who is happy in his job, with confidence in his management and cooperative relations with his co-workers, will spread his contentment throughout the community.[1]

"Doctor," said a corporation president to a neuropsychiatrist who had joined the medical department staff, "I believe that you have two functions with us, professional and educational. I'm not worried about your professional function, but I am worried about your educational function. I hope that as the years go by, you will be able to spend more of your time in educating me and all of us in management, down to the first line supervisor, in the area of knowing more about emotions, personality development, mental illness, the meaning behind behavior, and the development of healthy attitudes among all of us at work, towards ourselves, and towards our work, so that we might become more effective leaders and managers."

This educational function is in essence preventive psychiatry, in that leaders and managers can do much to prevent emotional upsets at work by understanding people more thoroughly, knowing what they want out of their jobs, developing the confidence of the employees in them as effective supervisors at any level of management, creating a mentally healthy climate at work and learning how one can be a better balanced person.

Throughout the years, the industrial psychiatrist has acquired the further functions of advisor and investigator. The neurologist and psychiatrist who labors in any work situation, whether it be a department store, a bank, a governmental agency, a business or an industry, usually has patients referred by occupational or community physicians, or by self referrals by employees. It is true that a supervisor at any level of management who has been well trained will have had some teaching in human

---

[1]Ralph T. Collins, M.D., *in* Think Magazine, Feb., 1961, Vol. 17, No. 2.

nature, in the early detection of emotional upsets among his employees, in interviewing techniques, and, hopefully, in handling worried employees. The supervisor then becomes another source of referral to the neuropsychiatrist, but only indirectly, because the supervisor should first refer the employee to the medical department. The occupational physician then will have the opportunity of taking a history, examining the employee and deciding if the employee should see the psychiatrist. This procedure prevents the supervisor from becoming a diagnostician.

Occupational physicians usually are able to handle most of the minor emotional problems that occur at the work place. These may accompany the physical disorders or occur separately. The psychiatrist is asked to see only the more difficult emotional and mental illnesses. This is as it should be, as the occupational physician functions more effectively in any occupational setting if he practices like the family physician. The occupational psychiatrist, in his educational role, meets with the physicians in a training program to discuss many topics which will aid them in understanding, diagnosing and treating disorders of behavior, thinking and feeling. Specifically, the following areas may be discussed: personality development, the etiology and meaning of symptoms, neurotic and psychotic reactions, disorders of character, anxiety and defense against anxiety, the sociopathic personality, alcoholism, drug addiction, depression and suicide. The occupational physician should learn something about interviewing techniques, brief psychotherapy, and the placement and management of employees with psychiatric disabilities.[2]

Occupational medicine has changed its focus within the past forty years from one of aspirin dispensing, throat spraying, finger wrapping and first aid, to one of total health maintenance through prevention and education. Management has also changed its focus from one of management-centered thinking to employee-centered thinking.

Occupational psychiatry is also social psychiatry. As McLean and Taylor point out,[3]

> "The psychiatrist's job is not so much the treatment of mental illness as the stimulation of mental health. Psychiatry, in this role, helps management in the understanding of its employees and of itself, helps it to understand the hopes, fears, gripes and wants of its people. Causes of employee tension can frequently be rooted out before serious trouble results. For the psychiatrist, industry provides an area of operation with real challenge. The challenge is the opportunity to forestall the develop-

[2]A Manual of Neurology and Psychiatry in Occupational Medicine: Collins, Ralph T., M.D., New York, Grune and Stratton, 1961.

[3]Mental Health in Industry, McLean, A. A., M.D., and Taylor, G. C., M.D.: New York, McGraw-Hill, 1958.

ment of serious mental illness through reduction of unnecessary emotional stress, through mental health education, and, where necessary,
through early, prompt and adequate treatment."

Actually, a large percentage of the people we see on the job are people
who have brought their off-the-job troubles to the job. They don't check
their troubles at the time clock.

Long term psychotherapy, as it is customarily understood, is seldom
used in the occupational setting. If the psychiatrist believes, after one or
two sessions with an employee, that long-term psychiatric therapy is in
order, he will refer the employee to his family physician, or, lacking any
family physician, to a community psychiatrist. The psychiatrist should
contact the family physician in any case. Group therapy has been used in
some industrial settings, but it is still in the experimental stage.

Employees become maladjusted because of many reasons stemming
from on-the-job problems, off-the-job problems, and from personality and
behavior disturbances. These maladjustments may lead to absenteeism,
alcoholism, accidents, tardiness, indifferent or unproductive work, troubles
with co-workers and supervision, and lowered morale. It has been esti-
mated that all of this costs business and industry about three billion dollars
a year. According to the National Fund for Medical Education,[4]

> "A well-rounded industrial health program which draws on the psy-
> chiatric knowledge presently available can materially reduce human
> discord by helping troubled workers overcome their difficulties and re-
> establish their usefulness; its cost can be recovered many times over
> through increased efficiency and greater productivity."

Business and industry spend billions of dollars on the purchase and
maintenance of machinery. How much is spent on the maintenance of the
human machinery? As one national business association member said to
me "America's number one problem in industry today is not production—
it is people. People are our unfinished business." Since work must be done
by people, it is a wise organization and a human one also which develops
and utilizes personnel policies which give cognizance to the importance of
human maintenance, the preservation of human dignity, the conservation
of human energy and the prevention of human breakdowns at work. We
should all remember that we hire the whole man and not just a hand.

The psychiatrist, in his advisory role, is able to advise management
about policies which affect employees. Many instances occur in which the
occupational psychiatrist confers with the personnel representative, the
supervisor, the employee counselor, or any other management person,
about a particular problem surrounding a particular employee. One must

---

[4]Medical Advance, The National Fund for Medical Education. New York,
May-June, 1954.

also consider other people involved in the department, the office or the laboratory, and manipulation of the environment may also be necessary in the solution of some personnel problems. The psychiatrist is often asked to advise about material to be used in the training of supervisors in the area of human nature. Companies, banks, and governmental agencies have trained their supervisors in this area through conferences on topics such as: the will to produce, understanding people, individual adjustment, the human factors in accidents, causes of absenteeism, job satisfaction, the meaning of work, the nature and effects of harmful worry, the executive's mental health and decision making, etc.

It would be helpful for all of us who deal with people anywhere to remember the following quotation from Charles Dickens' *Christmas Carol*:

> " 'But you were always a good man of business, Jacob,' faltered Scrooge, who now began to apply this to himself.
> " 'Business!' cried the Ghost, wringing his hands again. 'Mankind was my business; charity, mercy, forbearance, and benovelence were, all, my business. The dealings of my trade were but a drop of water in the comprehensive ocean of my business.' "

Day Hospital Treatment of Acute Psychiatric Illness

by Leon A. Steinman, M.D., and Robert C. Hunt, M.D.*

THE DAY HOSPITAL concept has blossomed out into such a variety of forms all over the world, with so many different kinds of experimentation that there is no uniformity of concepts, no general agreement as to definition, role, function, treatment programs, or types of patients to be treated. Bierer identifies his day hospital with "social groups," emphasizing and advocating "situational and group treatments." Others call their facilities "rehabilitation centers" or "recreational centers." Others are still more specialized in service offered and select groups served. The term "day hospital" is used so broadly as to have little meaning. The fact that patients attend the facility during the day and return home in the evening is the only common feature in the majority of "day hospitals," and only a few of them provide the type of comprehensive treatment usually expected of a hospital.

One of the units which does offer such a comprehensive program is the Poughkeepsie Day Care Center of the Hudson River State Hospital. Since opening in 1956, this facility has fulfilled the treatment functions of a psychiatric hospital geared to meet the needs of the severely mentally ill. It has focussed on those acute mentally ill who would have to be admitted to a hospital bed if these day services were not available.

In the five years since its opening, 724 patients out of 1,155 applicants processed have been admitted to the Center. The majority of these patients were ill enough to justify treatment on an inpatient basis. The 431 screened out as not requiring the full program were referred to appropriate sources of assistance in the community. Hospital admission was recommended for only 2 per cent of referrals, mostly because of grossly disturbed, highly aggressive or greatly destructive behavior; 12.8 per cent were admitted to day care on an emergency basis requiring immediate attention; 36.7 per cent evidenced dangerous tendencies. The age groups treated were mostly young and middle aged adults, with 78 per cent between 20 and 50 years of age. Some 37.9 per cent of all referrals were made by physicians, while 30.9 per cent were referred by clinics, agencies and state hospitals, and 31.2 per cent were self-referrals.

Criteria for admission are age 18 or older, psychiatric illness considered too severe for treatment on a fully ambulatory basis, and absence of a predominantly organic component. Patients also need residence and transportation arrangements which make possible the commuting involved. Patients with suicidal or aggressive tendencies are accepted when they have families who appreciate the dangers and agree to take necessary precautions. Acceptance of such risks is facilitated by the fact that the day hospital is part of the state hospital, so that crises can be dealt with by immediate admission to inpatient care when necessary. This is rarely resorted to, but its availability lends confidence to staff and families in giving day care a trial. It is our impression that day hospital treatment is especially prophylactic against suicide by offering hope of successful outcome, and doing so in a setting which does not add to the trauma and the extra burden of despair so likely to be felt on admission to hospital.

Of the 641 discharged patients, 74.4 per cent were returned to the community with various degrees of improvement. Half the patients complete their treatment in less than three months, one-quarter in three to six months, and the remainder in six months to a year with only an occasional patient being carried for more than a year for some special reason. Approximately 12 per cent of discharged patients have been readmitted to day care.

The Poughkeepsie day hospital is equipped and staffed to accommodate patients suffering from the widest range of psychiatric disorders, including the suicidal, agitated and mildly disturbed patients. The schizophrenic group comprising 27.3 per cent is running a close second to the neurotic group (33.6 per cent), while the involutionals (14.6 per cent) constitute the third largest. The remaining 24.5 per cent of patients consist of transient situational personality disorders, chronic brain pathology, affective reactions, etc.

The Center is able to offer the patients practically all types of therapy, with particular stress on individual and group psychotherapy. The possibility of combining various forms is one of the salient features of the facility. The therapeutic milieu of the Center—professional, social and interpersonal—is also considered of great significance. The planned and structured program appears to be of great benefit to the patient and speeds up his recovery.

Flexibility is another important factor in the program, with much individual variation in treatment and scheduling. Most patients attend the Center five days a week from 8:30 A.M. until 4 P.M. Attendance becomes less frequent as the acute disorder subsides.

Most patients are given some form of somatic therapy. While tranquilizers, and more recently safe and effective antidepressant drugs, have decreased the number of somatic treatments by older methods, still 16 per cent of the patients have been given ECT and 13 per cent sub-coma insulin (multiple insulin dosage method). While insulin therapy has lost its vogue in many places, it still appears to be of some value, particularly where other types of treatment have been unsuccessful. Coma insulin therapy should certainly not be administered on a day hospital basis, but sub-coma has proven safe. The multiple dosage method also appears safer and more economical than the single dosage sub-coma method. This method has been used over a period of five years and there has been no case of delayed hypoglycemia. The patients receive sub-coma insulin treatment in the morning, and in the afternoon are ready for psychotherapy and other therapeutic activities.

The psychotherapeutic program is a wide and comprehensive one, using diverse techniques. The full time professional staff of two psychiatrists, one clinical psychologist and one psychiatric social worker carry full case loads for individual and group therapy. Additional services are provided by psychiatrists and psychologists assigned for training on a part time basis. It has also been found feasible to place a number of patients with nonmedical staff members sufficiently skilled to provide supportive therapy and counseling under the supervision of the psychiatrists.

The group psychotherapy program is structured primarily to strengthen interpersonal relationships. Forty-three per cent were involved in group sessions twice a week.

The occupational and recreational programs are considered as therapeutic tools and are ordered by prescription. They are supervised by skilled, professional therapists. The patient finds there a range of activities tailored to his needs. They offer him the opportunity to release his anxiety, to divert his preoccupation with irrational fears, to overcome uncontrolled feelings, and at the same time to express his creative abilities and gain reassurance. Most activities are designed to promote group identification and socialization .

There has been developed a very successful program of individual and group sessions with relatives of patients. The understanding of the patient by his family and their interpersonal relationships appear of paramount importance. The adjustment of the attitude of the family toward the patient is as important as the treatment of the patient himself. The frequent visits of relatives to the Center, to bring the patient and to return him home, creates an atmosphere of constant mutual exchange on matters concerning the patient's life and fosters a favorable setting for good case work.

It is most difficult to get reliable data on the costs of treating the mentally ill in a day hospital as compared with an inpatient service. A 1959-60 research project sponsored by Manchester University and Nuffield Provincial Hospitals Trust showed that there was a little saving in day care centers. "Capital cost of a day hospital may be relatively smaller, but the running costs of a high quality treatment center may equal those or even be more expensive than inpatient care." In the Poughkeepsie experience, the daily operating cost per patient averages about seven dollars in the day hospital. This is substantially higher than the per capita cost in most state hospitals, which include large numbers of patients who get little active treatment. This, of course, does not constitute a valid comparison because the intensive treatment inpatient services in public mental hospitals are much more costly than the average for the entire institution. No accurate studies have been made, but we estimate that the cost of intensive treatment in the inpatient service averages $12.00 per patient day; thus the cost for patient day in a day hospital is in the neighborhood of one-half that of the comparable inpatient service.

Community acceptance of the Center has exceeded the most optimistic expectations. Patients and their families react to the illness and to the treatment regime with almost complete absence of the feelings of stigma which so handicap hospital treatment. The unit has earned a great deal of public recognition and the referrals by private psychiatrists, general practitioners, and agencies are increasing steadily. Thus the case load has reached an average of 120 patients at any one time, with daily attendance averaging around 50 to 60 patients.

In summary, the psychiatric day hospital of the type described can deal with a large number of severely sick people and is a valuable addition to the therapeutic resources of the community. The treatment of the mentally ill on a day basis, with avoidance of legal proceedings, eliminates the stigma on the patient and his family, prevents him from experiencing additional feelings of separation and loneliness or rejection by his family and society, and preserves his self esteem—all factors of paramount importance to the morale of the patient and his family. By enabling the patient to remain in close contact with his family and society, and to uphold his dignity, his social readaptation and rehabilitation can be better achieved. The psychiatric day hospital thus offers a new tool in combatting the staggering and growing problems of mental disorders.

Day Hospital Treatment for Psychotic Patients*

by Israel Zwerling, M.D., Ph.D., and Jack F. Wilder, M.D.

Introduction

THE FIRST PSYCHIATRIC day hospital was established in Moscow in 1932 and this treatment modality appears to have been limited to the Soviet Union until 1946 when Cameron,[3] in Montreal, and Bierer,[2] in London, independently inaugurated similar units within a few months of each other. The rapidity of growth, in both numbers and in diversity of function, of the day hospital in the past 15 years has been truly extraordinary; Farndale,[9] in his survey of day hospitals in England two years ago, visited a total of 65, of which 38 were general psychiatric day hospitals. No reliable estimate of the number of such units in the United States is known to the authors; but the rate of growth is so rapid, that there can be little disagreement with the conclusion of the World Health Organization Expert Committee on Mental Health[8] that the day hospital ". . . represents a distinct and important addition to the means of treating psychiatric patients, and one which every community mental hospital should consider establishing."

The emergence of the day hospital as a treatment modality for patients with mental illness is the resultant of a confluence of several diverse forces in contemporary psychiatry. First, perhaps, has been the growing awareness of the unintended but powerful antitherapeutic effects of traditional mental hospitals. Particularly in the last decade, sociologic studies of hospitals and wards as large and small communities (Stanton and Schwartz,[14] and Caudill[5]) have exposed the necessarily bureaucratic organization which develops and which, almost without regard to the stated purposes of the unit, then comes to impose its own laws of structure and function on the life of the unit. Goffman[10] introduces his contribution

---

*Division of Social and Community Psychiatry, Department of Psychiatry, Albert Einstein College of Medicine—Bronx Municipal Hospital Center.

with the wry comment that, "Whatever else psychiatry and medicine tell us, their happy way of sometimes viewing an insane asylum as if it were a treatment hospital does not help us very much in determining just what these places are and just what goes on in them," and he proceeds to develop a brilliant summary of the inevitable characteristics of what he aptly terms "total institutions." These considerations are the more relevant in the light of the purely custodial functions which most hospitals tend to perform outside of weekday and daytime hours. To the degree that total reliance for survival does not come to rest with the hospital staff, these institutional influences are significantly diluted; conversely, to the degree that realistic daily contact is maintained with the family and community during treatment, the need for the preservation of social skills continues, and regressive phenomena are consequently less frequent and less severe. A second focus in the development of the day hospital emerges from the vantage point of family psychodynamics. The closing of family ranks behind a member who has been extruded as a "sick patient" is a familiar problem in the hospital treatment of psychiatric patients. Not only are these difficulties obviated, but the continued residence of the patient at home forcibly brings to the treatment situation awareness of the family forces tending towards illness and towards recovery, so that these may be appropriately dealt with in the total treatment plan. A third pressure towards the emergence of day hospitals has been the patent economic advantage it offers; estimates of the cost per patient per day[9] range from two to three times as much for the traditional over the day hospital. Initial construction costs are of the same order of difference, since a considerable fraction of the space of a traditional hospital is required for dormitories and custodial care. In some instances, day hospital costs exceed the daily cost per patient of most state hospitals; here it has been pointed out by Goshen[11] that more intensive therapeutic efforts are made, and that in turn less time may be demanded directly from the psychiatrist. Another need which the day hospital appears to have been created to serve is the greater ease it offers of having patients accept hospitalization; one corollary of this is the beneficial impact upon the adverse attitude towards large geographically remote, state mental hospitals assumed by the general population when instead, the hospital is in the community, and when patients in hospital treatment are seen coming and going.

It must be emphasized that, however compelling the considerations which have determined the development of day hospitals, their utility remains uncertain. It is almost inevitable and perhaps even desirable that the pioneer contributors to a new direction should approach their work with a missionary zeal; it would, however, be unfortunate if this were not tempered by more objective and systematic appraisals. Unsubstantiated claims for day hospitals already may be found in some profusion. Thus, the W.H.O. Technical Report Series No. 73 states, in connection with the psychiatric day hospital, that: "First, it can enable patients to be discharged from the hospital at an earlier stage than before;" and Harris[12] states similarly that, "Treatment tends to be shortened, for it is no longer necessary to test the patient's reaction to his normal environment by sending him home for half-days and then weekends." These statements appear to go beyond reliable evidence. Craft[7] has reported a retrospective study, from existing records, of depressed patients treated in the day and the inpatient hospital services at Maudsley, which indicates that in presumably matched groups, day hospital treatment is equally effective in a shorter period of time than is inpatient treatment. While Craft's report is suggestive, it is not conclusive, and the ultimate value of the day hospital modality remains to be elucidated.

The greatest number of day hospitals accommodate between 20 and 30 patients daily, although Carmichael[4] and Kris[13] have described a much larger unit. In the absence of the traditional standard of reference for hospital size—i.e., beds—the unit of size for day hospitals has not been standardized. Some report their "capacity"; others the average daily attendance; others still the number of individual patients cared for each week. Most are open five days each week, from 9 A.M. to 4 or 5 P.M. The administrative location of day hospitals has varied among three principal positions: some have been established as separate and independent units, generally in the geographic center of the communities they intend to serve; some have been set up as units within a traditional mental hospital; and some have been organized as part of a parent general hospital containing a psychiatric division.

Selection of Patients

Perhaps the key issue to the future role of the day hospital in treatment of mental illness is the determination of which patients are or are not suitable for this modality. The earliest reports on psychiatric day hospitals reflect their widest use in the treatment of (a) patients with mild to moderate psychoses, or severe psychoneuroses; (b) geriatric patients with mild to moderate chronic brain syndromes; and (c) patients treated for acute psychotic states in traditional inpatient services and continued in treatment in day hospitals serving as halfway houses. Winick[16] reflects the general agreement that "Day centers tend not to accept patients (1) whose families cannot or will not cooperate in treatmen, (2) with a record of repeated suicide or homicide attempts, (3) unable to come regularly or who require special nursing care, (4) some psychopaths and sexual delinquents, alcoholics or addicts, and mental defectives. Some centers will not accept severely depressed patients, especially those with involutional melancholia. Sadism, masochism and 'injustice collecting' may be especially disruptive characteristics in day center patients." However, the more recent literature reflects a greater latitude in the selection of patients: Harris,[12] for example, writes,

> "In selecting patients one of our chief criteria has been that the patient must be so ill as to need admission to a hospital bed if the day hospital did not exist. We have closely adhered to this: all our patients are so far incapacitated by their illness as to be unable to work or lead their normal lives and most are unfit to be left alone at home during the daytime. On the other hand the patient must not be so disturbed as to be too difficult for his family to manage at night or for them to bring him and fetch him. He should not live much more than half an hour's journey away; for arrangements will break down if too much travelling is involved. Sensible, stable relatives, with affection and concern for the patient, who are willing to play an active, supporting role, are a very great help, and in their absence day hospital treatment is likely to prove difficult, though success has been achieved in some unfavorable family situations. With experience we have found that a very large proportion of potential inpatients can be treated on day hospital lines, and the pressure of recommended admissions is now greater on the Maudsley day hospital than on the wards."

Steinman and Hunt[15] similarly note,

> "The project has demonstrated that it is possible to treat effectively and safely in a day hospital many patients so ill that they would be hospitalized, were this service not available. It has unquestionably prevented many an admission to the state hospital."

However, the same authors continue to screen patients in advance of admission, but the criteria for screening patients in or out are not described. Craft[7] reports that the annual transfer rate from the day to the traditional inpatient service is 16 per cent for the Menninger Day Hospital and 14.7 per cent for the Maudsley Day Hospital; without detailed description of the criteria for initial selection, and the criteria for transfer, these data are of limited value. There has been no report of a systematic attempt to admit all patients requiring psychiatric hospitalization to a day hospital, and to define the nature and frequency of the circumstances which make it impossible to treat patients in the day hospital. This is the specific research objective of the Day Hospital of the Division of Social and Community Psychiatry, Department of Psychiatry, Albert Einstein College of Medicine–Bronx Municipal Hospital Center, described below.*

*Support for this project has been provided by the Health Reseach Council of New York City.

The Westchester Square Health Center Day Hospital

The Day Hospital is located approximately a mile away from the medical school–municipal hospital complex. It is open on weekdays, from 9 A.M. to 4 P.M. The building in which it is located is a district health center operated by the Department of Health of New York City; it houses the traditional preventive and public health service units of this department. Personnel staffing the Day Hospital are employees of the municipal Department of Hospitals and of the medical school, and are administratively responsible to the Albert Einstein College of Medicine–Bronx Municipal Hospital Center complex. The Day Hospital staff includes the following personnel; parenthetic designations indicate time devoted to Day Hospital duties:

Psychiatrists: 1—Ward Director (FT); 2—1st year residents (FT); 2—3rd year residents (2/3); 2—4th year fellows (½).

Psychiatric Nurses: 1—Head Nurse (FT); 2—RN (FT); 1—PN (FT); 3—Nurse's Aides (FT).

Psychology and Social Work: 2—Psychiatric Social Workers (1/3 time); 1—Clinical Psychologist (FT).

Ancillary Therapists and Supporting Personnel: 1—Art Therapist (¼ time); 1—Dance Therapist (⅛ time); 1—Ward Clerk (FT); 1—Stenographer (FT); 1—Typist (FT).

Patients admitted to the Day Hospital are randomly selected from among all patients judged in need of psychiatric admission by the Admitting Psychiatrist at the Bronx Municipal Hospital Center. Between 8 A.M. and 2 P.M., on weekdays, half of all admissions, in accordance with a previously arranged random sequence, are designated as Day Hospital patients and the remaining half are inpatient controls. Criteria for admission are severe, since (a) there is a very limited number of beds, and (b) alternative facilities exist through the Emergency Clinic[6] for outpatient care without preliminary screening procedures and without a waiting list. In effect, patients are admitted only when, in the clinical judgment of the Admitting Psychiatrist, they are so severely ill that they cannot be permitted to remain at home. The flow of psychiatric patients is such that the random selection procedure results in the admission of 3 to 5 new patients each week to the Day Hospital, and maintains a census in the Day Hospital of between 25 and 30 patients.

When the Admitting Psychiatrist is notified that the random order has designated an admitted patient as "Day Hospital," he notifies the Day Hospital director. The resident "on call" goes to the Admitting Room, explains the Day Hospital program to the patient and whatever family members have accompanied the patient, and all are then transported to the Day Hospital by hospital ambulance.

In the case of admitted patients who are designated as "Day Hospital" patients, and who cannot, in the judgment of the Day Hospital resident, be brought to the Day Hospital for treatment, approval for the admission of this patient in the Jacobi Hospital psychiatric inpatient service must be obtained from the Day Hospital director. Similarly, at the close of the Day Hospital at 4 P.M., approval for the transfer of a patient from the Day Hospital to the Inpatient Service must be obtained from the Day Hospital director. In each case, a thorough documentation of the reason for the action is required, with special emphasis upon (a) the physical disability which precludes the travel of the patient to and from home each day; or (b) the nature of the family objection to the care of the patient at home; or (c) the nature of the symptoms (overwhelming suicidal ideation; uncontrollable assaultive behavior; gross confusion) which necessitate the assignment or transfer of the patient to the inpatient service.

Therapy in the Day Hospital is conceived of as occurring at three levels —individual, family, and group. Therapists treat each patient individually a minimum of twice each week, and interview the patient together with the family at least once weekly. Drugs, and ECT, are used when indicated. Each new admission is reviewed after intake processing is completed with a supervising psychiatrist or at an Intake Conference, where a genetic-dynamic formulation is offered and a treatment plan for individual and family therapy set up. Individual treatment principles derive from a psychodynamic framework; the goal is the most rapid resolution of the disorganizing psychotic process. Family therapy reflects a number of contributions to the rapidly growing literature in this field, but most consistently flows from the theoretic model proposed by Ackerman.[1] Perhaps the most distinctive aspect of the therapeutic regimen of this Day Hospital is that which reflects the utilization of group processes for treatment and recovery.

Patients are assigned upon admission into activity groups; there are three such groups, each with an assigned census of 10 patients. To expedite communication among staff an attempt is made to assign all patients of an individual doctor to the same group. The group to which a patient is assigned is therefore determined by the doctor who is "on call." Upon learning of the sex of a new admission, the Day Hospital director may alter who is "on call" to balance disproportionate sex ratios in any one group. Otherwise, there has been no attempt to organize groups on the basis of diagnosis, age, level of socialization, or other criteria. The individual doctors meet twice a week with the group leaders to correlate individual, family, and activity group therapies. Each group has a group doctor and a nurse as an activity leader. The group doctor tends to be with his group only for short periods during the day; the nurse, who wears civilian clothes, is with her group for the greatest part of the day. The groups meet with their leaders each morning for the first hour. Group members may discuss over coffee their problems, their experiences at home or on the ward, or their reactions to each other in the meeting itself. The last part of the hour is usually devoted to planning the activities for the current day. The group leaders attempt to promote group cohesiveness by citing common concerns, needs, reactions, defenses, expectations, and fears—particularly around the focus of anxiety concerning separation from the Day Hospital—and by promoting democratic decision making. We are constantly impressed with the strong idealized group identification which occurs in a brief hospital stay among all diagnostic categories, even in a setting in which patients are assigned to individual psychiatrists. A moderately structured weekly activity program is also aimed at fostering group cohesiveness through the maintenance of group solidarity in the activities of the group. These are planned both within the Day Hospital or outside the community at large. A typical group activity schedule may be:

	MONDAY	TUESDAY	WEDNESDAY	THURSDAY	FRIDAY
A.M.	Group Art Activity (e. g. group murals)	Group Work Activity (e.g., making toys, framing pictures, clerical and light factory work for hospital and charities, operating ward canteen)	Group Lunch Preparation (selection, preparation, and serving for entire ward)	Group Work Activity	Ward Dance Therapy or Individual Optional Activities
P.M.	Group Optional Activity	Individual Optional Activities (e.g., art, crafts, beauty culture, vocational counselling, current events, household repairs, woodwork)	Group Optional Activity	Ward "Therapeutic Community" Meeting ——————— Ward Recreation	Ward Entertainment, Dance, and Recreation

As in other Day Hospitals we are constantly trying to combat the feminine atmosphere of most hospital activities. To this end, two of our three aides are male and one is an expert carpenter.

Patient stay is limited to two months, and patients are made aware of this from the very start. Experience has been that only infrequently has a consultation with the Day Hospital director been requested in order to prolong a patient's stay beyond the two month limit. Follow-up care, after discharge, is left to the discretion of each individual doctor and his supervisor; a separate research project is in the planning stages, to evaluate alternative patterns of post-discharge care of mentally ill patients.

Results

Preliminary experiences, with 72 "dry run" patients admitted under research conditions for the purpose of testing the suitability of the data gathering procedures, is summarized on table I. The following observations are of note:

(1) Out of 72 admitted patients for whom the Day Hospital resident was called, 17 were not actually accepted by the Day Hospital; 10 were males and 7 females. Of the 17, 5 (1 with psychotic depression, 4 with organic brain syndromes) were judged to be treatable in the Day Hospital and manageable by their families, but no means for transporting the patients between home and the hospital could be arranged; 3 (1 with chronic brain syndrome, 1 with schizoaffective psychosis and 1 with psychotic depression) were judged to be treatable in the Day Hospital, but this was not accepted by their families because of their refusal to care for the patients evenings and weekends; 4 (2 with acute brain syndromes, 1 brought by the police for molesting children, and 1 in a catatonic stupor) were not accepted because of the nature of the symptoms. The remaining 5 were admitted prior to the requirement of a report on all patients seen in the Admitting Room, and data are therefore inadequate. Thus, 23.6 per cent of patients requiring psychiatric hospitalization could not be admitted to or treated in the Day Hospital. It is the writers' opinion that this number will tend to remain constant for the larger study in progress.

(2) Of the 55 patients treated in the Day Hospital, 19 were males and 36 females; 17 required 1 or more days on the Inpatient service at Jacobi Hospital. Eleven of the 17 were transferred to the Inpatient service for the first night or two of hospitalization; 6 were transferred at a later date. Of the 17, six were transferred because the severity of their symptoms required 24 hour care. Of these, two were returned to the Day Hospital after 3 and 5 days respectively, and completed treatment there; the other 4 patients were transferred to state hospitals. Of the 17, ten were transferred by their families, or by the Day Hospital Director because of adamant family refusal to care for the patient evenings or weekends. In three instances, the family permitted the return of the patient to the Day Hospital within a week; one patient showed a remarkably rapid recovery on the Inpatient Service and was discharged home after a few days; the remainder completed treatment in state hospitals. Thus, in addition to the 23.6 per cent of all admitted patients who did not receive any treatment in the Day Hospital, 23.6 per cent required treatment for some time on the Inpatient Service; 16.7 per cent of these patients remained on the Inpatient Service or were transferred to state hospitals, and 6.9 per cent returned to the Day Hospital and completed treatment there. It is the opinion of the present writers that these figures will be substantially reduced for the patients currently being studied; these data reflect the earliest period of the Day Hospital service after it was geographically removed from the Jacobi Hospital, during which time considerable construction

was in progress, and treatment was conducted by residents newly assigned to the Day Hospital unit.

(3) Of the 72 admitted patients designated for Day Hospital treatment, 38, or 52.8 per cent were treated entirely within the Day Hospital. Diagnoses, and duration of Day Hospital treatment are listed in table I.

TABLE 1

DURATION OF HOSPITALIZATION FOR 38 PATIENTS TREATED ENTIRELY IN THE DAY HOSPITAL

Diagnosis	Less Than One Week	One To Three Weeks	Four To Six Weeks	Seven To Ten Weeks	Eleven To Twelve Weeks	Total
Chronic Brain Syndrome	0	0	0	1	0	1
Involutional Psychotic Reaction	2	0	0	1	1	4
Psychotic Depressive Reaction	0	0	0	4	2	6
Schizophrenic Reaction, Catatonic Type	0	0	0	1	0	1
Schizophrenic Reaction, Paranoid type	1	1	2	4	2	10
Schizophrenic Reaction, Other	3	0	0	0	0	3
Hysterical Psychosis	0	0	0	1	0	1
Depressive Reaction	1	0	2	0	0	3
Character Disorder	0	0	2	5	0	7
Alcoholism	2	0	0	0	0	2
TOTAL	9	1	6	17	5	38

The "less than one week patients" (12.5 per cent of the total sample) pose a special problem. None left on the advice of an individual doctor; however, only 1 of these has sought alternative hospitalization within a month after discharge. It is of interest to note that an independent study revealed that 10 per cent of all inpatients are discharged home within one week of hospitalization.

A number of clinical impressions are emerging from the Day Hospital experience which will require careful study for ultimate confirmation:

(1) Only 1 of 10 patients with chronic brain syndrome was treated on the Day Hospital, and this one patient required a brief stay on the medical ward. It is our feeling that at the present, by the time a family brings an aged person to a psychiatric hospital, the severity of the organicity presents extreme home management, travel, and medical problems, and the expectation of the family is that the psychotic person will be committed. Where hospital care is more readily sought by families early in this illness process, the Day Hospital has proved extremely useful in the treatment of patients with chronic organic brain syndromes.[16]

(2) In all patients with psychotic depression, there is initial concern and resistance on the part of the family to the treatment of the patient on the Day Hospital. This is appreciably more marked in the case of patients with involutional depressive psychoses, where the spouse is the critical family member involved, than in the depressive psychoses of older patients living with their children.

(3) We are particularly impressed with the outcome of day hospitalization in the case of patients diagnosed as having paranoid schizophrenia. Of the 13 such patients admitted and designated as Day Hospital patients, 10 were treated entirely within the Day Hospital. Day hospitalization appears to be not only feasible as a therapy modality but perhaps is even to be preferred to traditional inpatient hospitalization. Resistance to a group identification is usually evident during the first week, which is often stormy and is marked by lateness, absences, and threats of leaving. By the second week most paranoid schizophrenics appear to become the most conscientious and enthusiastic Day Hospital patients. The apparent "good results" with this diagnostic category is especially significant, since 85 per cent of all patients coming to the Jacobi Hospital Admitting Room with the diagnosis of paranoid schizophrenia are normally hospitalized on an inpatient service.

(4) Among patients whose initial symptoms include marked agitation or aggressive behavior, several problems are likely to be encountered in day hospital treatment. Families require considerable support in order to retain the patients at home; we have observed that with some frequency, the families of such patients seem particularly likely to remove the patient from the Day Hospital precisely at the time there is evidence of some significant improvement, and it may be that the tacit family attitude of extrusion which the patient senses to begin with accounts for the symptoms of agitation and aggression. In addition, other patients appear to have the geratest difficulty in accepting such patients, particularly if any overt sexual elements are present in the initial symptom picture. The challenge to a Day Hospital posed by such patients is then both to support the family, and to support the other Day Hospital patients. That we are some distance from a solution is reflected in the fact that of 18 acutely agitated schizophrenic patients other than paranoid schizophrenics, only 4 were treated entirely

in the Day Hospital and 3 others completed treatment in the Day Hospital after a brief stay in the inpatient service.

(5) As has been reported by other day hospitals, patients with severe neuroses and with character disorders are readily treatable in a day hospital setting.

The present structure of the Day Hospital does not permit conclusions concerning the relative efficacy of this modality for the treatment of psychiatric patients in contrast with traditional hospitalization; such a study is planned to follow upon the present effort to determine the extent to which the day hospital can be expected to provide treatment for acutely psychotic patients in a community. Certainly from the veiwpoint of the theoretic perspective of the writers—i.e., that knowledge of family dynamics and of community group life, added to the knowledge of the intrapsychic dynamics of the patient, significantly enlarges knowledge concerning the processes of mental illness and recovery—the Day Hospital is an ideal modality for the study, diagnosis and treatment of psychotic patients.

REFERENCES

1. ACKERMAN, NATHAN: The Psychodynamics of Family Life. New York, Basic Books, 1958.
2. BIERER, JOSHUA: The Day Hospital, London, H. K. Lewis & Co., Ltd., 1951.
3. CAMERON, D. EWEN: The Day Hospital, Mod. Hosp. 69:3, 1947.
4. CARMICHAEL, DONALD M.: A Psychiatric Day Hospital for Convalescent Patients, Ment. Hosps. 11:7, 1960.
5. CAUDILL, WILLIAM: Psychiatric Hospital as a Small Society, Cambridge, Mass., Harvard Univ. Press, 1958.
6. COLEMAN, M. DONALD, AND ZWERLING, I.: The Psychiatric Emergency Clinic: A Flexible Way of Meeting Community Mental Needs. Am. J. Psych. 115:981, 1959.
7. CRAFT, MICHAEL: Psychiatric Day Hospitals, Am. J. Psych. 116:251, 1959.
8. Expert Committee on Mental Health: WHO, Tech. Report #73, 1953.
9. FARNDALE, JAMES: The Day Hospital Movement in Great Britain, Pergamon Press, 1961.
10. GOFFMAN, ERVING: Characteristics of Total Institutions; Symposium in Preventive and Social Psychiatry, Walter Reed Army Institute of Research, Washington, D.C., 1957.
11. GOSHEN, CHARLES R.: New Concepts of Psychiatric Care with Special Reference to the Day Hospital. Am. J. Psych. 115:808, 1959.
12. HARRIS, ARTHUR: Day Hospitals and Night Hospitals in Psychiatry, The Lancet. 729, 1957.
13. KRIS, ELSE B.: Intensive Short-Term Therapy in a Day Care Facility for Control of Recurrent Psychotic Symptoms. Am. J. Psych. 115:1027, 1959.
14. STANTON, A. H. AND SCHWARTZ, M. S.: The Mental Hospital, New York, Basic Books, 1954.
15. STEINMAN, LEON A., AND HUNT, ROBERT C.: A Day Care Center in a State Hospital, Am. J. Psych. 117:112, 1961.
16. WINICK, CHARLES: Psychiatric Day Hospitals: A Survey, J. Social Issues, 8, 1960.

Fountain House: A Psychiatric Rehabilitation Program

by SAUL H. FISHER, M.D. AND JOHN H. BEARD, M.S.W.

A MONG THE NUMEROUS problems besetting modern psychiatry, one of the most pressing is that of the discharged mental hospital patient: his management and his treatment. This has always been a problem, but it has become more of one since the introduction of ataractic and antidepressant drugs, as well as intensified hospital care of the patient, for these have led to an increased rate of discharge, hence an increase in the number of post hospital patients in our population.[1]

The problem is two pronged: first, to prevent relapse and rehospitalization; second, to assist in the rehabilitation of the patient so that he can function in a reasonably constructive way in society. To achieve these goals, a variety of facilities and programs have developed, including day hospitals, night hospitals, after-care clinics, sheltered workshops, half way houses, hostels, social clubs, vocational programs, etc.[2] The purpose of this communication is to describe one such facility and program called Fountain House.

Fountain House, started officially in 1948, although it was preceded by a self help group organized in 1945 by patients discharged from Rockland State Hospital, a group called WANA—We Are Not Alone. Originally both WANA and Fountain House were social groups, with no defined program, in which patients supported one another, or were helped by a group of humanitarian individuals under the guidance of a social worker. In 1955, with a change of administration and a re-evaluation of program, Fountain House changed and evolved, so that today its program is professionally directed[3, 4] and is concerned not only with social and vocational rehabilitation, but training and research as well.

Fountain House, a four story brick building on the west side of Manhattan, possesses a courtyard and a running fountain from which the name is derived. Its facilities include a modern kitchen, dining room, a main lounge, a library, a T.V. room, a repair shop, and several other rooms for various group activities. Fountain House is a voluntary, non-fee charging agency, governed by a 38 member Board of Directors. The 1960 budget of $200,000 was derived from private foundations, the federal government, donations of Board members, the New York City Community Mental Health Board, benefit performances and parties, and individual contributions.

The members (ex-patients) come from middle and lower socio-economic groups. About half have completed high school. Eighty percent are diagnosed schizophrenia, 13 percent have other psychoses, while seven percent are nonpsychotic. Active membership numbers about 550. Two out of every three members have had more than one psychiatric hospitalization. Men outnumber women three to two. Two-thirds of the membership are in their twenties and thirties. Only one out of twenty is currently married.

Members are referred to Fountain House by psychiatric hospitals (24 percent), after-care clinics (19 percent), friends (16 percent), other agencies (15 percent). The remaining referrals (26 percent) were attributed to publicity, family, and professionals not in agencies. Fountain House in turn uses the services of the New York State After-care Clinics, the Division of Vocational Rehabilitation, the special placement section of the State Employment Service, and other community resources.

Most patients (about 75 a month) who apply are accepted, with the exception of those who have a long history of chronic alcoholism, narcotic addiction, overt homosexuality, convulsive disorders, severe physical handicaps, or aggressive behavior which precludes functioning in a group setting. Only two percent of the applicants fall in those categories. Most come to Fountain House within six months of their release. About 12 percent come while still hospitalized and on short term leave.

The full-time staff consists of eight social workers, a vocational counselor, and a sociologist engaged in research. A psychiatrist serves as part-time consultant, and there are about 100 active volunteers who have undergone a course of orientation and training prior to program assignment. Finally, there are four lay employees (housekeeper, etc.), and five administrative-clerical workers. The program may be divided into various categories:

(1) *Field Group Program*

A field group consists of 20 to 25 members, six or eight volunteers, and a staff worker. The members represent varying levels of community adjustment. Some are still hospitalized, others are successfully employed and making a good community adjustment, and a few are homebound. The primary function of the group is to enable the individual patient, regardless of level of adjustment, successfully to achieve membership in a small social unit so that the process of isolation and rejection is significantly reversed.

The field group engages in a wide variety of activities. Personal contact with homebound and hospitalized members is regularly maintained. Emphasis is placed on helping the marginally adjusted patient to become active in the Fountain House Day program so that essential work habits and motivation for productive work can be reinstituted. Leadership roles are available for members who have been successful in achieving primary rehabilitative goals. Regular group meetings are held in community facilities at which time the current life situation of each member is discussed. Approval and recognition are given to successful efforts or accomplishments. Concern for a member's current difficulties is expressed and a plan of assistance formulated. The cohesive quality of the group provides a non-threatening atmosphere which makes it possible for even the most withdrawn member to have an accepted role in the group. The atmosphere is a confident and optimistic one, fortified by the achievement by successful members of realistic personal goals.

(2) *The Day Program*

The first objective of the Fountain House Day program is to attract into the club house during the day men and women who are making only a marginal adjustment in the community. Initially the involvement is on a passive level: sitting, reading, talking, eating, watching television. Members at this stage are not employed and tend to be socially isolated. Their initial passivity occurs in an atmosphere in which many productive activities are proceeding. Members, volunteers, and staff are mutually engaged in the various operations of the day program, including the operation of the office, the housekeeping and maintenance of the center, and the preparation and serving of food. The newcomer, over a period of time, slowly becomes involved in these activities at his own pace, on the basis of the motivation stimulated by the setting. The term "assignment" would not adequately describe the process through which members take on responsible duties in the day program. Some members are attracted to the program and ask to be included. Sometimes professional workers will set up situations designed to attract a member. In some instances a direct assignment is made. What the member does is not significant, rather the fact that he expresses a desire to engage in constructive activities, cooperating with others, is important.

The day at Fountain House begins at 8:45 A.M. with the serving of

breakfast to about 35 members. Most of these and some 30 others who
arrive later are regularly involved in the day program. Members work at
planning the luncheon menu, shopping for food, setting tables, cooking,
serving, clearing the tables, and dish washing. Mid-afternoon and evening
refreshments also are served. Members work, too, at housekeeping and
clerical tasks.

(3) *Transitional Employment Program*

One out of three Fountain House members get jobs on their own, or
through public and private employment agencies. Some members are
referred for vocational training through the State Department of Vocational Rehabilitation. Others, who have had a lengthy hospitalization or
long periods in the community during which time they were not self-
supporting, come into the Fountain House day program. Experience has
shown that after three to nine months in the day program, many members
can go on to jobs in the community. Some, however, after doing well in
the day program, are still unable to move on to regular jobs. For this
group, a transitional employment program was developed by involving
commerce and industry in the rehabilitation process. This is in contrast to
the sheltered workshop concept for convalescent patients.

To date, twelve business firms have been enlisted in this program
through individual effort on the part of the staff. These include a large
women's clothing department store, a Wall Street brokerage firm, a
commercial printer, and a small duplicating (mimeo) service. Arrangements are made for a staff worker to do each job before placement of a
member. This permits the staff worker to determine the standards
necessary on the job, to get to know other employees and gain their
cooperation, to learn the interpersonal problems which might arise, and
thus be able to deal more realistically and effectively with the member
when he starts on the job. Arrangements are made for a member to work
as little as one hour a day at the going salary rate. During periods of stress,
the staff worker is permitted to work alongside the member. Placement is
limited to three to four months duration. In this way the same job can be
used again for a new member.

Successful completion of the job is ego building. But equally important,
from a practical point of view, is the fact that the member can go out into
the normal labor market with an absolute essential: a good reference from
a recent employer. In its small way, this program contributes to the
lowering of the resistance of employers to hiring previously hospitalized
people.

(4) *Social Recreational Program*

Informal recreational activities are an integral part of the Fountain House day program: visits to museums, sport events, television shows, etc. The organized program is largely an evening and weekend activity. Included are volunteer-directed classes in such varied activities as group singing, social and folk dancing, bridge, typing, sewing, dramatics, photography, languages, etc. Visiting artists and lecturers are regular features on the program.

(5) *Housing Program*

Since Fountain House is not a residential center, and since some members have no families or cannot live with their families, Fountain House has rented a number of low cost apartments which are available to members for temporary residence, and are supervised by one of the professional workers. This was done instead of establishing a hostel because it provides a more realistic setting in the community.

(6) *Individual Therapy*

While Fountain House is not primarily intended for this, problems arise which demand attention, often of an emergency nature. The psychiatric consultant is called in on many of these problems, and perhaps a few remarks about them would be of interest.

(a) *Hostile-aggressive Behavior.* It has been a source of wonder that so few cases of aggressive acting-out and violence have occurred. The physical plant of Fountain House is not large, and on occasion the house is quite crowded, with members standing or sitting on the stairs, and there are many reasons or occasions for irritation or frustration; yet these rarely erupt into open anger or violence. Where this has occurred, it usually has been provoked by a member who has been drinking before coming to the house.

One of the members, a non alcoholic, engaged in several violent outbursts, all of them directed at the head of Fountain House. In each episode he would make an unreasonable demand for action or time, then explode and threaten to destroy the house or its director. In each of these episodes the psychiatric consultant was called and he arranged to see the member that very day. Several sessions of psychotherapy in addition to chlorpromazine were effective in ameliorating the crisis and permitting the member to continue his job.

Of crucial importance in these emergencies is the immediate availability of the consultant. By immediate is meant contact by phone, being permitted to sit in the psychiatrist's waiting room and seen between hours until time is available to the member. The immediate availability of the psychiatrist, and for that matter all of the professional workers at Fountain House, is facilitated by 24 hour telephone service.

(b) *Depression and Suicide.* Discharge from a psychiatric hospital is by no means based on "cure", and the road back to a reasonably normal life for the ex-mental hospital patient is not an easy one. The obstacles, the failures, the frustrations, the rejections, both internal and external, real and imagined, lead to frequent depressions. Most of these are managed by a dedicated and often perceptive professional staff, as well as by the existence of a supportive social structure and program such as is offered by Fountain House. The more severe and persistent depressions are seen by the psychiatric consultant and are dealt with by psychotherapy and anti depressive drugs. Electro shock therapy has never been necessary in our members while they were still part of the program.

It might be expected that in a population so basically ill, suicidal attempts, whether successful or unsuccessful, would be a frequent, or at least a not uncommon, problem. The fact is, that since 1955, and having had several thousand members in our program, suicide as a problem has been virtually nonexistent. We have no record of any members dying of suicide. It may be that they have occurred and we have not heard of it, but this is unlikely. Families and friends notify us of deaths by illness or accident, of anything unusual occurring, yet we have never heard of suicide. If a member fails to show up, one of our staff is assigned to seek out the reason.

There have been a few suicidal attempts since 1955, but none of these has been of a serious nature. Usually it represents an attempt to get to sleep, or a gesture to arouse the concern of the staff. For example, one patient took thirty 10 mg. Librium capsules; another took six Miltown tablets. We have no examples of more serious attempts, as by gas or hanging. The total number of such attempts since 1955 amount to about one-half dozen.

It is not uncommon, however, for members to express death wishes. These are always taken seriously by other members and the staff who will spend time with the depressed or desperate member, listen to him, encourage him, etc. It is rare, as has been emphasized, for such problems to reach a point of action either for the patient or for the psychiatric consultant.

This surprising rarity of suicide as a problem in a psychiatric rehabilitation center is similar to the rarity of suicide among the severely physically disabled in a physical rehabilitation center.[5] Sociologic studies have indicated a correlation between incidence of suicide and social disintegration and isolation. It may be that a rehabilitation setting, representing an organized and positive social structure, provides even the most deprived and desperate patient with a feeling that someone really cares for him. This is a potent antidote to the isolation which apparently is a predisposing factor in suicide. In addition, the availability of emergency service may serve a preventive function in forestalling the acting out of suicidal impulses.

(c) *Withdrawal and Negativism.* On occasion a patient discharged from the hospital goes home and regresses immediately, much to the distress of the family. He stays in bed all morning or all day, refusing to do anything. This problem is of particular importance to Fountain House because it is antithetical to rehabilitation. If Mohammed won't come to the mountain, then the mountain goes to Mohammed. Either a professional worker or an active member or group of members visit the recalcitrant patient and are often successful in getting the member to at least visit the house. Force and firmness never seem to work, but merely showing that much interest in going to the patient's home, in sitting there for hours, often in silence, seems to work far better.

(d) *Acute Psychotic Episodes.* As would be expected, some patients experience relapses, developing hallucinations, paranoid delusions, bizarre behavior and dress, withdrawal, change in sleep patterns, mounting tension, etc., often representing a complex of symptoms which led to their previous hospitalizations. All such patients are seen by the psychiatric consultant. In most cases it is possible to uncover an external stress situation which can be altered, and in combination with ataractic drugs and psychotherapy, the process can be reversed. It is often surprising how rapidly this can be effected. It is our conviction that the ready availability of the facts in the situation, provided by the professional worker who has become part of the life of the member, as well as the absence of fear of the psychiatrist on the part of the member, contribute to this quick and dramatic result. The psychiatrist can get to the heart of the matter without groping, and the member knows that the psychiatrist, part of the Fountain House team, is motivated toward keeping him out of the hospital if it is humanly and medically possible.

(e) *Rehospitalization.* Not all such episodes can be reversed, of course, and rehospitalization becomes indicated. While some may see this as a failure, we at Fountain House do not.[7] Given the nature of the problems and the present state of the art, it is inevitable that this be so. What is important, however, is that *this* hospitalization is different from others. In most instances the patient enters voluntarily. His social worker usually will be with him on readmission. The psychiatric consultant will visit him at the disposition center (Bellevue), and Fountain House workers and members will visit him and write to him at the State hospital. He is never rejected by Fountain House, and when he is discharged again, he resumes his program. The entire experience is not nearly as traumatic as the previous ones have been, and it is seen as an episode which has reasons and from which the patient and staff try to learn. It is not unlike a diabetic or cardiac who, because of infection or other undue stress, must go back to the hospital until his equilibrium is re-established.

REFERENCES

1. GREENBLATT, M., AND SIMON, B.: Rehabilitation of the Mentally Ill. Publication No. 58, American Association for the Advancement of Science, Washington, D. C. 1959.
2. SCHWARTZ, C. G.: Rehabilitation of Mental Hospital Patients. Public Health Monograph No. 17, U. S. Dept. of Health, Education and Welfare. Superintendent of Documents, U. S. Gov't. Printing Office, Washington 25, D. C.
3. FISHER, S. H., BEARD, J. H., AND GOERTZEL, V.: Rehabilitation of the mental hospital patient: the Fountain House program. Int. Journ. Soc. Psychiat. 4:295-298, 1960.
4. GOERTZEL, V., BEARD, J. H., AND PILNICK, S.: Fountain House Foundation: case study of an expatient club. J. Soc. Iss. 16:54-61, 1960.
5. RUSK, H.: Rehabilitation Medicine, The C. V. Mosby Co., St. Louis, 1958, pp. 226-227.
6. SAINSBURY, P.: Suicide in London. Maudsley Monograph No. 1, New York, Basic Books, Inc., 1956.
7. FISHER, S. H.: The recovered patient returns to the community. Ment. Hyg. 42:463-473, 1958.

Psychotherapy in the Hospital (1740 -1840)

by ERIC T. CARLSON, M.D. AND NORMAN DAIN, PH.D.

PSYCHIATRY EMERGED as a medical specialty in the late eighteenth century. Its source was the Enlightenment, an era which regarded man as a component part of the entire physical universe and which optimistically believed that, by means of reason and scientific procedure, man could immeasurably improve both his understanding and his existence. This optimism extended to mental illness: the Enlightenment considered mental illness the result of natural causes and, as such, a condition which could eventually be cured if these causes could be determined. In the meantime, it felt, the mental patient should be treated as an unfortunate fellow creature deserving of humanitarian concern and care.

Between 1740 and 1840, the severely ill psychiatric patient submitted to a variety of therapies, each inspired by some contemporary physiological theory of the cause of mental illness. At first pharmaceutical therapy predominated, but, although it never entirely disappeared, its use decreased as various nonmedical methods of treatment emerged. There was a variety of names for these nonmedical methods, but the one most often used was "moral treatment," a term made popular by Philippe Pinel in his 1801 treatise on mental illness.[1] This phrase, in which "moral" meant "psychological," emphasized the fact that nonmedical procedures were not designed out of simple benevolence towards all humanity, but were employed for their undeniable therapeutic effectiveness.

Perhaps the major philosophical influence upon early nineteenth century medical psychology was associationism, a product of the psychological concepts of Locke and Condillac. In this epoch psychiatry consid-

---

*An occasional historical paper will be included in this series for the purpose of putting our current methods of psychiatric therapy in proper perspective.—Ed.

ered insanity entirely a disorder of the intellect. Consequently it valued as potentially useful in therapy a theory like associationism, which explained intellectual functioning and non-functioning in psychological terms. According to associationism, human thought developed from repeated primary sense perceptions which were gradually brought together and synthesized in patterns. Since insanity was a disorder of the higher intellectual levels of the mind, sanity might be reestablished by means of psychological rebuilding through basic sense perceptions. Reil (1803) was one of the first to attempt to apply this theory in therapy; he instructed his patients to describe various fundamental experiences of touch, smell, and hearing "to reeducate the imagination of the patient and his relationship to reality."[2]

A principal therapeutic goal of associationally-oriented nineteenth century psychiatry was the elimination of associations which contributed to the patient's illness. Hospitalization was thus essential for the severely ill person, and almost all physicians recommended it, despite the reputation some hospitals had for cruelty and brutality. Because they might reawaken unpleasant memories and emotions the hospital restricted and controlled visits from relatives and friends.

Once sheltered within the hospital the patient found himself classified and separated according to his sex and degree and type of illness. Such an arrangement made possible more efficient treatment and also provided the support of the group for each of its members. As his condition improved the patient progressed to new groups and received more privileges, and this progression contributed an added incentive to recover. The patient felt accepted as a fellow human being, albeit ill, in a setting where the staff cared about him and understood him. This situation in itself stimulated hope, an emotion recognized as therapeutically useful early in the nineteenth century, and the sight of other patients in a convalescent state reinforced this hope.

Influenced by association psychology, hospital physicians stressed the need to divert the patient from his painful thoughts and break up his ill associations. Harper recommended in 1789 that the doctor avoid all mention of ideas pertaining to the original cause of the patient's illness, and substitute instead appropriate new ideas.[3] He also stated that the physician should refuse to indulge the patient's disturbed whims and should attempt to break up his undesirable habit patterns, but he did not give any directions about how best to accomplish this retraining.

In order to divert the patient's attention the hospital also established a routine similar to that of the modern psychiatric hospital in its number of activities. The amusements available to the nineteenth century mental patient ranged from chess to horseback riding, and rivaled in number and variety the best recreational programs of today. The nineteenth century counterpart of modern occupational therapy was more limited in scope; most common were farming, for men, and household duties, for women. Religious programs varied from hospital to hospital, and educational instruction as therapy appeared only towards the 1840's.

A major element of nineteenth century psychiatric hospital treatment was the relationship between the physician and his patient. In this era learning self control was considered the first step towards cure, if not synonymous with it, and the physician was responsible for teaching the patient this control over his unacceptable thoughts and behavior. He tried to do so by gaining ascendancy over him, by rewarding or punishing him, and by utilizing his emotions.[4]

At first the physician was conceived of as an active agent working upon an essentially passive subject. This attitude is especially apparent in the discussions about how to achieve ascendancy over a patient. At first a certain brutality was evident in the methods of gaining this ascendancy— William Cullen (1790) sanctioned the use of blows provided the patient understood their purpose—but these methods soon gave way to milder techniques.

A classic example of this milder but still forceful techinque is the approach used in the 1790's by Pargeter, an advocate of the idea that all treatment would be ineffective unless the physician gained complete supremacy in his first encounter with the patient.[5] Suddenly flinging open the door of a patient's room, he would burst inside, catch the patient's eye, and thereby stare him down; he frequently achieved complete dominance without uttering a word. Pargeter asserted this method had never failed for him, but pointed out that as it might not always work the physician should first obtain a complete case history. Having obtained dominance Pargeter perpetuated it by treating the patient kindly and by trying to gain his confidence. He stressed the fact that too severe coercion would be both cruel and misguided, arousing violent reactions in the patients and thereby making them less manageable.

Other advocates of a less authoritarian approach included Monro (1758),[6] Daquin (1791),[7] Chiarugi (1793),[8] and Pinel (1801). These men held that firmness should be tempered with kindness and that control was possible without abuse. Pinel, for instance, believed in using coercion when necessary, but preferred the psychological effect of a show of force to its actual application.

After 1800 physicians began to suggest that it was possible to achieve ascendancy without hurting or frightening the patient. In 1806 Cox stated that firmness and tenderness should be the rule, although he acknowledged that threats would influence some patients.[9] He asserted also that kindness bred confidence, and that by releasing a patient from mechanical restraint the doctor might well win his devotion. In the same year Trotter pointed out that the patient needed to feel the physician's trust in him.[10] In 1809, moreover, Haslam voiced his doubts about the actual effectiveness of the "penetrating eye," remarking that he had yet to see anyone willing to test this technique on a violent maniac.[11] He maintained that the physician could more readily achieve ascendancy over his patients by treating them with sympathy and understanding, since patients tended to respect those who understood their illness. Although on occasion he permitted the use of force or coercion, especially in setting an example for other patients, he asserted that one should never threaten a patient beforehand, but act immediately.

Later years saw a recognition of the need for more active participation in therapy by the patient, and a consequent shift in the doctor-patient relationship to one which was based on friendship and which stressed the therapeutic value of tact. Chiarugi (1793) and Heinroth (1818)[12] both mentioned the usefulness of tact, and Burrows (1828)[13] especially commended its use. In 1838 Ellis argued that women were more successful than men in treating mental patients because they were more generously endowed with this trait.[14]

Another method of teaching the patient self control was the use of rewards and punishments. In 1795 Ferriar suggested setting aside a special room exclusively for those patients who had learned to behave acceptably.[15] A few years later Haslam suggested that punishing the rational but uncooperative patient by denying him privileges might induce him to control his behavior. Haslam stated that the punishments should be immediate and public because the patient would then connect the punishment with the offense and, being awed by the presence of onlookers, would give in more readily. Haslam considered such coercion indispensable, since self control was essential to recovery and since fear of punishment would deter both the rational and irrational person.

The punitive technique was widely used. The Friends' Asylum in Philadelphia used it in the 1820's; there a patient could lose his privileges if he failed to control himself, but would immediately receive them again as soon as he showed regret for his misdemeanors and promised to do better.[16] In 1833 Allen emphasized the effectiveness of shaming a patient and thereby motivating him to correct himself.[17] He acknowledged that this procedure might lead the patients to hide their aberrations, but felt that, so long as the doctor fully understood their illness, such deceptions would not be harmful. In 1835 Prichard advanced the idea that an individual other than the physician should be the punitive agent, so the physician himself could remain a protective figure, kind and sympathetic.[18]

Physicians also attempted to utilize their patients' emotions in order to teach them self control. At times the therapist himself would arouse certain emotions to induce the patient to behave. In 1813, for example, Samuel Tuke cited the effectiveness of mild fear, as in the training of children; he preferred, however, the encouragement of such feelings as hope and self esteem.[19]

Psychiatrists also attempted to use emotions in therapy in another way: by counteracting one emotion with another, a technique known as the use of "contrary passions." Battie illustrated this method in 1758, when he pointed out that the physician might use fear to combat anger, and joy to dominate sorrow.[20] Battie insisted, however, that only the physician was qualified to order this treatment, since the results were unpredictable. In 1789 Harper warned against attempting to check the patient's violent passions suddenly, recommending instead gradually replacing them with other, more pleasant emotions. He suggested that the doctor should arrange amusements for the grief-stricken or depressed patient and should trust and console the jealous one. Pinel wanted pleasant surroundings and a cheerful atmosphere for his melancholic patients, and Georget, Pinel's pupil, thought that the physician should try to impart courage to this type of patient.[21] In later years there was a definite shift to the use of milder emotions; Allen stated that if one must use fear one should do so only by denying the patient sympathy, and Cox advocated never using fear at all.

The medical writers before 1800 were skeptical about the therapeutic value of appeals to the insane patient's reason. Cullen considered such an approach generally useless in cases of hypochondriasis, Perfect felt the same regarding treatment of religious melancholy,[22] and all physicians united in maintaining the futility of reasoning or arguing with a patient about his delusions and hallucinations. Of the various alternative methods which might serve to banish such symptoms, one of the most popular was a form of suggestive trickery called "pious frauds" by Cullen and "strategems" by Pinel. An example of this technique is the case of a Frenchman who firmly believed that he was under suspicion for having criticized the Revolution. Pinel had him brought before a group of men masquerading as a board of inquiry, and after questioning the patient closely the "board" pronounced him exonerated. With the burden of his guilt lifted, the patient soon regained his sanity. Pinel recognized, however, that there were certain risks involved in using this technique—a complete relapse followed this initially-successful strategem when the patient learned it was a hoax.

Discussion about how to conduct the doctor-patient transactions—a subject of great importance in the history of psychotherapy—appears infrequently and generally later in the nineteenth century psychiatric literature. Physicians apparently did not codify and publish their conclusions about this relationship, probably because they believed, like Haslam, that this skill could not be taught and must therefore perish with the individual practitioner. They undoubtedly thought much about this aspect of therapy, however, and there is enough literature available to provide a basic understanding of their precepts.

Around 1790 medical writers began to agree that the physician should, by spending as much time as possible with them, come to know his patients intimately and individually. In 1792 Hahnemann, for example, devoted two weeks to studying a patient before attempting treatment.[23] Several outstanding physicians— Chiarugi, Pinel, Cox and Heinroth—emphasized the importance of complete case histories. Heinroth insisted that therapy should be adapted to the individual patient, since psychopathology varied with age, sex, and temperament.

Physicians after 1790 recognized the usefulness in treatment of conversation with the doctor. Ferriar (1795) and Allen (1838) both cited cases in which the patient recovered after reflecting on ideas implanted by the physician's remarks, and in 1818 Hallaran referred to the importance of "the business of conversation,"[24] but unfortunately the early physicians published few specific rules about how to conduct such therapy through conversation. In 1809 Haslam suggested that in order to learn more about the patient the doctor should not interrupt him too often, and most doctors agreed that one should avoid irritating the patient or bringing up painful ideas; for example, Burrows (1828) recommended that the physician refrain from pointing out to the patient his defects in memory or speech.

After 1830 medical writers devoted more space to the techniques of conversational therapy. Conolly (1830) asserted that the doctor's main purpose was to instruct, amuse, soothe, converse with, and advise his patients.[25] Allen (1833), who wrote more extensively than most physicians on what he called "intellectual therapy," saw his goal as one of making "truth visible" to the insane, a purpose previously mentioned by Chiarugi and Reil. Allen maintained that with intelligence and insight the doctor could trace his patient's peculiarities to their origin.

The development in the early nineteenth century of phrenological theory, which emphasized the study of the individual personality, introduced another concept into psychotherapy. In 1825 Gall asserted that close attention to a patient's actions and his remarks about his past life could provide the physician with valuable insight into the patient's illness.[26] Six years later Combe discussed phrenology's relevance to psychiatric treatment, stating that the phrenologist–physician should first achieve a knowledge of human nature in general and then use phrenology to understand the personality of the individual patient.[27] This approach introduced a type of psychiatric analysis, in which the doctor tried to help the patient understand that he had become ill because some of his motivations and faculties (associated in theory with specific areas of the brain) were over- or underdeveloped. With the aid of his physician the patient was to repress the overactive faculties and at the same time strengthen the weaker ones, so that his personality would come back into balance and he would recover his health.[28]

Like this interest in the patient's fundamental personality structure, recognition of the importance of the physician's own personality was a relatively late development. There were numerous statements about how he should behave towards his patients: he should be intelligent, courageous, firm but kind, understanding, hopeful, tender, cheerful, and upright. Haslam, however, who admitted that he lacked the lightning in his eye, the thunder in his voice, and the majestic bearing that some considered essential to the ideal psychiatrist, was one of the few to point out the inevitability of personality variations between psychiatrists, and the relevance of such variations to treatment.

Physicians generally acknowledged that therapeutic acumen was an art. Both Cox and Haslam emphasized that the physician must learn to remain calm and never show agitation; unless he did so he could not hope to win his patients' confidence and respect. Trotter observed that the young physician needed extensive knowledge of human nature and man's behavior before he could hope to achieve such self-control. Burrows believed that tact was the pivotal factor in the doctor-patient relationship, and that it was an intuitive art which could never be taught, although it might be elicited by chance and then developed by experience. Burrows also stressed the need for delicacy and intelligence in all therapeutic attempts.

Allen seems to be the only doctor of this period to recognize and discuss the physician's own reaction to his patients. He cited a case of a woman who so exhausted him emotionally that he himself became depressed and was forced to transfer her to the care of his wife. This woman also overwhelmed his wife at times, so that Mrs. Allen was compelled to threaten her with separation and transfer unless the patient stopped her difficult and demanding behavior.

In this century between 1740 and 1840 we can discern, therefore, a trend towards increasingly complex but more explicit psychotherapeutic methods which are meaningful to the psychotherapy we practice today.

REFERENCES

1. PINEL, P.: Traité Médicophilosophique sur L'Aliénation Mentale, Paris, Richard, Caille and Ravier, 1801.

2. HARMS, E. J.: Modern psychotherapy—150 years ago. J. Ment. Sci., 103:804-809 (Oct.), 1957.

3. HARPER, A.: A Treatise on the Real Cause and Cure of Insanity, London, C. Stalker and J. Walter, 1789.

4. CARLSON, E. T., AND McFADDEN, R. B.: Dr. William Cullen on Mania. Am. J. Psychiat. 117:463-465 (Nov.), 1960.

5. PARGETER, W.: Observations on Maniacal Disorders, Reading, The Author, 1792.

6. MONRO, J.: Remarks on Dr. Battie's Treatise on Madness, London, John Clarke, 1758.

7. DAQUIN, J.: La Philosophie de la Folie, Chambéry, Gorrin, 1791.

8. MORA, G.: Vincenzo Chiarugi (1759-1820)—his contribution to psychiatry. Bull. Isaac Ray Med. Library, 2:50-104 (April), 1954.

9. COX, J. M.: Practical Observations on Insanity. Philadelphia, Thomas Dobson, 1811. 2nd ed.

10. TROTTER, T.: A View of the Nervous Temperament. London, Longman, Hurst, Rees and Orme, 1807. 2nd ed.

11. HASLAM, J.: Observations on Madness and Melancholy. London, J. Callow and G. Hayden, 1809. 2nd ed.

12. HARMS, E.: An attempt to formulate a system of psychotherapy in 1818. Am. J. Psychotherapy 13:269-282 (April), 1959.

13. BURROWS, G. M.: Commentaries on the Causes, Forms, Symptoms, and Treatment, Moral and Medical, of Insanity. London, Thomas and George Underwood, 1828.

14. ELLIS, W. C.: A Treatise on the Nature, Symptoms, Causes, and Treatment of Insanity. London, Samuel Holdsworth, 1838.

15. FERRIAR, J.: Medical Histories and Reflections, London, Cadell and Davies, 1795. Vol. II.

16. DAIN, N., AND CARLSON, E. T.: Milieu therapy in the nineteenth century; patient care at the friend's asylum, Frankfort, Pennsylvania, 1817-1861. J. Nerv. & Ment. Dis. 131:277-290 (Oct.), 1960.

17. ALLEN, M.: Essay on the Classification of the Insane. London, John Taylor, 1833.

18. PRICHARD, J. C.: A Treatise on Insanity and Other Disorders Affecting the Mind. London, Sherwood, Gilbert and Piper, 1835.

19. TUKE, S.: Description of the Retreat. Philadelphia, Isaac Peirce, 1813.

20. BATTIE, W.: A Treatise on Madness. London, J. Whiston and B. White, 1758.

21. GEORGET, E.: De la Folie, Paris, Grevot, 1820.

22. PERFECT, W.: Select Cases in the Different Species of Insanity. Rochester, W. Gillman, 1787.

23. BRADFORD, T. L.: The Life and Letters of Dr. Samuel Hahnemann. Philadelphia, Boericke and Tafel, 1895.

24. HALLARAN, W. S.: Practical Observations on the Causes and Cure of Insanity. Cork, Edwards and Savage, 1818.

25. CONOLLY, J.: An Inquiry Concerning the Indications of Insanity. London, John Taylor, 1830.

26. GALL, F. J.: Sur les Fonctions du Cerveau, Paris, J. B. Baillière. 1925. 6 vols.

27. COMBE, A.: Observations on Mental Derangement. Edinburgh, John Anderson, 1831.

28. CARLSON, E. T.: The Influence of phrenology on early American psychiatric thought. Am. J. Psychiat. 115:535-538 (Dec.), 1958.

Occupational Therapy in the Psychoses

by WILLIAM R. CONTE, M.D.

P SYCHIATRIC OCCUPATIONAL THERAPY is a treatment procedure based on an interpersonal relationship between patient and therapist and facilitated by tools which aid in bringing the participants together. Although occupational therapy is essentially a noninterpretive treatment procedure, the relationships established, together with the symbolic character of the tools employed, provide the necessary avenues for the working through of many problems. Thus it is that occupational therapy has a legitimate role in the treatment of the psychoses.

Historical considerations are always of value in understanding current practices. A few brief comments referable to the development of occupational therapy as a treatment procedure in the psychoses may be helpful. Four observations are outstanding:

    a. In the past, occupational therapy has been viewed as recreational and diversionary.

    b. The craft utilized by the occupational therapist has been looked on as providing a specific therapeutic effect.

    c. Occupational therapists have been seen as educators.

    d. The need for improving the communication between occupational therapists and physicians has been recognized.[1]

While originally occupational therapy was considered to be a recreational and diversionary procedure, this concept is now embraced by only a few.[2] The reason for this change is that the long recognized benefits derived are now understood to stem from the satisfactions of deprived needs accomplished through the close interpersonal relationship between patient and occupational therapist.

Likewise, the idea of the specific therapeutic effectiveness of the craft in occupational therapy is losing support. Previously, some had hoped that a specificity would be developed which would not be unlike the specificity of digitalis. The occupational therapist in the role of educator is also less rigidly adhered to, but is maintained to a degree in that therapists do much to assist the learning process of their patients. The long sought specificity in the craft has been replaced by a "specificity" in the self, and the role of the occupational therapist has been extended from educator in the traditional sense to "therapist" in its broadest meaning.

The need to communicate with physicians, an ever present problem, is historical in origin and even now is only partly accomplished. An improvement here will ultimately secure the recently attained position of the occupational therapist on the treatment team.

In an extensive opinion survey[3] recently conducted by the subcommittee on occupational therapy of the American Psychiatric Association, a group of psychiatrists, selected because of a high level of sophistication in the field of occupational therapy, saw the relationship aspect of the procedure as a more important factor in the treatment than the craft. This view was supported by the occupational therapists who were questioned. The group activities characteristic of occupational therapy were seen to provide a learning experience in socialization. The survey also revealed profound communication difficulties between occupational therapists and physicians as reflected in consultation services, inservice training programs, and the utilization of the reports prepared by occupational therapists.

To be effective in the psychoses, occupational therapists must acquire a sound knowledge of the signs and symptoms of the psychiatric disorders, must have a working understanding of the unconscious, and should be able to recognize the symbolization of behavior as well as to appreciate the symbolic significance of the tools with which they work. Schools of occupational therapy and clinical training centers are dedicated to this concept.

At the risk of oversimplification, the function of occupational therapy in the psychoses may be divided into three specific areas:

   a. The diagnostic function
   b. The prognostic function, and
   c. The specific therapeutic effect.

While diagnosis is the art and responsibility of the physician and the appraisal of prognosis is likewise in his domain, it happens that both of these functions are being shared with an ever increasing psychiatric team. This is also true in the treatment, for today only a few patients are receiving individual psychotherapy from the psychiatrist. A much greater number of psychotic patients are being treated by a team of workers— a team which is headed by a physician and includes nurses, occupational therapists, and others.

In diagnosis and evaluation of prognosis, the occupational therapist is a respected member of the psychiatric team. As such he is concerned with basic observations of the behavior of the patient—observations which may point to the patient's abilities to relate or to his difficulties in establishing contact with others, as well as with observations of the specific signs and symptoms of the individual psychiatric disease entities.

By the same token, the appraisal of the patient's comprehension, his degree of cooperation, his manifest resistances and his dependencies are legitimate functions of the occupational therapist, and all serve as valuable consideration in the team's effort to arrive at a diagnosis.

As the work with the psychotic patient continues, all members of the psychiatric team become concerned with prognosis. Any signs which reflect changes in the symptom complex, or in the ability of the patient to relate with comfort are important. The subjective experiences of the occupational therapist, together with the clinical setting in which he works, provide an excellent arena to observe behavior, to make controlled observations, and to conduct treatment.

The third function of occupational therapy is that of treatment. To understand the treatment role however, one must first consider certain aspects of the psychotic process in which the occupational therapist will be involved.

It can be stated with conviction that the psychotic patient has found the world unresponsive to his needs and as a result has withdrawn from it. The reasons for the lack of satisfaction, and his particular ego reaction to it, are numerous and varied. However, the major problem seems to lie in impaired interpersonal relationships with those important people around him on whom he might have depended for love, appreciation, and respect.

Freud's theory of the psychosexual development of the child and the concept of fixation at the various levels is pertinent here. The psychosis represents an ego defense against anxiety which, in turn, stems from problems arising in one or another of the stages of psychosexual development and carries symptoms symbolic of it. Also important in this concept are the many problems which impair the learning of integrity and responsibility and which may lead to inappropriate sexual identification.

As the ego struggles with continuing conflict and meets repeated frustration there is a faltering of ego strength accompanied by a loss of identity, new anxiety, and regression to much earlier levels of adjustment. Object relations are lost—partly from the original denial of needs, but the loss is enhanced by the fracturing of ego function and the failure to perceive reality.

With this background as a frame of reference, the specific treatment functions of the occupational therapist in the psychoses can be divided into four major categories. These are: (a) the establishment of supporting relationships; (b) the augmentation of defenses; (c) the therapeutic use of controls; (d) social retraining. Some comment on each is in order.

The Establishment of Supporting Relationships

Treatment of the psychotic patients is dependent in part on supplying them with a warm and supporting relationship which, unfortunately, has been denied them. This relationship, however, must be something different than the patient has known before if, indeed, the treatment is to help the patient reject his world of unreality. The parents on whom the patient might have depended for love and support have often been self-centered, domineering individuals whose children have been mere extensions of themselves, rather than independent growing human beings. Thus, the occupational therapist in the role of the supporting "parent" must be one who can graciously stand by and watch his patient become an independent worker in whatever project he might be employed. He must be able to support him when he is depressed or when his hostilities overwhelm him and when he is critical and otherwise hostile. To support, to love, to encourage, and to convey the message that the patient is understood and accepted is part and parcel of the relationship role of the occupational therapist.

Many occupational therapists are unwilling to assume this role with their patients in the same way that some psychiatrists are unwilling to be as supporting as their patients need them to be. Some occupational therapists can be taught a great deal about providing this care while others cannot. Obviously, the more self-understanding which the occupational therapist can acquire, including the kind of self-understanding that comes from a personal analysis, the greater is his opportunity to be effective in dealing with patients.

The Augmentation of Defenses

The most commonly employed and easily understood defense mechanism utilized in occupational therapy is that of expression. There are countless opportunities to express hostilities and aggressiveness as well as those emotions which appeal to the more esthetic senses. Play therapy and the creative arts are frequently utilized. Since the occupational therapy clinic is recognized as a place where this type of expression may take place, aberrant behavior is often more readily accepted there than in other treatment areas.

The relationship with the occupational therapist and the setting in which he works provides the proper climate for regression and rationalization to be recognized, understood, and reflected when appropriate.

Needless to say, the relationship also provides the patient the opportunity for close identification with the therapist. This, hopefully, may be a learning experience moving the patient toward a more appropriate understanding of his own identity and sex role.

Many of the tools of the occupational therapist have symbolic significance. The mud and the clay and the paint as well as the hammer and brush may be related to early fixations in the psychosexual development of the patient. The understanding of these symbolizations and their effective utilization in the relationship which the therapist establishes with his patient may serve a therapeutic advantage. It has been postulated that gratification of basic needs by symbolic realization in some patients with severe emotional disturbances may lead to better contact with reality.[4]

This point is beautifully illustrated by Schaefer and Smith.[5] They report an interesting clinical research study utilizing a group of schizophrenic patients. Members of the treatment team served as substitute parents and siblings. Objects similar to the "original needed infant objects" (wet clay, milk, toys, candy, etc.) were provided and patients were encouraged to utilize these objects for the gratification of their own frustrated needs. The investigators observed that "patients seem to leave fixation positions after gratification of needs that had been frustrated . . . Patients thus treated establish a better contact with reality and a higher ego integration resulting in better functioning in and out of the hospital."

The significance of the use of the tools in occupational therapy as the subject of object relationships is greatly enhanced when the symbolic nature of these tools is more clearly defined.

THE THERAPEUTIC USE OF CONTROLS

The boundless ego of the regressed psychotic patient, like that of the child, is in need of controls which define the acceptable and the unacceptable. The occupational therapy clinic with its necessary rules and regulations, together with the personality of the occupational therapist, create the opportunity to exercise controls and to set the much needed limits.

SOCIAL RETRAINING

The relationship to the occupational therapist and the group setting in which the occupational therapy is frequently practiced, provide an unusual experience in group living. Working with an understanding therapist and fellow patients may provide the patient his first opportunity to learn the true significance of interpersonal relationships, to work out problems, and to test newfound strengths.

SUMMARY

The contribution of occupational therapy to psychotic patients is clearly defined by Fiddler when she points out that occupational therapy makes vital contributions to the milieu of the hospital community, augments formal psychotherapy, provides factual data, and that occupational therapy assists patients to assume their economic and social responsibilities.[6]

Occupational therapists do not operate as independent agents, nor do their tools hold a specific therapeutic effect. Rather they are team members and active participants in the total treatment effort. Their several functions provide much needed support, symbolic gratification, and the opportunity for a safe, understood, and accepted expression of feeling.

REFERENCES

1. CONTE, WILLIAM R.: The occupational therapist as a therapist. Am. J. Occupat. Ther. 14 (Jan.-Feb.), 1960.
2. WITTKOWER, E. D., LA TENDRESSE, T. D.: Rehabilitation of chronic schizophrenics by a new method of occupational therapy. Brit. J. M. Psychol. 28:42, 1955.
3. Subcommittee on Occupational Therapy, American Psychiatric Association: An Opinion Survey Concerning Occupational Therapy: on file with the Council of the American Psychiatric Association, not yet published.
4. SECHEHAYE, MARGUERITE: A New Psychotherapy in Schizophrenia. New York, Grune and Stratton, 1956.
5. SCHAEFER, DONALD L., AND SMITH, JANE J.: A dynamic therapy for schizophrenia. Am. J. Occupat. Ther. 7:5, 1958.
6. FIDDLER, GAIL S.: The role of occupational therapy in a multi-discipline approach to psychiatric illness. Am. J. Occupat. Ther. 6:1, 1957.

Recent Advances in Veterans' Administration Psychiatry

by J. F. CASEY, M.D., AND CLYDE J. LINDLEY, M.A.

D URING THE PAST DECADE there have been significant changes in the psychiatric treatment program of the Veterans Administration.[1] Brief descriptions of these developments will be made in relation to physical facilities, staffing, treatment programs, and research and education activities.

Very early there was recognition of the important role that modern concepts of psychiatric hospital architecture have in total treatment.[28, 29] In its hospital construction program model facilities have been provided for predominantly psychiatric hospitals, based on the concept of smaller wards and nursing units.[2, 4, 26] Eight new type, 1000 bed psychiatric hospitals have now been constructed*

In the initial phases of its modernization program the VA recognized the value of the general hospital in the treatment of acute psychiatric patients. Therefore, when a new or replacement general hospital was built, provision was made for psychiatric services as an integral part of the hospital. This became the standard pattern not only in the VA but also much more common in civilian hospitals.[6]

Currently, VA's long-range plans have been further refined to embrace a concept of general hospitals which provide facilities for treating all types of patients, including the long term as well as the acute psychiatric patient. One such hospital is now under construction at Washington, D. C. (710 beds), and three others are being planned for Miami (800 beds), Gainesville (480 beds), and Memphis (1000 beds). Each of these hospitals has 240 beds, for psychiatric patients. The psychiatric beds have

---

*VAH Salt Lake City, Utah, 1952, 687 beds, has 410 psychiatric beds of modern design, but is designated a general medical and surgical hospital; VAH Brockton, Mass., 1953; VAH Salisbury, N. Car., 1953; VAH Sepulveda, Calif., 1955; VAH Jefferson Barracks, Mo., 1957; VAH Topeka, Kans., 1958; VAH Palo Alto, Calif., 1960; VAH Brecksville, Ohio, May 1961.

all of the facilities generally provided in a predominantly psychiatric hospital. To foster a family living atmosphere, there are 30-bed nursing units, with each unit having its own solarium, sitting room, dining room and physical medicine and rehabilitation activities. Facilities for outpatient care, including space for a mental hygiene clinic and day care center, are available.[5]

The VA does not plan to build any more psychiatric hospitals. However, because of the obsolescence of many of its present predominantly psychiatric hospitals, it will be necessary to renovate existing facilities to meet total responsibilities for the treatment of the psychiatric veteran patient. Many of the older hospitals are larger than 1000 beds. In renovating these hospitals the plans call for smaller units for psychiatric patients, and additional general medical and surgical facilities, so that all types of medical care will be available. When practicable, these hospitals will be no larger than 1000 beds, 720 of which will be psychiatric. However, recognizing the importance of smaller facilities, there will be three separate buildings of 240 psychiatric beds which can be operated administratively as independent units. The plans also include one foster home preparation cottage for 40 patients. The general medical and surgical building will have 240 beds, which will include beds for neurological patients.

In some instances renovated hospitals will necessarily be larger than 1000 beds because of the size of existing hospitals. Some of the disadvantages of large size will be overcome by dividing the psychiatric services into several functionally independent units. This concept of functionally independent psychiatric units has already been adopted by several of VA's predominantly psychiatric hospitals. This change toward professionally autonomous smaller units is proving to be successful, particularly with reference to continuity of care. It is expected that many other hospitals will adopt this method of operation.

The VA operates one of the largest medical programs in the nation. There are now 171 hospitals, 40 of which are classified as predominantly psychiatric,* 8 tuberculosis, and 123 general medical and surgical. Seventy-one of the 123 general medical and surgical hospitals have neuropsychiatric services. The average daily patient load (fiscal year 1961) in all VA hospitals was 111,351. Fifty-six per cent (62,280) of these patients are classified as neuropsychiatric (57,816 psychiatric, 4486 neuro-

---

*VAH Salt Lake City, Utah, and VAH Augusta, Georgia, are designated as general medical and surgical hospitals, but have large psychiatric services, and are usually included as psychiatric for statistical reporting purposes about patient loads.

logical†). Almost 90 per cent of all psychiatric patients are classified as psychotic.

The VA also operates 67 mental hygiene clinics in its outpatient program. As of June 30, 1961, over 35,000 patients were receiving treatment in a VA mental hygiene clinic, and another 16,000 from non-VA physicians (on a fee basis) in the community. The VA also has 85 neuropsychiatric examination units which provide medical examinations for determining compensation and other awards. Many of these units render minimal supportive type treatment services to many of the 100,000 veteran patients they examine each year.

Although the VA has not attained the number of professional staff recommended by various standards, it has achieved a relatively favorable staffing ratio. The greatest shortages are in terms of psychiatrists, and, to a lesser extent, psychologists. Recruitment has been much better for other professional specialists. A rough indication of the increase in staff–patient ratios can be obtained by comparing the per diem figures for psychiatric hospitals of $7.22 per day, fiscal year 1951, to $13.40 per day for fiscal year 1961. A similar increase has occurred in general medical and surgical hospitals, from $16.47 per day to $25.89 per day. Although these figures reflect other factors than staffing, this makes up the greatest part of the total increase.

In order to procure professional staff in its hospitals, a psychiatric residency program was established in connection with the Deans Committee system operating within the VA. In 1954 this training program was extended to include the training of career physicians as well as regular residents. Career residents are full-time staff physicians, who receive identical training as the regular resident, but who agree to serve a period of obligated service upon completion of their residency. The VA (1961) has 192 regular and 118 career residents in training in psychiatry. There are 43 approved 3 year residency programs and 3 approved for 2 years. Currently, there are 62 career physicians serving obligated service at locations designated by the VA; approximately 40 career physicians will become available in 1962 for obligated service. To date, 89 of the career residents who have completed their obligated service have remained in continued employment with the VA for at least one year. A number of these physicians now occupy key positions in VA hospitals. Thus the career residency program has made it possible to staff isolated hospitals with some well-trained psychiatrists.

The VA Psychology Training Program also continues to serve as the

---

†VA's program for the neurologic patients will not be discussed in this article.

most important source of recruitment for staff positions.[22] During fiscal year 1961 there were 675 trainees receiving training while they were performing valuable services to patients. Fifty-eight universities offer training in the fields of clinical and counseling psychology which leads to the doctoral degree. This degree is a requirement for staff positions in psychology. Indicative of the high recruitment potential of this training program is the fact that over two-thirds of the present VA staff psychologists were recruited from the VA training program.

Concurrently with the development of modern hospital facilities, increased attention has been given to the design of furniture for psychiatric day-rooms, the use of equipment to promote habits of independence, and the development of "therapeutic community" atmosphere, the "open door" hospital, and after-care programs. Special attention has been given to the better utilization of staff, and particularly the importance of staff attitudes, staff communication, and the administrative organization of the hospital, to encompass a total therapeutic program.[54] During this period the VA initiated a member employee program. Under this program the patient has a new status as a paid employee, and lives in employees' quarters at the hospital. Thus, long term, chronic schizophrenics are able to make the first step in community living by a realistic work experience in the protected atmosphere of the hospital.[55, 56] This led to the development of a foster home preparation cottage on the grounds of the hospital. Patients can now learn to adjust in a non-hospital homelike setting prior to being released to a foster home.[57]

The VA has had a foster home program operating for a number of years. This program has progressed so that 2400 patients were placed in homes in calendar year 1960, a 22 per cent increase over the previous year. Patients in foster homes are given supervision by their foster parents as well as social service, and, when needed, by a physician. Patients in foster homes are on trial visit and can be brought back to the hospital at any time.

Many psychiatric patients are placed on a trial visit status prior to receiving a final discharge. The patient may be on trial visit for a year and during this period may be readmitted to the hospital if he needs treatment. Trial visit patients receive supervision through social service. The number of patients on trial visit has steadily increased from 7186, June 30, 1956, to 11,413, June 30, 1961.

In order to keep abreast of the most modern developments, a planned review was made of the significant psychiatric treatment programs in Europe.[16] The major emphasis was directed toward studying the treatment of long term and the elderly psychiatric patient, and evaluating the techniques of retraining and reeducation in the areas of social living and vocational adjustment.[12] Intensive efforts have been made to encourage and stimulate the development and further improvement of VA's psychiatric treatment program through a series of conferences about European psychiatric treatment with VA psychiatrists through the United States. Although the VA has initiated similar programs, there had not been the same emphasis upon development of after-care resources.[11] The half way house is an example of a program which has received encouragement as a result of these conferences.

The half way house provides a residence in the community where many former patients can live in one place. The patients are independent, and assume some degree of responsibility for themselves. Many leave the half way house when they have finally gained self-confidence to be entirely on their own. Supervision, when needed, can be provided by the staff from the hospital. At the end of the calendar year 1960 there were 16 half way houses in operation, associated with VA hospitals. These houses had received 187 patients during the year, with 117 remaining at the end of the year.

In January 1957, an extensive survey was made in 79 of VA's hospitals to determine the over-all effects of the use of the tranquilizers on the total treatment program.[43] There was a significant decrease in electroshock and insulin coma therapy, marked reduction in need for neutral packs and tubs, and an increase in the use of individual and group psychotherapy, and the granting of more privileges and independence to patients. Many of the hospitals indicated that these changes in therapies were not due to the tranquilizers alone, since many hospitals were beginning to eliminate shock therapies before the appearance of tranquilizers. However, there was general consensus that many patients were now more available for increased therapeutic activities, were more responsive and could function at a higher level. The decrease in use of shock therapies has continued to the present (1961), so that this therapy is used relatively infrequently. Likewise, group psychotherapy has continued to increase (1961), along with such modifications as group methods, patient self-government, and other group-social approaches to patients.

In VA's mental hygiene clinics, individual and group psychotherapy are the main therapeutic approaches of the treatment team, composed of a psychiatrist, psychologist, and social worker. However, since many psychotic as well as psychoneurotic patients began to request treatment in mental hygiene clinics, personnel began to explore new approaches for the effective treatment of these patients. This led to the development of a new concept of treatment: psychiatric day care treatment centers as

an integral part of VA mental hygiene clinics. There are now 12 day
care centers in VA mental hygiene clinics and a total of 36 is planned
by 1966.

Some of the aims of a day care program are (1) to assist the patient
to make a wholesome and satisfactory transition from hospital to normal
community existence; (2) to help the patient resume normal activities
in community and family living; and (3) to prevent regression of the
patient with resultant readmission to the hospital.[62] The day care treatment center represents an intermediate step toward integration into
normal community living. Emphasis is placed on re-learning of basic
habits of socialization in the therapeutic atmosphere of the day care
center. This is accomplished through the use of group therapy, occupational therapy, manual arts therapy, recreational therapy, and active
participation in community activities through the assistance of trained
volunteers from the community. The patients spend the major part of
each day at the day center, rather than being limited to the conventional
psychotherapy hour. The program does not duplicate the type of treatment offered either in full time or day hospitals,[47] but offers a milieu
type therapy in an outpatient setting, emphasizing the relearning of social
skills required for community living.

Another program which appears unusually effective is operating at
one of the smaller psychiatric hospitals located at Fort Meade, South
Dakota.[18] This program has been designed to make the psychiatric aide
an active participant in the patient's hospital life. He becomes involved
in the decision-making process of granting privileges, planning activities,
assignment, recommending ward transfers, etc. The entire hospital staff
became committed to this approach. At the end of 30 months, a significantly higher number of "hard core" patients had been discharged
to the community and are making a satisfactory adjustment there.

At the VA Hospital in Palo Alto, California, an experimental approach
in group cohesion in the rehabilitation of psychiatric patients has had
noteworthy results.[19] Patients are assigned to small task groups and
remain in this group until they leave the hospital. The group as a unit
is responsible for its individual members. The patients progress through
four steps to complete the program. Four hours a day are spent in the
small task group with the remainder of the time spent on individual job
assignments. The first step level is that of personal care, punctuality on
assignments and orientation of new members. When in this step the
patient receives $10 per week (non-Government funds) and a one day
pass. In progress to step four the patient receives increasing amounts of
money and passes commensurate with progression at that step level, until
step four when he can have unlimited amounts of money. Four out of

every five days the task group meets without staff members present. The members evaluate each other and prepare recommendations for the staff when they meet with them on the fifth day. The staff communicates with the task group by notes, and the task group has the expectation of taking appropriate action on the notes. The action taken is a decision by the task group and not by the staff. The initial evaluation of this program reveals that the discharge rate is between 50 and 60 per cent higher for these task groups as compared to control groups.

In 1956 the VA initiated large scale cooperative studies to evaluate the effectiveness of psychopharmacologic agents with psychiatric patients.[3, 41] Five studies in hospitals[13, 14, 15, 51] and one in mental hygiene clinics have been completed.[45] The studies have been carefully developed in conferences involving both clinical and research experts representing a number of different professional disciplines. Special scientific personnel at VA central research laboratories assumed responsibility for the final development of the protocols for each study, and an executive committee gave guidance and direction. The studies are double-blind and generally include an inert or active placebo or a drug of known effectiveness. Special attention is given to criteria for the selection of patients who are assigned randomly to each study treatment. Dosage strengths are carefully planned and have included both fixed and flexible dosage patterns, as well as combinations of drugs. Criteria of change have been evaluated by objective rating scales. The principal method to determine the variables having prognostic significance was analysis of covariance. Sandifer,[59] in comparing the reporting and design of research publications on psychiatric drug treatment, concluded that "the methodological quality of VA research is clearly superior." Caffey[8] has summarized the main findings of these studies. He indicates that all phenothiazines were effective in reduction of symptomatology, but there were no similar benefits as a result of administering inert substances or phenobarbital.[7] Energizing drugs, added to a maintenance phenothiazine produced no significant improvement in chronic, withdrawn and apathetic male schizophrenics.[14] The incidence of side effects and complications with phenothiazines was less than had been expected from other studies. There were no cases of agranulocytosis or jaundice with the phenothiazines in the patients studied. Extrapyramidal syndromes, seizures, and skin eruptions were relatively infrequent. On the other hand, weight gain was consistently noted with the phenothiazines, alone or in combination with an energizer.[35] Hollister, Caffey and Klett[30] report that some of the observed effects may in actuality be manifestations of spontaneous variations in the behavior of schizophrenic patients.

In the completed outpatient psychiatric study, the effects of two tranquilizers on psychotherapy were evaluated. Neither tranquilizer had an advantage over the other or the controls, and was no more effective in reducing anxiety and hostility than psychotherapy alone. Some therapists observed that patients receiving phenobarbital are slowed down in their recovery.[45]

These VA cooperative chemotherapy studies have been a major stimulus to the development of improved methods of assessing behavior change in patients,[23, 24, 36, 38, 40, 44, 50] the use of special approaches such as sequential analysis,[37] the investigation of a number of related matters, such as attitude toward medication,[25, 46] the development of medical models,[34, 48, 49, 52, 53] and the development of techniques for detection of phenothiazine compounds and others in the human system.[17, 20, 21, 31] Members of the Executive Committee, VA Cooperative Chemotherapy Studies in Psychiatry, wrote a medical bulletin (1960) giving general guidelines regarding the use of tranquilizing and antidepressant drugs in psychiatry and in non-psychiatric practice.[9]

The VA encourages a wide variety of research approaches ranging from the biological and neurophysiological to the psychological, sociological and anthropological studies of behavior. Studies concerning the biological correlates of behavior, the relationship of the central and autonomic nervous systems and the effects of biochemical, neurochemical and neurophysiological reactions on behavior are under way in many VA hospitals. Studies are also being conducted to measure the effects of sensory deprivation, the reactions to stress and conflict, and the ability to learn new habits of behavior. Many current studies focus on the relationship of electro-cortical stimulation of the brain to perception and learning, and one investigator has developed an electronic device for measuring cortical reception of sensory impulses. Psychological, sociological and anthropological studies are also under way which focus upon interpersonal relationships, the studies of attitudes and how they change, the behavior of persons in groups, the effects of environmental variables upon behavior, and the significance of communication in the process of adjustment. Several studies are under way to determine the relative effectiveness of current therapeutic modalities such as individual psychotherapy, group psychotherapy, patient government and member employee programs, and other rehabiliative measures.[42]

A broader approach to evaluation is represented by The Psychiatric Evaluation Project. This project is a long term, five year program, initiated in 1955, to determine the relative effectiveness of differing staffing patterns, treatment programs and hospital designs in the improvement or recovery of schizophrenic patients. The study includes twelve hospitals located throughout the country, which are almost equally divided between high staffing and low staffing criteria. The whole range of per diem costs in psychiatric hospitals is covered; some very small (less than 1500 patients), others were large (more than 1500 patients), and some represented the latest in hospital architectural design (new, smaller hospitals), while others were old style hospitals. Every effort has been made to solve the methodological difficulties relating to insuring that patients selected for the study at different hospitals will be essentially similar in their clinical condition. One of the many devices which has helped these efforts is the development of a symptom rating scale.[33] Preliminary results suggest that both high over-all staffing ratios and small hospital size favor early return to the community of patients with functional psychoses.[32] It is expected that subsequent analysis will provide a wealth of data in terms of hospital and nursing unit size, types of staffing patterns (personnel) and relative influence of differing treatment program emphases.* The Psychiatric Evaluation Project is now in Phase II, investigating factors critical in the employment of the mentally ill.[27]

In any large hospital system there is an occasional unpredicted death by suicide. In 1958, the VA established a Central Research Unit for the Study of Unpredicted Deaths, at VA Center, Los Angeles. All clinical records of suicides, and a non-suicidal control, since 1950 (and those occurring presently), are sent to this Center for intensive analysis and inter-group comparisons (suicide versus controls). Consultative services are also available to hospitals upon request to disseminate information to hospital staff about clues to suicide. The Unit is now engaged in a study of suicides in psychiatric and general hospitals, a follow-up study of attempted suicides, a cancer study, a social case history analysis, a depressive study, and has already published a first medical bulletin, "Suicide —The Problem and its Magnitude."[60] Two other bulletins will be released soon dealing with research findings about suicide in psychiatric hospitals and in general medical and surgical hospitals.

A medical audit plan for psychiatric hospitals is under way at VAH Perry Point, Maryland.[61] This research is designed to develop methods for appraising the effectiveness of the significant elements of performance of psychiatric hospitals. The term "medical audit" refers to procedures for obtaining information about a hospital which are often used as a standard in determining whether the hospital is meeting or deviating from standards.[58] No criteria of performance for psychiatric hospitals was available, so the medical audit is developing these criterion measures. Next it seeks to measure hospital resources, programs and policies. Much

---

*A psychologist, social worker and clerk are assigned to each of the 12 hospitals to carry out this extensive evaluative study. Followup in the community to determine adjustment status is an integral part of the Psychiatric Evaluation Project.

of this area of work is relatively uncharted and deals with over-all goals of psychiatric hospitals. One area of investigation that appears promising is the assessment of the record system and the purposes it serves, and the development of a system to make the records dynamically useful in the treatment of patients.[39]

SUMMARY

The VA psychiatric program has developed new concepts of hospital construction that embody the philosophy of complete facilities for the treatment of all types of patients. Psychiatric treatment facilities are no longer isolated, but are an integral part of the total medical center. The general hospital includes psychiatric services that treat both the long term and acute psychiatric patient.

The career training program in psychiatry has been of great assistance in obtaining essential psychiatric staff for all hospitals, and especially those that are isolated and in which recruitment is difficult. The psychology training program (clinical and counseling) has provided a steady source of VA career psychologists.

Advances have been made in the treatment program of patients in the hospital. The importance of staff attitudes, communication and group-interrelationships have been stressed. Group therapy is used more extensively. Experimental programs are under way evaluating the effectiveness of new roles for employees, new social structures, patient self government programs, and different approaches in staff–patient interrelationships. Increased emphasis has been given to the development of programs bridging the gap between hospital life and community life. The VA has studied European psychiatric practices and has been especially stimulated by their achievements in after-care programs. After-care has been stressed through member employment, foster home placement, trial visit procedures, and half-way houses. The day care center in mental hygiene clinics is a treatment innovation that represents a significant advance in the re-education and re-socialization of psychiatric patients for community living. Broad evaluative studies such as the Psychiatric Evaluation Project and the Medical Audit should give new insights into the relative value of different treatment programs and establish substantive criteria for the development of more realistic treatment goals.

The advent of the tranquilizing drugs gave impetus to the development of research programs in the field of mental illness. The Cooperative Research Program was developed to evaluate the effectiveness of the tranquilizing drugs, and later was broadened to include all research efforts relating to the discovery of the causes and most effective treatment methods for mental illness.

REFERENCES

1. Action for Mental Health, Final Report of Joint Commission on Mental Illness and Health. New York, Basic Books, Inc., 1961.

2. BAKER, A., DAVIES, R. L., AND SIVADON, P.: Psychiatric Services and Architecture. Public Health Papers 1, World Health Organization, Palais Des Nations, Geneva, 1959. 59 pp.

3. BENNETT, I. F.: Cooperative VA Study of Chemotherapy in Psychiatry— Project No. 1. Psychopharmacology, Problems in Evaluation. Edited by Cole, J. O. and Gerard, R. W. Washington, National Academy of Sciences —Science Research Council, 412-420, 1959.

4. BLASKO, JOHN J.: Action for intensive treatment: III. Intensive treatment centers, private psychiatric hospitals and other facilities needed for those with major mental illnesses. Ment. Hosp. 12:24-26, 1961.

5. ———, AND MILLER, V. P.: New concepts in general hospital psychiatry. Address by Dr. Blasko, American Hospital Association Annual Convention, Atlantic City, Sept. 28, 1961.

6. BRACELAND, FRANCIS J.: Psychiatry in general hospitals. Hosp. Prog. 41:58-61, 1960.

7. CAFFEY, E. M., JR.: Controlled studies of tranquilizing and antidepressant drugs in 2000 hospital patients. Paper read at Third World Congress of Psychiatry, Montreal, Canada, June 4-10, 1961.

8. ———: Experiences with large scale interhospital cooperative research in chemotherapy. Amer. J. Psychiat., 117:713-719, 1961.

9. ———, HOLLISTER, L. E., POKORNY, A. D., AND BENNETT, J. L.: Tranquilizing and Anti-Depressant Drugs. DM&S Medical Bulletin MB-6, Veterans Administration, Washington, D. C., Sept. 12, 1960.

10. ———, AND KLETT, C. J.: Side effects and laboratory findings during combined drug therapy of chronic schizophrenics. Dis. Nerv. Syst. 22:370-375, 1961.

11. CASEY, J. F.: The care and treatment of the elderly, chronically ill psychiatric and neurologic patient in the Veterans Administration. South. M. J. 51:31-34, 1958.

12. ———: The care of the psychiatric patient in Europe. Georgetown Med. Bull. 14:179-192, Feb. 1961.

13. ———, BENNETT, I. F., LINDLEY, C. J., HOLLISTER, L. E., GORDON, M. H., AND SPRINGER, N. N.: Drug therapy in schizophrenia: A controlled study of the relative effectiveness of chlorpromazine, promazine, phenobarbital and placebo. A.M.A. Arch. Genl. Psychiat. 2:210-220, 1960.

14. ———, HOLLISTER, L. E., KLETT, C. J., LASKY, J. J., AND CAFFEY, E. M., JR.: Combined drug therapy of chronic schizophrenics: A controlled evaluation of placebo, dextro-amphetamine, imipramine, isocarboxazid, and trifluoperazine added to maintenance doses of chlorpromazine. Am. J. Psychiat. 117:997-1003, 1961.

15. ———, LASKY, J. J., KLETT, C. J., AND HOLLISTER, L. E.: Treatment of schizophrenic patients with phenothiazine derivatives: A comparative study of chlorpromazine, trifluopromazine, mepazine, prochlorperazine, perphenazine and phenobarbital. Am. J. Psychiat. 117:97-105, 1960.

16. ———, AND RACKOW, L. L.: Observations on the treatment of the mentally ill in Europe. Veterans Administration, July 1960, Washington 25, D. C.

17. EIDUSON, SAMUEL: Relation of phenothiazine excretion to patient improvement. *In* Chemotherapy in Psychiatry, Transactions of Third (1958) Research Conference, Vol. 3, 163-165, April 1959. Veterans Administration, Washington 25, D. C.

18. ELLSWORTH, ROBERT B.: The psychiatric aide as an active participant in patient rehabilitation. Paper presented at VA Psychology Research Meeting, Aug. 1961, New York City.

19. FAIRWEATHER, GEORGE W.: The social psychology of mental illness: An experimental approach. Paper presented at VA Psychology Research Meeting, Aug. 1961, New York City.

20. FORREST, F. M., FORREST, J. S., AND MASON, A. S.: A rapid urine color test for triflupromazine (Vesprin). Am. J. Psychiat. 115:1114-1115, 1959.

21. ——, ——, AND ——: A rapid, semiquantitative urine color test for piperazine-linked phenothiazine drugs (Compazine, Trilafon and analogous compounds). Am. J. Psychiat., 116:549-551, 1959.

22. GINSBERG, S. T. AND HOUTCHENS, H. MAX.: Training of psychologists in mental hospitals. Ment. Hosp. 8:14-15, April 1957.

23. GORHAM, D. R., AND OVERALL, J. E.: Drug action profiles based on an abbreviated psychiatric rating scale. J. Nerv. & Ment. Dis. 131:528-535, 1960.

24. ——, AND ——: A short psychiatric rating scale for evaluating treatment change in schizophrenic patients. Am. Psychol. 15:387, 1960.

25. ——, AND SHERMAN, L. J.: The relation of attitude toward medication to treatment outcomes in chemotherapy. Am. J. Psychiat. 117:830-832, 1961.

26. GOSHEN, CHARLES E. (ed.): Psychiatric Architecture. American Psychiatric Association, Washington, D. C., 1959.

27. GUREL, LEE: Phase II: Psychiatric evaluation project: employment of the mentally ill. In Chemotherapy in Psychiatry and Broad Research Approaches to Mental Illness, Transactions of Sixth (1961) Research Conference, vol. 6, Dec. 1961, 366-367. Veterans Administration, Washington 25, D. C.

28. HAUN, PAUL: A program for a psychiatric hospital. Architect. Record, 108:136-141, 1950.

29. ——: The modern mental hospital. Am. J. Psychiat. 109:163-167, 1952-3.

30. HOLLISTER, L. E., CAFFEY, E. M., JR., AND KLETT, C. J.: Abnormal symptoms signs and laboratory tests during treatment with phenothiazine derivatives. Clin. Pharm. & Therapeut. 1:284-293, 1960.

31. HOLLISTER, L. E., MARRAZZI, A. S., AND CASEY, J. F.: Serum oxidase in chronic schizophrenics treated with tranquilizing drugs. Am. J. Psychiat. 116:553-554, 1959.

32. JENKINS, R. L., AND GUREL, L.: Predictive factors in early release. Ment. Hosp., 10 (9): 11-14 (Nov.), 1959.

33. ——, STAUFFACHER, J., AND HESTER, R.: A symptom rating scale for use with psychotic patients. A.M.A. Arch. Genl. Psychiat. 1:197-204, 1959.

34. KLETT, C. J.: Modern concepts and techniques in research design and analysis (symposium). Transactions of Fifth Research Conference on Chemotherapy in Psychiatry., Vol. 5., 294-298, 1961. Veterans Administration, Washington 25, D. C.

35. ——, AND CAFFEY, E. M., JR.: Weight changes during treatment with phenothiazine derivatives. J. Neuro. Psychiat. 2:102-108, 1960.

36. ——, AND LASKY, J. J.: Agreement among raters on the multidimensional scale for rating psychiatric patients. J. Consult. Psychol. 23:281, 1959.

37. ——, AND ——: A clinical trial of five phenothiazines using sequential analysis. J. Clin. and Exper. Psychopath. 21:89-100, 1960.

38. ——, AND ——: A patient progress scale, Psychol. Rep. 9:415, 1961.

39. KLETT, S., AND SEWALL, L. G.: Automatic data processing of patient records. Ment. Hosp., 12 (5): (May) 1961.

40. LASKY, J. J.: Veterans Administration Cooperative Chemotherapy Projects and Related Studies; chap. 44 In: Drugs and Behavior, ed. by Uhr, L., and Miller, J. G., New York, Wiley, 540-554. 1960.

41. LINDLEY, CLYDE J. (ed.): Chemotherapy in Psychiatry, Transactions First (1956) Research Conference, Vol. 1, Veterans Administration, Washington 25, D. C.

42. —— (ed.): Chemotherapy in Psychiatry and Broad Research Approaches to Mental Illness. Transactions of Fifth (June 1960), and Sixth (Mar. 1961) Research Conferences, Veterans Administration, Washington 25, D. C. Vol. 5, Dec. 1960, Vol. 6, Dec. 1961.

43. ——: VA Hospital survey of tranquilizing drugs. In Chemotherapy in Psychiatry, Transactions of Second (1957) Research Conference, June 1958, Vol. 2, 29-34. Veterans Administration, Washington 25, D. C.

44. LORR, MAURICE: Rating Scales, Behavior Inventories, and Drugs. In Drugs and Behavior. Ed. by Leonard Uhr and James G. Miller, New York, John Wiley & Sons, chap. 43, pp. 519-539, 1960.

45. LORR, M., McNAIR, D. C., WEINSTEIN, G. J., MICHAUX, W. W., AND RASKIN, A.: Meprobamate and chlorpromazine in psychotherapy: Some effects on anxiety and hostility of outpatients. A.M.A. Arch. Genl. Psychiat- 4:381-389, 1961.

46. MASON, A. S., AND SACKS, J. M.: Measurement of attitudes toward tranquilizing drugs. Dis. Nev. Syst. 20:1-3, 1959.

47. MELTZOFF, J., AND RICHMAN, A. A.: Therapeutic rationale of a psychiatric day center. Psychiat. Quart. 35:295-305, 1961.

48. OVERALL, J. E.: Formulating the multivariate hypothesis, Symposium: multivariate approaches to research in mental illness. Transactions of Sixth VA chiatry and Broad Research Approaches to Mental Illness. Transactions Sixth Research Conference, Veterans Administration, Washington 25, D.C., Vol. 6, Dec., 1961.

49. ——, AND GORHAM, D. R.: Factor space D² analysis applied to the study of changes in schizophrenic symptomatology during chemotherapy. J. Clin. & Exper. Psychopathol. 21:187-195, 1960.

50. ——, AND ——: Basic dimensions of change in the symptomatology of chronic schizophrenics during chemotherapy. J. Abnorm. & Soc. Psychol. (in press).

51. ——, HOLLISTER, L. E., POKORNY, A. D., CASEY, J. F., AND KATZ, G.: Drug therapy in depressions: controlled evaluation of imipramine, isocarboxazid, detroamphetamine-amobarbital, and placebo. (In press.) J. Clin. Pharmacol. & Therapeut. (Submitted: October 1961).

52. ——, AND WILLIAMS, C. M.: Models for medical diagnosis. Behav. Sci. 6:134-141 (April), 1961.

53. ——, AND ——: Models for medical diagnosis: factor analysis, Part I,

theoretical, Medical Documentation: Medizin. Dokumentat. 5:51-56, April 1961.

54. OZARIN, LUCY D.: A positive approach to psychiatric patients (film) [Rev. by Martha J. Thomas] Ment. Hosp. 7, 4:28, 1956.

55. PEFFER, PETER A.: Money, a rehabilitation incentive for mental patients. Amer. J. Psychiat. 110:84-92 (August), 1953.

56. ——: Motivation of the chronic mental patient. Am. J. Psychiat., 113:55-59 (July), 1956.

57. ——, AND GLYNN, J. FREDERICK: Foster home cottage—a new approach to discharge. Ment. Hosp. 8, 14, 1957.

58. RICE, C. E., BERGER, D. G., SEWALL, L. G., AND LEMKAU, P. V.: Measuring social restoration performance of public psychiatric hospitals. Publ. Health Rep. 76:437-446, May 1961.

59. SANDIFER, MYRON G.: The reporting and design of research on psychiatric drug treatment: a comparison of two years. Psychopharmacology Service Center Bulletin, 6-10, July 1961. U. S. Department of Health, Education, and Welfare, Public Health Service.

60. SCHNEIDMAN, EDWIN S., AND FARBEROW, NORMAN L.: Suicide—The Problem and Its Magnitude. Medical Bulletin (MB-7), Veterans Administration Department of Medicine and Surgery, March 1, 1961.

61. SEWALL, LEE G., AND BERGER, DAVID G.: The medical audit plan for psychiatric hospitals. Ment. Hosp., 10 (9), (Nov.) 1959.

62. WEINSTEIN, GEORGE J.: Pilot programs in day care. Ment. Hosp. 11:9-11, 1960.

Mental Hospital Therapy: A Review and Integration*

by JOHN H. VITALE

N O PREVIOUS AGE has so keenly understood the problem of the care and rehabilitation of the mental patient and underwritten its cost, even though steps toward its solution are as yet tentative and incomplete (Joint Commission on Mental Illness[1]).This evaluation of current mental hospital practices and results has been organized to touch upon the following key topics in an effort to clarify this point: (1) historical factors, as they have affected the concept of the mental hospital and patient status; (2) the realization that the reduction of the chronic resident mental patient population and the elimination of factors in the system which produce chronicity are the major problems confronting the American mental hospital system, (3) an assessment of early and current efforts to carry out the treatment function assigned to mental hospitals, together with a delineation of promising theoretical and experimental leads; (4) consideration of the adequacy and value of aftercare facilities complementary to mental hospital efforts; and (5) general conclusions growing out of this assessment.

HISTORICAL PERSPECTIVES

In the era of moral treatment (1820-1860), physicians believed that mental hospitals could provide the necessary environmental conditions for early rehabilitation and release of its residents. In the custodial phase (1860-1930), on the other hand, the character and policies of the institutions were important forces which so molded the way of life of a large segment of their populations that many patients failed to be released. In the custodial phase mental hospitals were regarded as the responsible agency for the protection of society from the unpredictable and rejected behavior of individuals suspected of suffering from incurable brain lesions,

---

*Mrs. Helen Pearson contributed her special competence in checking and organizing the references and typing the manuscript.

a theory that contrasted sharply with the moral treatment doctrine that the disturbed behavior of such individuals was primarily social and psychological in origin, and treatment required societal measures.

An early asylum, established in Valencia, Spain, in 1409, probably as an influence from Arabic thought which had preserved Greek enlightenment, removed chains from the insane, established the use of psychological procedures in treatment, and emphasized the value of rehabilitative procedures during and after recovery (Bassoe[2]). This promising start was a victim of the bitter quarrel between the Christian and Moslem worlds. It remained for the modern world to explore the theory of therapy in greatest depth, first during the moral treatment period (Bockoven,[3, 4] Deutsch,[5] Malamud[6]) and again during the present era. Toward the end of the eighteenth century, experiments in psychological treatment occurred first in Italy, to be followed shortly by more persuasive developments in France, England, and in the remainder of Europe, illustrating Snow's[7] point that technologically similar societies produce similar inventions. The changes consisted of profound alterations in the psychological and physical environment for accommodating psychologically disturbed individuals in accordance with the changed concept of the patient as a disabled human rather than a criminal, animal, or demon.

Chiarugi, who preceded Pinel by five years, opened St.Boniface in Florence in 1788, which was regarded as a model asylum where commitment procedures protected the patient's interests, diagnosis and treatment were technically based, and a schedule of social, recreational, vocational, and pharmaceutical measures was offered in an atmosphere of liberty and order. Curiosity seekers were forbidden, physical restraint was limited, chaining was abolished. Chiarugi improved the status of the patient at a time when Pinel had just proposed his solution for reforming the French mental hospitals to the new, militant French Government (Livi[8]). Pinel's stature and influence outweighed the originality of Chiarugi's efforts, perhaps because the latter worked in isolation from his contemporaries, so Pinel has been accorded the reputation of the founder of "purposeful psychological treatment" (Walk[9]). Almost concurrently, Tuke organized an asylum in England upon the concept of improved patient status and self regulation in place of coercion. These reforms in theory and method, which replaced physical coercion with psychological procedures, were not uniform and absolute (Walk[9]). Nevertheless, in many American mental hospitals the status of the patient changed to that of a disordered but responsible individual for whom asylum methods permitted temporary restraint during the acute phase but were followed by convalescent care and social rehabilitation as soon as recovery permitted (Malamud,[6] Meijering,[10] Robinson[11].)

The moral treatment period in American mental hospitals achieved results comparable to modern recovery rates for the acute psychoses; yet this experiment in treatment failed because of the combined effect of several factors such as increased hospital size for purposes of economy, the contention that the release rates were illusory, the emergence of the organic theory of mental disorder, and an absence of qualified successors to early moral treatment leaders (Bockoven,[3, 4] Rees and Glatt,[12] Solomon[13]). Release figures dropped precipitously as custody and security concerns replaced treatment, and did not rise until a theory of treatment had been developed (by 1930) which placed physiological, psychological, social, and cultural factors in the forefront of attention. Prior to that development, the status of the patient was that of a permanently disabled and dependent individual who required continuous close supervision, a status carrying vastly different implications from that accorded him under moral treatment which regarded the disability as temporary, and his dependence as partial. Chronicity had been institutionalized.

Early somatic therapies contributed a fresh approach—especially during the period 1936 to 1945 when ward milieu and interest in patient potential were important—and recoveries approximated the 75 to 85 per cent recorded for moral treatment (Bockoven,[4] Kramer et al.[14], Odegard[15]). Despite these encouraging tends, it soon became clear that hospitalization introduced a factor of unknown dimensions which created a chronic, static population. One inquiry (Vitale[16]) revealed that patient conformity to hospital norms and methods was enforced, that a loosely organized but powerful patient system existed and that the staff and patient systems erected mutual barriers despite the importance of human relations in treatment. The over-all outcome of these factors placed most patients in the impossible situation of so constricting their psychological reality to themselves and their immediate environment that attachment to external realities became impossible. Consequently, only the most ·intact groups were able to pursue a hospital course that terminated in early release (Caudill et al.,[17] Goffman[18].)

The problem of chronicity could be avoided no longer when release rates for those confined longer than a year showed little change over previous figures despite the transformation of the hospital from a custodial to a treatment agency (Jones[19]), the implementation of aftercare programs, efforts toward better public acceptance of released mental patients, and the new chemotherapies. Interestingly, it was discovered that the most potent factors associated with release and relapse rates were the demographic characteristics of (1) length of hospitalization, (2) diagnosis, and (3) age (Ellsworth,[20] Fairweather et al.,[21] Lindemann[22].)

Studies in other countries indicated clearly that mental hospitals are not essential to the care, treatment, and rehabilitation of chronic mental patients (Eaton and Weil,[23] Meijering,[10] Lemkau and Crocetti[24]), even though such care is considered essential in America. As Bockoven[4] states, "Medicine and law have rendered committed patients (in this country) almost impotent to obtain a hearing in their own behalf. In spite of their relative helplessness, they have made themselves felt, for by their very increase in numbers and failure to recover they have come to cost our society more than we like to pay. The time is hard at hand when we cannot afford to continue managing their lives as if they all had structured brain defects." By contrast, Europe, England, and Scandinavia have relied on social and legislative reforms (Freeman and Farndale,[25] Kalinowsky,[26] Muth,[27] Rees and Glatt[12]).

THE PROBLEM OF CHRONICITY

Physiological, biochemical, and psychodynamic models have proved inadequate because they focus on deficit behavior (Foulkes,[28] Masserman[29]), but they have provided important assistance by their contribution to knowledge of deficit behavior (Winder[30]), to the recovery of the partially disabled, and by promoting objective inquiry. Their failure to affect a large segment of the mental disorders emphasizes the futility of employing a narrow theoretical model to furnish answers for a broad, complex problem (Brady and Fishman,[31] Chapanis,[32] Garner,[33] Martin,[34] Morison,[35] Rees,[36] Rees and Glatt[37]). The patient is regarded as dependent and put in an unrealistic situation which he cannot readily escape (Goffman;[18] Appleby, Scher, and Cumming;[38] Stanton;[39] Joint Commission on Mental Illness[1]). The final deterioration of resident psychotic patients under an extremely impoverished psychological though physically benign environment can be found carefully described by Arieti[40]. As a result, basic assumptions regarding the purposes, methods, organization, practices, and effects of hospitalization have been questioned (Clark;[41] Ellsworth;[42, 20] Hyde;[43] Main;[44] Rees and Glatt;[45] Appleby, Scher, and Cumming;[38] Weinberg;[46] The Joint Commission on Mental Illness;[1] Sanders et al.;[47, 48, 49] Fairweather et al.[21]), and new techniques are being attempted in order to transform the mental hospital system into a treatment agency (Sanders et al.;[47] Fairweather*). The preponderance of evidence suggests that large numbers of psychotic patients cannot successfully oppose the dependent situation created by the mental hospital and that while this dependency has been too readily legalized and sanctioned by theory and practice, it can be altered by a vitalized, interested staff.

---

*Fairweather, G. W.: Personal communication, 1961.

Older methods, such as the somatotherapies (Staudt and Zubin[50]) and total push (Galioni,[51, 52] Sines et al.[53]), which contributed to shortening length of stay for acute patients and raised the within-hospital behavioral level of chronic ones, have been replaced by chemotherapy and the therapeutic milieu (Jones,[19] Main,[44] Rees,[36] Greenblatt and Simon,[54] Denber,[55] Sivadon[56]). The most important change, however, is ideological and has occurred regarding the role and status of the patient, which is slowly being upgraded in theory from that of a dependent, carefully supervised and controlled inmate to that of a responsible, but inexperienced and partially disabled adult, who requires the kind of thoughtful asistance which succeeded in integrating the physically handicapped into the industrial fabric (Bell,[57] Bockoven,[3, 4] Brady and Fishman,[31] Clark,[41] Clark and Hoy,[58] Freeman and Farndale,[25] Jones,[19] Glass,[59] Main,[44] Rees,[36] Rees and Glatt,[45] Mental Hospitals,[60] Patton,[61] Stanton,[39] Wilmer,[62] Weinberg,[46] Scheerer,[63] Joint Commission on Mental Illness[1]). But, revision of hospital structure and practice to accommodate this change concept is only now beginning.

The value of tranquilizing drugs is not fully known; there is evidence that they do not affect relapse rates materially (Ellsworth and Clayton,[64] Fairweather, et al.,[21] Joint Commission on Mental Illness[1]); however, they have been judged to quiet wards, foster the staff—patient relationship, and improve release rates for acute and nonpsychotic categories (Odegard[65]), much as the somatotherapies (Staudt and Zubin[50]) had done earlier. Psychotherapy, as a treatment procedure for state and Veterans' Administration hospital patients, which account for more than 90 per cent of all mental patient beds (Kramer, et al.[66]), has been seriously questioned because (1) within-hospital improvement has been found poorly correlated with post-hospital behavior, and valid measures of efficacy of treatment have not been found (Astin,[67] Bandura,[68] Brady and Fishman,[31] Rotter,[69] Fairweather, et al.[21]); (2) it lengthens hospital stay without detectable post-hospital effects (Fairweather et al.[21]); and (3) it appears to be inappropriate to the socioeconomic level of most patients, except for the few who are motivated and capable (Hollingshead and Redlich,[70] Brady and Fishman[31]).

Despite ideological and technical changes, release rates for functional psychotic patients hospitalized two years or longer are little different today from what they were 40 years ago (Kramer,[14] Odegard,[65] Wright[71]) and relapse rates of the magnitude of approximately 70 per cent for that group have been shown by one carefully controlled study to appear within the first six months (Fairweather, et al.[21]). By contrast, those hospitalized less than two years relapsed at the rate of approximately 40 per cent in six months (Fairweather et al.[21]), but if the period of hospitalization was as little as three months on the average, only approximately 13 per cent relapsed in as long as three years (Bockoven et al.[72]).

Chronicity is, of course, a relative matter, but it appears after the first year of hospitalization when release probabilities drop from four-fifths for the first year to one-quarter for the second year, and continue to decline until after five years of hospitalization, the probability of release has dropped to about one-sixteenth under custodial practices (Ellsworth,[20] Kramer et al.,[14] Odegard,[15] Morgan and Johnson,[73] Giedt and Schlosser*). It is obvious that different treatment measures must be found if mental hospitals are to fulfill their primary function as treatment centers rather than custodial centers. The search, though uncoordinated among various hospitals, has started. Two major conceptual elements predominate; the concept of the hospital is being broadened, liberalized, and made continuous with society (Greenland[74]) and social measures are favored as a treatment concept for furthering gains associated with chemotherapeutic approaches (Scheerer,[63] Cooper[75]).

THE PROBLEM OF TREATMENT

The open hospital concept and the therapeutic community concept, which require a redefinition of the patient from a helpless and permanently damaged individual to a responsible regulated group member, and which have had an influence on the attempt to reorganize internal hospital relationships and structure, have succeeded in raising questions about hospital organization, patient status and role, staff relationships, and community attitudes toward mental patients (Jones,[19] Main,[44] Rees,[36] Wilmer[62]). American progress in this sphere, where changes are approached experimentally, has been slower than European and English, where changes have been made pragmatically (Kalinowsky,[26] Lemkau and Crocetti[24]).

The open hospital and the therapeutic community, which orginated in England and Europe, have not demonstrably improved release rates for chronic patients over other social measures (Sanders,[49] Wilmer,[62] Fairweather et al.[21]). However, comparisons are difficult since, for example, the powerful variable of commitment of patients, which establishes the relationship between the patient and the hospital is approximately 10 per cent in England and is between 60 to 90 per cent in America (Kalinowsky,[26] Pollock et al.[76]). Instead, the majority of studies, which will be reported more fully below, have concerned themselves with assessment of modification of elements of the patients' day such as work, staff-led groups, psychotherapy, self care, and carefully organized human relationships within the hospital.

*Giedt, F. H., and Schlosser, J. R.: Personal communication, 1961.

A few studies carried out in England have reported on the modification of ward structure to take advantage of the historically proved value of work for improving behavioral adjustment within the hospital, and uniformly suggest that staff expectations and support in this sphere of social behavior is accompanied by improved within-hospital chronic patient behavior and improved release rates for that category (Baker et al.,[77] Baker and Lond,[78] Carstairs et al.,[79] Collins et al.[80]). Similar findings occurred in a study reported by Connors[81] in America. These and other experimental methods have usually been organized within the restrictions of the medical—legal framework of mental hospitals by placing a staff member in charge of a series of small groups, ordinarily behaviorally homogeneous, for the purpose of teaching by example (Masserman[29]) and for social therapy (Appleby et al.,[38] Ellsworth,[20, 42] Rackow et al.,[82] Padula,[83] Sanders et al.,[47, 48, 49] Brooks,[84] Sines et al;[53] Spohn*). One study ignored direct patient contact by attempting to reorganize the total hospital system as a way of treatment, but succeeded only in altering relationships among departments without detectable effect on patients (James[85]). An early study by Schlosser et al.,[86] provided evidence that several chronic wards could be reorganized, if security precautions were sufficiently relaxed, to combat the inactivity and social withdrawal fostered by monotonous protective ward routines. Schlosser observed an improved release rate for chronic patients at a time when the chemotherapies had not yet quieted the wards and brought about a better relationship between the staff and patients. Fairweather et al.,[21] in a carefully controlled study, contrasted four treatment methods and three diagnostic groups, carefully equated and matched for age, diagnosis, and length of hospitalization. The treatment methods were individual therapy, group therapy, group living to resemble the therapeutic community concept, and work alone with traditional ward schedules. The diagnostic groups were the nonpsychotic, the acute psychotic, and the chronic psychotic. He found that work alone was just as effective for chronic categories, insofar as release rates were concerned, as other more complex methods and that neither drugs nor psychotherapy prevented the relapse rate among chronics from greatly exceeding that found in the acute and nonpsychotic categories. Fairweather and Simon[87] found, furthermore, that adjustment of all categories at 18 months was reliably predicted by adjustment at 6 months. Their results suggest that the greatest relapse rate occurs within the first 6 months for all categories, and slowly drops thereafter, pointing to the importance of community arrangements for sustaining the improvement of released patients and reducing relapse rates. In this connection, Bockoven et al.,[72] observed a pattern of breakdown resulting in

---

*Spohn, H. E.: Personal communication, 1961.

rehospitalization which consisted of (1) withdrawal from recreation and social activities; (2) difficulty on the job and cessation of work; (3) build-up of economic and familial difficulties; and (4) rehospitalization. They suggest the establishment of community arrangements to buffer patients from this stepwise progression. Sanders and his research team[47, 48, 49] de-vised an elaborate test of the efficiency of three different experimental social systems for chronic patients, all of which accented patient responsi-bility, self care, and social participation—as compared with a control ward, where these factors were minimal. All three experimental condi-tions were so organized that staff members were group leaders; thus, pa-tient responsibility was limited. Sanders concluded that the three experi-mental conditions, while not distinguishable from each other, were su-perior to the control situation on within-hospital behavior measures and on release rate.

Brooks[84] took an important ideological step when he devised a study to examine the utility of a self care system for chronic patients, which gave them considerable realistic personal responsibility independent of direct staff control, and Brooks and Wright[88] report much improved release rates for such patients. Ellsworth[20] carefully contrasted an experimental ward, where the aide was placed in charge of small groups of patients as a model, with a matched control ward, where the usual leadership patterns existed. He observed differential release rates according to prior length of hospital-ization, as did Fairweather et al.[21] In addition, the most chronic patients, defined as those with more than five years of prior hospitalization, were released at the slowest rate, and showed little improvement until they had been in the program for at least 12 to 14 months.

Cooper[75] contrasted a nurse-led group, a combination of nurse-led group and chemotherapy, and chemotherapy alone on a chronic ward, but was unable to detect a differential advantage for the group method or combined group-chemotherapy method over chemotherapy alone. It is significant, however, that all methods recorded significant within-hospital improvement for the duration of the study. His suggestion that chemother-apy alone is the most efficient method for chronic patients, in view of the simplicity of the procedure and the absence of strain on the personnel, is questioned by the data from Fairweather et al.,[21] and Ellsworth.[20] Perhaps, in retrospect, his failure to find an advantage for group methods over chemotherapy alone for this sample may have occurred because, as in so many other studies, the patient groups were of homogeneous composi-tion and were staff led (Hunt et al.[89]). In short, behavioral expectations may have been staff imposed and too lenient.

Most of these studies have demonstrated an ability to improve release rates for chronic patients over that expected by traditional custodial methods (which anticipate a 6 to 14 per cent release rate per year), their range being 20 to 88 per cent per year depending upon the interest shown by the staff. These studies and others (Hoch[90]) indicate, too, that acute and nonpsychotic categories can expect a high release rate (85 to 100 per cent) and a short hospital stay approximating 6 to 12 months with good results (27 to 50 per cent relapse), but that chronic populations can expect far poorer results in that, while release rates can be raised to 20 to 88 per cent depending upon discharge policy, behavioral improvement, and vocational assistance, relapse rates are invariably high within six months (approximately 65 per cent) and climb even higher after 18 months (approximately 70 per cent).

The next logical step in treatment planning may utilize the power of small groups as a therapeutic instrument. Usual ward structure and methods do not permit small group formation among patients because leaders may not stay long enough, homogeneity of wards prevents the type of situation which would permit role differentiation and the creation of adaptive group norms to which members might be expected to adhere, and the informal groups have no sanctioned existence or work (Brooks,[84] Rees,[36] Rees and Glatt,[37] Stanton,[39] Parker,[91]). In addition, small groups cannot be readily formed by the staff on the usual ward because of the individualization of treatment theory which emphasizes the doctor–patient relationship and makes all other relationships subordinate to it, even though the factors for their formation are present in latent form. Stanton[39] believes that small group formations, both formal and informal, can operate as the most powerful agent for education and discipline. These structures have been found to exist among patients when attention has been turned in that direction (Caudill et al.,[17] Parker,[91]) but they usually exist outside the awareness of the staff and their potential has been almost uniformly overlooked because hospital organization tends to regard them as destructive structures. Sivadon[56] has shown how their destructive potential can be diverted into constructive channels.

Considering the fact that mental patients, and particularly the chronic catgeory, are members of a rejected minority group who lack institutionalized means for protecting themselves from the effects of rejection, that their behavior is viewed unsympathetically, and that their life is totally organized by means of a system that exacts compliance and conformity (Goffman[18]), it is not surprising that they should exhibit the bitterness, rebelliousness, and indifference to societal norms repeatedly found associated with their behavior, beyond the usual intrapsychic disturbance (Joint Commission on Mental Illness[1]). It is understandable, then, that usual hospital practices have noted these destructive and oppositional qualities in spontaneously formed small group structures among patients and refuses them recognition or sanction. Perhaps it is true, as small group theory suggests, that they are capable of the loyalty to each other that generates efforts at self control, behavior change, discipline, and mutual assistance with problems and concerns, and can transfer this new confidence, based on identification with the group structure, to attempts at living independently of the mental hospital (Scheerer[63]). The findings of Eaton and Weill[23] as well as the work in England (for example, Freeman and Farndale[25]) strongly favor the notion that the chronic, partially recovered mental patient, whose confidence has been somewhat restored, can adapt to an accepting society and only occasionally require hospitalization for brief periods when symptoms become acute.

The change from staff-led to patient-led groups has been made by Fairweather (personal communication). He designed a rigorous study to examine the idea that cohesive, problem-solving small group structures can be formed among chronic patients who have daily responsibility for each other. In this study, they are expected to help each other through an orderly system of increased responsibility and personal freedom, and finally assist each other with discharge and disposition planning. They receive assistance and guidance, but not direction, from the staff, which insists on patient leadership for the groups. Preliminary results indicate fairly clearly that such groups can be formed and continued over time, and that they do exert a profound effect upon patient motivation, behavior, adaptation, and release rates for both chronic and nonchronic categories.

Several factors stand out clearly in this total body of work:

1. The patient's status within the hospital has been gradually altered conceptually from that of a dependent, somewhat irresponsible inmate to that of a disabled, but responsible adult, but the same cannot be said for his status outside the hospital.

2. Research programs affect release rates regularly. Rashkis[92, 93] has argued that this effect occurs because research imposes order and regularity, limits, and goals upon an otherwise neutral or mildly disorganized and restrictive environment. To this can be added the argument that perhaps research promotes small group formation unintentionally, with internal group norms and greater expectations. This small group formation may be an important factor in the occurrence of the Hawthorne effect, wherein the phenomena are affected by the process of observation and the enthusiasm arising from the special status accorded to the studied group (Brown,[94] Vitale[16]).

3. It seems fairly clear that staff discharge policy is the most potent factor determining release rate; patient condition within clinical diagnosis, at point of discharge, seems relatively unimportant (Ellsworth et al.,[95] Odegard[96]).

4. Improved release rates are not reflected in lower relapse rates. These methods can treat and discharge chronic patients at a better rate, but a community system for accepting and accommodating them must be devised to sustain their adjustment. Most of the programs reported in these studies did not have an organized after-care system to call upon to sustain their high release rates, but where such assistance has been explicitly made a part of the disposition planning, relapse rates have been reported significantly reduced (Brown et al.,[97] Greenblatt et al.,[98] Ullmann and Berkman[99]).

5. The idea of the patient as a therapeutic agent is gaining currency, although its implementation is in its infancy because the full realization of this idea requires a redefinition of the task and relationship of the staff. Their new task would require them to devise and support a system such that this element of patients' potential could be effectively harnessed for their therapeutic benefit both within and outside the hospital. Mental patients might then be able to organize in the usual minority group manner to combat rejective operations. In short, the usual staff–patient hierarchy and relationships would have to be drastically altered, but the difficulties are so great that no immediate progress can be expected.

The Problem of Aftercare

The existing aftercare system is uneven, scanty, and poorly coordinated between agencies and mental hospitals (Joint Commission on Mental Illness[1]); wherever they exist, despite their variation in theory, purpose, method and organization, these facilities are thought to prevent or reduce the incidence of rehospitalization. The functions and problems of aftercare facilities have been described in detail (Landy and Wechsler,[100] Muth[27]). The major established forms are: (1) Day and night hospitals (Bierer,[101, 102] Mental Hospitals,[60] Cameron,[103] Winick[104]); (2) Halfway houses (Wechsler[105]); (3) Family Care (Crutcher,[106] Patton,[61] Ullmann and Berkman,[99] Muth[27]); (4) Social clubs (Bierer,[107] Palmer,[108] Wechsler[109]); (5) Sheltered workshops (Black,[110] Hubbs,[111, 112] Meyer and Borgatta,[113] Olshansky[114]); and (6) Aftercare clinics (Muth[27]).

Estimates of patients served by existing facilities, derived from the reports above, suggest that these facilities reach not more than 10 per cent of those potentially requiring this service, and that of those 10 per cent the majority of cases constitute individuals judged to have the best prognosis and behavioral potential. Where studies have been made (Patton,[61] Ullmann and Berkman,[99] Meyer and Borgatta,[113] Hubbs[111, 112]), there is a fairly strong suggestion that these facilities do lengthen time out of the hospital and reduce relapse rate among the chronic populations. This is what one might expect, because aftercare facilities afford a protective function similar to that of mental hospitals, so that the gap between them is less difficult for chronic patients to bridge than the gap between mental hospitals and society at large. These trends provide some evidence that organized and continuous assistance at the adult level is important for sustaining hospital treatment effects for chronic populations.

However, until the contemplated extension of the above elements of aftercare can be effected, mental hospitals have no alternative but to improve their within-hospital treatment programs to reduce length of stay for all categories, especially the chronic, and by releasing higher proportions of patients yearly, gradually reduce the existing chronic population and the frequency of buildup of chronic cases. Estimates suggest that 20 per cent of the schizophrenic categories, which constitute 25 per cent of all admissions, admitted in any one year will have been continuously hospitalized 10 years later (Odegard[96]). Without aftercare to assist in maintaining treatment effects, and without employer confidence in hiring ex-mental patients, whose attitudes have been assessed more often as neutral (Olshansky et al.[115]) or occasionally positive (Linder and Landy[116]) rather than negative, mental hospital programs cannot expect treatment effects to last for the bulk of released chronic patients, and so must prepare for a high return rate.

Despite the paucity of reliable data concerning the results of these avenues of approach, aftercare facilities have noted the value of peer group formation and group membership for enforcing discipline and providing mutual assistance. Unfortunately, the usual structure of aftercare facilities requires continued dependence from the patient and a continuation of his patient role; neither of these requirements permits patients their full scope as therapeutic agents for each other. Greenblatt,[117] Pratt et al.,[118] and others (Joint Commission on Mental Illness,[1] Mental Hospitals[119]) have explained the need for a reorganized and coordinated hospital–community system as a solution to these problems. At the moment, this position is more an ideal than a possible reality because of chronic manpower and fund shortages (Albee,[120] Joint Commission on Mental Illness[1]).

It is tempting to think that it might indeed be possible that patients, especially in the chronic categories, can undergo a succession of steps from leaderless groups to sanctioned peer groups with a stable and cohesive structure, function, purpose, goals, and norms which reflect staff concerns and objectives but are not completely dependent upon staff action (Clark and Hoy[58]). Curle[121] and Curle and Trist[122] described a somewhat similar phenomenon among British prisoners of war who were deprived of their normally assigned leaders, but found leadership within their own ranks and developed a purpose and technique for sustaining group and individual integrity under psychologically deprived conditions. However, Curle noted that the newly created group structure fitted its environment so well that after the men were repatriated and deprived of this group membership, their adjustment to ordinary civilian routines was often seriously impaired. This conflict of realities faces every chronic patient who must quickly divest himself of laboriously learned behaviors appropriate to a mental hospital, and assume those expected in society at large.

Small group theory suggests that groups formed in this manner are able to assist materially in the many vexing problems connected with management, social withdrawal, resocialization, discharge and disposition planning, and post-hospital maintenance of treatment effects. An evaluation of the expectations of this theory is essential for perhaps then neither manpower nor fund shortages would be so critical.

CONCLUSIONS

These findings are hopeful, at least, for they indicate that the institutional process can be arrested and reversed, if only temporarily, when realistic patient participation can be obtained. They have provided, as well, a certain clarification of the social psychological status of the patient, with long overdue emphasis on remaining capacities rather than interfering disabilities, both within and outside the hospital. Beyond these two general factors, it must be conceded that little systematic progress has occurred that would make it possible to regard mental hospitals as a treatment instrument coordinate with the level of current technical excellence, as inferred from Schwartz in his preliminary report to the Joint Commission on Mental Illness[1] and Pratt et al.[118] For treatment to achieve its broadest scope, means must be found to expand and improve aftercare articulation and continuity with mental hospitals. The latter may have to examine their theoretical position to accommodate small group procedures to take full advantage of patients' capabilities for mutual assistance and support. Perhaps a combined within- and post-hospital revision of theory and practice along small group theory lines can reduce hospital stay further, improve release rates, lengthen stay out of the hospital, and reduce relapse rates for all categories. If this can be done, the problem of chronicity will slowly disappear as treatment failures during the first year of hospitalization decline from their current high proportions.

REFERENCES

1. Joint Commission on Mental Illness: Action for Mental Health. New York, Basic Books, Inc., 1961.

2. BASSOE, P.: Spain as the cradle of psychiatry. Am. J. Psychiat. 101:731-738, 1945.

3. BOCKOVEN, J. S.: Moral treatment in American psychiatry. J. Nerv. Ment. Dis. 124:167-194, 1956.

4. ——: Moral treatment in American psychiatry. J. Nerv. Ment. Dis. 124: 292-321, 1956.

5. DEUTSCH, A.: The Mentally Ill in America. Garden City, Doubleday, Doran, and Co., Inc., 1937.

6. MALAMUD, W.: History of Psychiatric Therapies, 100 Years of American Psychiatry. New York, Am. Psychiat. Assoc., 1944, pp. 273-323.

7. SNOW, C. P.: Science and Government. Cambridge, Harvard University Press, 1961.

8. LIVI, C.: Life of Chiarugi. Alienist & Neurologist 3:93-118, 1882.

9. WALK, A.: Some aspects of the "moral treatment" of the insane up to 1954. J. Ment. Sci. 100:807-837, 1954.

10. MEIJERING, W. L.: Recent Developments in Social Psychiatry in the Netherlands, In Symposium on Preventive and Social Psychiatry. Washington, D.C., Walter Reed Army Institute of Research, 1957, pp. 409-418.

11. ROBINSON, C.: Home treatment of the earlier stages of insanity. Lancet 2:724-725, 1863.

12. REES, T. P., AND GLATT, M. M.: Mental Hospitals, The Field of Group Psychotherapy; Slavson, S. R., (ed.). New York, International Universities Press, Inc., 1956, pp. 17-40.

13. SOLOMON, H.: Some historical perspectives. Ment. Hosps. 9:5-9, 1958.

14. KRAMER, M., GOLDSTEIN, H., ISRAEL, R. H., AND JOHNSON, N. A.: Application of life table methodology to the study of mental hospital populations. Psychiat. Res. Rep. 5:49-76, 1956.

15. ODEGARD, O.: Pattern of discharge and remission in psychiatric hospitals in Norway—1926 to 1955. Ment. Hyg. 45: 185-193, 1961.

16. VITALE, J.: The Therapeutic Community: A Review. In The Psychiatric Hospital as a Social System, Third Annual Conference. Social Science Institute Training Program for Research in Community Mental Health, Washington University, St. Louis, Mo., 1961, pp. 28-52.

17. CAUDILL, W., REDLICH, F. C., GILMORE, H. H., AND BRODY, E. E.: Social structure and interaction processes on a psychiatric ward. Am. J. Orthopsychiat. 22:314-334, 1952.

18. GOFFMAN, E.: Characteristics of Total Institutions; In: Symposium on Preventive and Social Psychiatry. Washington, D.C., Walter Reed Army Institute of Research, 1957, pp. 43-84.

19. JONES, M.: Intra and extramural community psychiatry. Am. J. Psychiat. 117:784-787, 1961.

20. ELLSWORTH, R. B.: Psychiatric Aide-Role Project, 2nd Interim Report. VA Hospital, Fort Meade, South Dakota, May, 1961, mimeographed.

21. FAIRWEATHER, G. W., SIMON, R., GEBHARD, MILDRED E., WEINGARTEN, E., HOLLAND, J. L., SANDERS, R., STONE, G. B., AND REAHL, J. E.: Relative effectiveness of psychotherapeutic programs: a multicriteria comparison of four programs for three different patient groups. Psychol. Mon. 74:1-26, 1960 (Whole No. 492).

22. LINDEMANN, J. E., FAIRWEATHER, G. W., STONE, G. B., SMITH, R. S., AND LONDON, I. T.: The use of demographic characteristics in predicting

length of neuropsychiatric hospital stay. J. Consult. Psychol. 23:85-89, 1959.

23. EATON, J. W., AND WEILL, R. J.: Culture and Mental Illness. Glencoe, Ill., The Free Press, 1955.

24. LEMKAU, P. V., AND CROCETTI, G. M.: The Amsterdam municipal psychiatric service: a psychiatric-sociologic review. Am. J. Psychiat. 7:779-783, 1961.

25. FREEMAN, H. L., AND FARNDALE, W. A. J.: Current aspects of psychiatry in Great Britain, II. Recent developments in British mental health services. Ment. Hyg. 44:475-487, 1960.

26. KALINOWSKY, L. B.: Advances in management and treatment in European mental hospitals. Am. J. Psychiat. 113: 549-556, 1956.

27. MUTH, L. T.: Aftercare for the Mentally Ill—A World Picture. Philadelphia, The Mental Health Education Unit, Smith, Kline, and French Laboratories, 1957.

28. FOULKES, S. H.: Psychotherapy. Brit. J. M. Psychol., 34:91-102, 1961.

29. MASSERMAN, J.: Norms, Neurotics, and Nepenthics—In: Biological Psychiatry: Masserman, J., (ed.) New York, Grune & Stratton, Inc., 1959, pp. 90-112.

30. WINDER, C. L.: Some Psychological Studies of Schizophrenia; In: The Etiology of Schizophrenia: Jackson, D. D., (ed.) New York, Basic Books, Inc., 1960, pp. 191-247.

31. BRADY, E. D., AND FISHMAN, M.: Therapeutic response and length of hospitalization of psychiatrically ill veterans. AMA Arch. Gen. Psychiat. 2:175-181, 1960.

32. CHAPANIS, A.: Men. machines, and models. Am. Psychol. 16:113-131, 1961.

33. GARNER, A. M.: Abnormalities of Behavior—In: Annual Review of Psychology: Farnsworth, P. R., and McNemar, Q., (eds.) Palo Alto, Annual Reviews, Inc., 1958, pp. 391-418.

34. MARTIN, D. V.: Institutionalization. Lancet 2:1188-1190, 1955.

35. MORISON, R. S.: Gradualness, gradualness, gradualness. Am. Psychol. 15:187-197, 1960.

36. REES, T. P.: Back to moral treatment and community care. J. Ment. Sci. 103:303-313, 1957.

37. ——, AND GLATT, M. M.: The organization of the mental hospital on the basis of group participation. Int. J. Group Psychother. 5:157-161, 1955.

38. APPLEBY, L., SCHER, J. M., AND CUMMING, J. (eds.): Chronic Schizophrenia. Glencoe, Ill., The Free Press, 1960.

39. STANTON, A. H.: Problems in Analysis of Therapeutic Implications of the Institutional Milieu—In: Symposium on Preventive and Social Psychiatry. Washington, D.C., Walter Reed Army Institute of Research, 1957, pp. 493-502.

40. ARIETI, S.: Interpretation of Schizophrenia. New York, Robert Brunner, 1955.

41. CLARK, D. H.: Functions of the mental hospital. Lancet 271:1005-1009, 1956.

42. ELLSWORTH, R. B.: Psychiatric Aide-Role Project, 1st Interim Report. VA Hospital, Fort Meade, South Dakota, May, 1960 (mimeographed).

43. HYDE, R. W.: Current Developments in Social Psychiatry in the United States—In: Symposium on Preventive and Social Psychiatry. Washington,

D.C.: Walter Reed Army Institute of Research, 1957, pp. 419-429.

44. MAIN, T. F.: The hospital as a therapeutic institution. Bull. Menn. Clin. 10:66-76, 1946.

45. REES, T. P., AND GLATT, M. M.: The management of a chronic ward in a hospital Practitioner 175:62-65, 1955.

46. WEINBERG, S. K.: Social Psychological Aspects of Schizophrenia—In: Chronic Schizophrenia: Appleby, L., Scher, J. M., and Cumming, J. eds. Glencoe, Ill., The Free Press, 1960, pp. 68-88.

47. SANDERS, R., FITZGERALD, B. J., HOBKIRK, JANICE, SMITH, A., SMITH, R. S., AND WEINMAN, B.: Social Rehabilitation of the Chronic Mental Patient; 1st Interim Report. Philadelphia State Hospital, Philadelphia, 1959.

48. SANDERS, R., FITZGERALD, B. J., HOBKIRK-KENNY, JANICE, SMITH, A., SMITH, R. S., AND WEINMAN, B.: Social Rehabilitation of the Chronic Mental Patient; 2nd Interim Report. Philadelphia State Hospital, Philadelphia, 1960.

49. SANDERS, R.: Social Rehabilitation of the Chronic Mental Patient, 3rd Interim Report, Philadelphia State Hospital, Philadelphia, Pa., 1961.

50. STAUDT, VIRGINIA, AND ZUBIN, J. A.: A biometric evaluation of the somatotherapies in schizophrenia. Psychol. Bull. 54:171-196, 1957.

51. GALIONI, E. F., ADAMS, F. H., AND TALLMAN, F. F.: Intensive treatment of back-ward patients—a controlled pilot study. Am. J. Psychiat. 109:576-583, 1953.

52. ——: Evaluation of a Treatment Program for Chronically Ill Schizophrenic Patients & A Six Year Program—In: Chronic Schizophrenia: Appleby, L. et al., eds. Glencoe, Ill., The Free Press, 1960, pp. 303-324.

53. SINES, J. O., LUCERO, R. J., AND KAMMON, G. R., A state hospital total push program for regressed schizophrenics. J. Clin. Psychol. 8:189-193, 1952.

54. GREENBLATT, M., AND SIMON, B. (eds.): Rehabilitation of the Mentally Ill. Washington, D.C., Am. Assoc. for Advancement of Science, 1959, Pub. No. 58.

55. DENBER, H. C. B. (ed.): Research Conference on Therapeutic Community. Springfield, Ill., Charles C. Thomas, 1960.

56. SIVADON, P.: Techniques of Sociotherapy—In: Symposium on Preventive and Social Psychiatry. Washington, D.C., Walter Reed Army Institute of Research, 1957, pp. 457-464.

57. BELL, G. M.: A mental hospital with open doors. Internat. J. Soc. Psychiat. 1: 42-48, 1955.

58. CLARK, V. H., AND HOY, R.: Reform in the mental hospital: a critical study of a programme. Int. J. Soc. Psychiat. 3:211-223, 1957.

59. GLASS, A. J.: Observations upon the Epidemiology of Mental Illness in Troops during Warfare—In: Symposium on Preventive and Social Psychiatry. Washington, D.C., Walter Reed Army Institute of Research, 1957, pp. 185-198.

60. Proceedings of the Ninth Mental Hospital Institute. Ment. Hosps. 9, 1958.

61. PATTON, G. O.: Foster homes and rehabilitation of long-term mental patients. Canad. Psychiat. Assoc. J. 6:20-25, 1961.

62. WILMER, H. A.: Social Psychiatry in Action. Springfield, Ill., Charles C. Thomas, 1958.

63. SCHEERER, M.: The Unsettled and Unsettling Question of Chronic Schizophrenia—*In*: Chronic Schizophrenia: Appleby, L., et al. (eds.). Glencoe, Ill., The Free Press, 1960, pp. 326-360.

64. ELLSWORTH, R. B., AND CLAYTON, W. B.: The effects of chemotherapy on length of stay and rate of return for psychiatrically hospitalized patients. J. Consult. Psychol. 24:50-53, 1960.

65. ODEGARD, O.: Current Studies of Incidence and Prevalence of Hospitalized Mental Patients in Scandinavia—*In*: Comparative Epidemiology of the Mental Disorders: Hoch, P. H., and Zubin, J., eds. New York, Grune & Stratton, Inc., 1961, pp. 45-55.

66. KRAMER, M., GOLDSTEIN, H., ISRAEL, R. H., AND JOHNSON, N. A.: A Historical Study of the Disposition of First Admissions to a State Mental Hospital. Public Health Mon., No. 32, 1955.

67. ASTIN, A. W.: The functional autonomy of psychotherapy. Am. Psychol. 16:75-78, 1961.

68. BANDURA, A.: Psychotherapy as a learning process. Psychol. Bull. 58:143-159, 1961.

69. ROTTER, J. B.: Psychotherapy—*In*: Annual Review of Psychology: Farnsworth, P. R., and McNemar, Q., (eds.). Palo Alto, Annual Reviews, Inc., 1960, pp. 381-414.

70. HOLLINGSHEAD, A. DEB., AND REDLICH, F. C.: Social Class and Mental Illness: A Community Study. New York, John Wiley & Sons, Inc., 1958.

71. WRIGHT, M. E.: Abnormalities of Behavior—*In*: Annual Review of Psychology: Farnsworth, P. R., and McNemar, Q., (eds.). Palo Alto, Annual Reviews, Inc., 1957, pp. 269-308.

72. BOCKOVEN, J. S., PANDISCIO, ANNA R., AND SOLOMON, H. C.: Social adjustment of patients in the community three years after commitment to the Boston Psychopathic Hospital. Ment. Hyg. 40:353-374, 1956.

73. MORGAN, N. C., AND JOHNSON, N. A.: The chronic hospital patient. Am. J. Psychiat. 113:824-830, 1957.

74. GREENLAND, CYRIL: The Dymond Report and chronic patients in Ontario hospitals. Canad. Psychiat. J. 6:37-44, 1961.

75. COOPER, B.: Grouping and tranquillizers in the chronic ward. Brit. J. M. Psychol. 34:157-162, 1961.

76. POLLACK, E. S., PERSON, P. H., KRAMER, M., AND GOLDSTEIN, H. G.: Patterns of Retention, Release, and Death of First Admissions to State Mental Hospitals. Public Health Mon. No. 58, 1959.

77. BAKER, A. A., THORPE, J. G., AND JENKINS, V.: Social status after 5 years in a mental hospital. Brit. J. M. Psychol. 30:113-118, 1957.

78. BAKER, A. A., AND LOND, M. D.: Factory in a hospital. Lancet, 1:278-279, 1956.

79. CARSTAIRS, C. M., O'CONNOR, N., AND RAWNSLEY, K.: Organization of a hospital workshop for chronic patients. Brit. J. Prevent. Soc. Med. 10:136-140, 1956.

80. COLLINS, S. D., FLYNN, S. J., MANNERS, F., AND MORGAN, R.: Factory on a ward. Lancet 2:609-611, 1959.

81. CONNORS, J. E.: A new step in the rehabilitation of the chronic mental patient. J. Counsel. Psychol. 5:115-119, 1958.

82. RACKOW, L. L., SPOHN, H. E., ROSENBERG, G., AND KLEBANOFF, S. G.: Opportunities and Problems in the Treatment of Hospitalized Schizo-

phrenics. Montrose VA Hospital, Montrose, New York: Paper delivered to the Amer. Psychiat. Assoc., 1959.

83. PADULA, HELEN: Social Service Rehabilitation Wards. Spring Grove State Hospital, Baltimore, Md., Sept., 1957 (mimeographed).

84. BROOKS, G. W.: Rehabilitation of Hospitalized Chronic Schizophrenic Patients—In: Chronic Schizophrenia: Appleby, L., et al. (eds.) Glencoe, Ill., The Free Press, 1960, pp. 248-257.

85. JAMES, J.: Summary of Final Report of the Oregon Study of Rehabilitation of Mental Hospital Patients. Salem, Oregon, June, 1960 (mimeographed).

86. SCHLOSSER, J. R., SANDERS, R., BUEHLER, R. E., AND McGREEVY, JOAN: The Chronic Patient Pilot Study—A Preliminary Report. Veterans Administration DM&S Information Bulletin 10-78, 1954, pp. 3-9.

87. FAIRWEATHER, G. W., AND SIMON, R.: An 18 Month Follow-up Evaluation of the Relative Effectiveness of Four Psychotherapeutic Programs. VA Hospital, Palo Alto (unpublished manuscript).

88. WRIGHT, F. H.: The Exit Unit Program for Psychiatric Patients. J. Counsel. Psychol. 6:116-120, 1959.

89. HUNT, R. C., GRUENBERG, E. M., HACKEN, E., AND HUXLEY, M.: A comprehensive hospital-community service in a state hospital. Am. J. Psychiat. 117:817-821, 1961.

90. HOCH, P. H.: Interim Annual Report. Department of Mental Hygiene, State of New York, 1959-1960 (mimeographed).

91. PARKER, S.: Leadership patterns in a psychiatric ward. Human Relat. 11:287-301, 1958.

92. RASHKIS, H. A.: Cognitive restructuring: why research is therapy. AMA Arch. Gen. Psychiat. 2:612-621, 1960.

93. RASHKIS, H. A.: Does clinical research interfere with treatment? AMA Arch. Gen. Psychiat. 4:105-108, 1961.

94. BROWN, J. A. C.: The Social Psychology of Industry. Baltimore, Md., Penguin Books, Inc., 1954, pp. 69-97.

95. ELLSWORTH, R. B., MEAD, B .T., AND CLAYTON, W. H.: The rehabilitation and disposition of chronically hospitalized schizophrenic patients. Ment. Hyg. 42:343-348, 1958.

96. ODEGARD, O.: A statistical study of factors influencing discharge from psychiatric hospitals. J. Ment. Sci. 106:1124-1133, 1960.

97. BROWN, G. W. CARSTAIRS, G. M., AND TAPPING, G.: Post-hospital adjustment of chronic mental patients. Lancet 2:685, 1958.

98. GREENBLATT, M., LANDY, D., HYDE, R. W., AND BOCKOVEN, J. S.: Rehabilitation of the mentally ill: impact of a project upon hospital structure. Am. J. Psychiat. 11:986-992, 1958.

99. ULLMANN, L. P., AND BERKMAN, VIRGINIA C.: Efficacy of placement of neuropsychiatric patients in family care. AMA Arch. Gen. Psychiat. 1:273-274, 1959.

100. LANDY, D., AND WECHSLER, H.: Common assumptions, dimensions, and problems of pathway organizations. J. Soc. Issues 16:70-78, 1960.

101. BIERER, J.: Day Hospital. London, H. K. Lewis, 1951.

102. ——: Theory and practice of psychiatric day hospitals. Lancet 2:901-902, 1959.

103. CAMERON, D. E.: Day Hospital. Mod. Hosp. 69:60-62, 1947.

104. WINICK, C.: Psychiatric day hospitals: a survey. J. Soc. Issues 16: 8-13, 1960.

105. WECHSLER, H.: Halfway houses for former mental patients: a survey. J. Soc. Issues 16:20-26, 1960.

106. CRUTCHER, HESTER B.: Foster Home Care—*In*: American Handbook of Psychiatry: Arieti, S., ed. New York, Basic Books, Inc., 1959, pp. 1877-1884.

107. BIERER, J. A new form of group psychotherapy. Proc. Roy. Soc. Med. 37:208-209, 1943.

108. PALMER, MARY: Social rehabilitation for mental patients. Ment. Hyg. 42:24-28, 1958.

109. WECHSLER, H.: The ex-patient organization: a survey. J. Soc. Issues 16:47-53, 1960.

110. BLACK, B. J.: The protected workshop in the rehabilitation of the mentally ill. Psychiat. Quart. Suppl. 33:105-118, 1959.

111. HUBBS, R.: The Sheltered Workshop. Ment. Hosp. 11:7-9, 1960.

112. ——: The sheltered workshop for psychiatric patients. Ment. Hosp. 12:47, 1961.

113. MEYER, H. J., AND BORGATTA, E.: An Experiment in Mental Patient Rehabilitation. New York, Russell Sage Foundation, 1959.

114. OLSHANSKY, S.: The transitional sheltered workshop: a survey. J. Soc. Issues 16:33-39, 1960.

115. ——, GROB, S., AND EKDAHL, M.: Survey of employment experiences of patients discharged from three state mental hospitals during period 1951-1953. Ment. Hyg. 44:510-521, 1960.

116. LINDER, MARJORIE P., AND LANDY, D.: Post-discharge experience and vocational rehabilitation needs of psychiatric patients. Ment. Hyg. 42:29-44, 1958.

117. GREENBLATT, M.: The transitional hospital: a clinical and administrative viewpoint. J. Soc. Issues 16:62-69, 1960.

118. PRATT, S., SCOTT, G., TREESH, E., KHANNA, J., LESTER, T., KHANNA P., GARDINER, G., AND WRIGHT, W.: The mental hospital and the treatment-field. J. Psychol. Studies 11:1-179, 1960.

119. Proceedings of the 12th Mental Hospitals Institute. Ment. Hosps. 12: 1961.

120. ALBEE, G. W.: Mental Health Manpower Trends. New York, Basic Books, Inc., 1959.

121. CURLE, A.: I. Transitional communities and social reconnection: a follow-up study of a civil resettlement of British prisoners of war. Hum. Relat. I:42-68, 1947.

122. CURLE, A., AND TRIST, E. L.: II. Transitional communities and social reconnection: A follow-up study of civil resettlement of British prisoners of war. Hum. Relat. I:240-288, 1947.

Psychiatric Therapy In France*

by HENRY EY

SINCE FRANCE was among the first of all countries to organize its mental institutions, our progress in psychotherapy may interest our American colleagues.

MODERNIZATION OF PSYCHIATRIC HOSPITALS AND OUTPATIENT CLINICS

Thirty years ago, we possessed the only type of "asylum" then known: closed hospitals of penitentiary style in which admissions and controls were—and still are—regulated by the law of 1838. In some of these hospitals, a few psychiatrists adopted the "open door" system, but this was infrequent until 1930, when Edouard Toulouse organized it at the "Asile St. Anne" in Paris. This policy has since become generalized, until now about 100 psychiatric hospitals with an average capacity of 800 to 1000 beds are "open-door." Of the 50,000 to 60,000 patients admitted, about 20,000 come voluntarily and it is more and more the exception to be committed under the law of 1838. All of these psychiatric hospitals are new or "modernized." Many additional psychiatric services have been created in general hospitals and especially in the Psychiatric Departments of the Universities (13 throughout the country).

Further, the health insurance system called *"Securité Sociale"* permitted (1) the development of various special services, such as those of Dr. Sivadon and Dr. Le Guillant in Paris, and my own in Bonneval; (2) the payment of expenses for hospitalization and therapy of 85 per cent of all mental patients; and (3) the utilization of private clinics for psychiatric treatments.

We plan to give up the large hospitals (1000 beds or more) in favor of smaller therapeutic centers (200 to 300 beds), and to place the pre-

---

*Each annual volume will contain a review of psychiatric developments abroad as summarized by a leading authority in a selected country—ED.

vention, care and after-care of mental patients in the hands of one medicosocial team in charge of a given demographic sector of from 40,000 to 50,000 inhabitants.

BIOLOGICAL THERAPEUTICS

Convulsive

Insulin therapy has been used since 1934, and, although its vogue has declined in France as in other countries, it is still frequently utilized in schizophrenics and acute delusional psychoses. All the *shock therapies* (including ECT by the techniques of Lapipe and Rondepierre and of Delmas-Marsalet employing acetylcholin and amphetamins) have been extensively utilized with modifications for better results, less discomfort and less danger through the use of electronarcosis, intravenous injections of pentothal or amytal sodium, curarisation, etc. H. Baruk has been almost the only one opposed to these "psychiatric aggressions." Important investigations have been conducted by J. Delay and his school on the diencephalic mechanism of action of ECT and on the analogy of the therapeutic "stress" and the physiopathology of the defences to the theoretical model of Selye. The techniques of Egas Moniz and of Freeman and Watts were tried between 1945 and 1952, but have been supplemented by the topectomy of Scoville and the infiltration of procain in the frontal lobes (Abely and Guyot). Talairach has devised *stereotaxic methods* that produce localized coagulations of well defined structures or functional systems such as the thalamic nuclei, gyrus cingularis and thalamoparietal fibers. However, all of these methods are being seriously questioned and less frequently employed.

DRUGS

The discovery of promethazine in 1946 inaugurated in France and in the world the new biochemical era in psychiatry. This drug, studied as an antihistaminic derivative of phenothiazine (long known, but too toxic to be used in man), quickly displayed its hypnotic and antiallergic action and led to studies of its derivatives. In this way French chemists found Chlorpromazine, which was first utilized in anesthesiology, then in psychiatry (1952). With it and other drugs H. Laborit devised the techniques of *hibernation* applied afterwards in milder form, as *"hiberno-therapy."*

Almost at the same time, the chemists of Basel extracted the alkaloid reserpine from Rauwolfia serpentina, with a chemical structure and a neurophysiological activity entirely different from Chlorpromazine, but productive of similar therapeutic results. These drugs are still the basis of treatment in acute psychosis and states of agitation.

By modifying the nucleus and side-chain of Chlorpromazine simultaneously two new series of drugs were obtained which are widely used in France: (1) *Levopromazine* which is more sedative, hypnotic, hypotensive and analgesic, and (2) *Prochlorpemazine* which diminishes hallucinations in paranoid psychoses. *Thioproperazine,* probably the most powerful of all known neuroleptics, can control a manic state in a few days, but can cause severe neurological complications. A new chemical series, the *Butyrophenones,* equivalent in importance to the phenothiazines, has been discovered in Belgium; of these *R. 1625,* is a powerful but possibly dangerous ataractic. *Meprobamate* continues to be widely employed, but *Chlorodiaepoxide* may prove superior.

In the field of antidepressive drugs, French psychiatrists employ Imipramine in widely varying doses. Among the monoaminooxidase inhibitors, Iproniazine is the most frequently used, with the *Nialamide* considered less active. In the field of *hypnotics,* France has contributed *Hemineurine,* a derivative of *Aneurin* or vitamin B 1, and a steroid, *Hydroxydione* useful in the control of alcoholic delirium tremens.

Psychotherapy

Psychoanalysis has had difficulty in taking root, since most of our university faculties reject not only the "psychologie des profondeurs" but also the Adlerian and Jungian systems. There is no teaching of psychology and no obligation to study psychiatry in French medical schools. Nevertheless, there are now two Societies of Psychoanalysis: the first led by Nacht, Lebovici, Bouvet, Diatkine, etc., (Société de Psychanalyse de Paris), and the other by Lacan, Lagache and Mme. Boutonier-Favez (Société Française de Psychanalyse). The latter, with its review "L'Evolution Psychiatrique" of which E. Minkowski and myself are the editors, has for its mission the *reintegration of psychoanalysis with psychiatry.* This would include *narcoanalysis,* the techniques of wakeful dreaming of R. Desoille, and the *autogenic* training of Schultz.

But it is mostly in the direction of the *group psychotherapies* that the methods derived from psychodynamic concepts have found the most interesting applications. In this respect, *the analytic psychodrama* as practiced by Lebovici, Diatkine and their school provides a therapeutic community therapy. In my own service, we employ the collective sleeping cure associated with group psychotherapy.

Existential Analysis

This, as practiced by some psychiatrists with philosophical training (L. Binswanger et al.), has practically no following in France, except for the brief interest of J. P. Sarte.

REFERENCES

DELAY, J.: Méthodes Biologiques en Clinique Psychiatrique. Éd. Masson, Paris, 1950.

——: Symposium sur la Chlorpromazine. Encéphale 45:4, 1956.

DENIKER, P.: Hibernotherapie et Médicaments Neuroleptiques en Therapeutique Psychiatrique: Report to the 2d International Congress of Psychiatry. Zürich, Ed. Doin., 1957.

EBTINGER, R.: Aspects Psychopathologiques du Postélectrochoc. Thèse, Strassburg, 1958.

FAURE, H.: Cure de Sommiel Collectif et Psychotherapie de Groupe. Paris, Éd. Masson, 1958.

Fédération des Organismes de Sécurité Sociale: Nos. 3 & 4. Paris, La Technique du Livre (eds.), 1960.

GAYRAL, L., AND DAUTY, R.: Nouvelles Chimiotherapies en Psychiatrie: Report to the Congress of French-speaking Alienist Physicians and Neurologists. Lyon, 1957.

LABORIT, H., HUGUERRARD, P., et al.: Practique de Hibernotherapie en Chirurgie et en Médécin. Paris, Éd. Masson, 1954.

REVOL, L., et al.: La Therapeutique par la Chlorpromazine en Practique Psychiatrique. Paris, Éd. Masson, 1956.

TALAIRACH, J.: Rév. Neurol. 2:87, 111, 119. Also: Congress of Neurosurgury. Zürich, 1959.

The Therapy of Human Injustice

by Louis Jolyon West, M.D.

March 15, 1961

To The Editor of the Sunday Oklahoman:

Last Saturday afternoon I went downtown with a small group of distinguished Negro colleagues. Later, as I sat on the cold muddy marble outside a "service-to-whites-only" cafeteria, I couldn't help thinking of a line from Ibsen: "You should never wear your best trousers when you go out to fight for freedom and truth." Having committed this sartorial error, I am now called upon to state whether my becoming a white participant in a Negro "sit-in" demonstration was not wholly an error. Hostile anonymous telephonists and anxious personal friends ask the same question: "Why did you do it?"

That such a question should be put to a physician in this country nearly a century after Lincoln described us as a nation "conceived in liberty, and dedicated to the proposition that all men are created equal," is not so much astonishing as anachronistic. That it should happen in Oklahoma City, one of the most progressive and forward looking communities in the United States, is of only passing significance. In a few short years such incidents may be regarded as historical curiosities, and participants in these demonstrations will perhaps be considered as having been moved by the spirit of their time, rather than having themselves contributed significantly to progress. If this be the case, why bother to demonstrate? There are three major reasons for my doing so; three principles involved.

1. *Ethical reasons: the Christian Principle*

As a product of twentieth century American culture, with its great debt to the Old and New Testaments, I sometimes call myself a Christian. To

---

EDITORIAL NOTE: *As physicians and psychiatrists, we are committed by dedication and oath to the welfare of all humanity. When the editor, some months ago, read the following contribution by an esteemed colleague, he secured permission to reprint it.*

me this means a moral commitment to the ideal of the brotherhood of man. Am I my brother's keeper? I must try to be. However, like Voltaire, I am very fond of truth, but not at all of martyrdom. Well, do I love my neighbor enough to risk helping him when he is reviled, persecuted, demeaned or humiliated because of the color of his skin? If not, I fail to be true to myself; I violate the Christian Principle as I understand it, and my conscience bothers me. If another man's understanding of Christianity differs from mine, I cannot help it. Byron said man's conscience is the oracle of God. Mine may be neither prophetic nor divine, but it tells me to speak out in public against racial discrimination. To this voice I must respond; it speaks louder than all other voices because it is closest to my ear.

2. *Political reasons: the Democratic Principle*

At the dawn of the Republic, our first president prayed that all Americans would "entertain a brotherly affection and love for one another." Today a few individuals, by their persistent refusal to treat citizens of all races as brothers, impugn Washington's wisdom. My call openly to oppose their discriminatory practices, even when they are seemingly condoned by law, is as old as the call to democracy on this continent.

An encroachment upon the dignity of any man debases mankind. Nobody is entitled to "reserve the right" to violate the principles of human dignity on which our democracy is based and from which all our freedoms derive. Any such violation threatens to alienate those rights, including equality, declared inalienable by the founders of our political system. Therefore, by defending the rights of any citizen, one defends the rights of all. Can the responsibility for this be delegated by me to a Negro organization? No, because it is not only a struggle for the dignity and equality of the Negro in which I am engaged; it is for my own and every man's. If freedom is deserved only by those who are willing to fight for it, then I must take a personal part.

3. *National reasons: the Patriotic Principle*

Our country leads the free world in the most terrible struggle in the history of mankind, against a monstrous tyranny that would bury liberty forever. The battle is global; it is joined; men and women and children are suffering and dying in it in Europe, Asia, and Africa. We are numerically inferior to our opponents, and we are losing ground steadily. Today our best hope for preserving religious freedom, free elections, free speech, free press, free assembly, private property, private profit, and private cafeterias, is to persuade the uncommitted peoples of the world to join us in our fight for a free way of life. These people are of all races; whites are a small minority.

Already western civilization has reaped whirlwind after whirlwind of hatred from the seeds of racism it has sown. Now, tales of racial discrimination in the United States are being used against us by the communists with vicious effectiveness far and wide. These propaganda weapons, employed in the battle for the minds of men, can destroy us more surely than atomic weapons. Can freedom as a way of life survive, and with it our nation? If so, colored people in every land must come to know that democracy offers them something precious, worth winning and preserving. But we must exemplify democracy, proving its value by truly living it. Viewed in this light, any insistence upon prolonging racial discriminatory practices in the United States can be seen as giving aid and comfort to the enemy.

Whether it be treason or merely stupidity, cynically profitable or indignantly righteous, emotionally prejudiced or blandly traditional, northern or southern, public or private, racial discrimination in America serves the cause of communism everywhere. As patriotic citizens, and in the national interest, we must all work quickly to end racial discrimination in this country forever, and pray that it is not already too late.

Louis Jolyon West, M.D.
Oklahoma City

Or Shall We All Commit Suicide?

by JULES H. MASSERMAN, M.D.

M ANY THOUGHTFUL MEN, after reading a book such as this thus far, may feel strengthened in their opinion that we psychiatrists, though laudably concerned with our small groups of ill and troubled patients, are as dereistic and escapist as they in refusing to deal with the rapidly mounting danger of the destruction of our civilization and perhaps of humanity itself. This final chapter on psychiatry in our global crisis may therefore be considered appropriate.

A CONFERENCE ON PEACE

As fortuitously as similar bids to international thought and adventure had come on previous occasions,* a formal invitation was extended to me by R. M. Hutchins, President of the Center for the Study of Democratic Institutions, to participate as a guest of the Center in a Congress on World Order and Freedom to be held in the Senate Chamber of the Greek Parliament Building from October 23 to 27, 1961. It required little reflection to recognize the importance of this opportunity, and I of course accepted.

I cannot here acknowledge adequately the gracious welcome and unfailing hospitality accorded by the Greek people and government to the small group they honored as "world scholars," or enthuse overlong over the bright, serene eternity of the Attic landscape and the clean classic beauty in which we met nor can I detail delight in exploring the diversely brilliant minds of my colleagues during the land-bound week of the Conference and its extension aboard a cruise ship, which continued the intellectual argosy among the Aegean Islands. I must instead summarize only those proceedings of the Conference most closely relevant to our interests as psychiatrists—and as citizens of a darkly threatened world.

The opening comments by Chairman Hutchins made it evident that, with 20,000 megatons, some in 100-megaton missiles, cocked on either side of the Atlantic, there were no defenses against imminent genosuicide other than an exploration of every avenue that might return men to sanity: the recognition of universal law, progressive disarmament, the re-establishment of communications, the rectification of economic and

---

*Masserman, J. H.: Psychiatry in Latin America: In Masserman, J. H. and Moreno, J. L. (eds.) Progress in Psychotherapy, vol. III, New York, Grune & Stratton, 1958, pp. 282-310; Ibid: The Czechoslovak Congress of Psychiatry. Idem, vol. V, 1961, pp. 231-254.

cultural disparities, and the organization of a peaceful world. These topics were then explored in successive meetings of the Conference as follows:

The Law:

Justice William O. Douglas of the United States Supreme Court reviewed man's current efforts towards international arbitration and justice as exemplified by establishments such as the World Bank, the European Economic Union, the European Court of Human Rights and the International Court of Justice. Although the jurisdiction and power of these institutions depended on the previous assent of the litigants, it was highly significant that such tribunals could function without the prior existence of a World Constitution or a World Parliament; ergo, the current unavailability of these need not deter us from developing temporarily more limited and parochial approaches to international equity. As an initial, practical step, we could submit issues such as the Berlin question to the UN or to the World Court.

Professor Helmut Coing of the Institute of International Justice, Frankfurt, Germany, then took as his theme an historical extension of the Treaty of Westphalia of 1648. This judicial decision, after long negotiations, ended the Thirty Years War and made possible the enduring coexistence of Catholic and Protestant state systems previously regarded as irreconcilable. In the final paper of the day, Scott Buchanan, former Dean of St. John's, rang the changes on the concept that the verb *to persuade* had three Greek roots connoting *convince, believe* and *obey,* but that we had no certain means to persuade other nations to adhere to our beliefs and mores under any of these rubics except as it seemed to their advantage.

The Military Situation:

On Tuesday morning, the military historian Walter Millis restated the incontrovertible fact that there was no way to avert impending global destruction other than to abolish the "war system" under which the world now kept only an exceedingly precarious "balance of terror." Karl Marx had predicted that peace would evolve through the self destruction of capitalism and the emergence of a world proletariat, but had not foreseen the interposition of viable and powerful welfare states. Kennedy and Khrushchev, though equally opposed to world government, both wished to avoid war by limiting armies to small national police forces, but every disarmament conference since the first one called by Russia in 1899 had been undermined by a continuation of militarist thinking that had, after Hiroshima, become completely unrealistic. Warner Neal, Professor of

International Relations at Claremont, agreed that "we may all yet be killed by an anachronism," but that, since the West "would not accept a world government that was neither white nor Protestant", for the time being we would have to work within the confines of nationalistic thinking and conflicts of mobilized and militarized regional interests. With engaging wit, Denis Healey, M.P. and member of the British "Shadow Cabinet," then chided the Americans for a "false courage" born of their lack of experience in the destructiveness of war, and for their parochialism in reducing the world's problems to their self-righteous quarrels with Russia; indeed, so awry were the attitudes of some of our present leaders, "certain of whom seem to use the atom bomb as their virility symbol . . . that arrangements should be made forthwith to have them meet for individual and group therapy in Dr. Masserman's office."

Technology:

On the second afternoon of the Conference, Professor Jacques Ellul of the University of Bordeaux and Robert Theobold of the Foreign Policy Association, in separate addresses, warned that "technology is getting out of hand," i.e., with the geometric rise of labor-saving inventions, unemployment and social discord would soon overwhelm the world unless new demands for goods were created. A system of freer global trade was therefore imperative, and was indeed practicable if the industrialized countries would devote the $3\frac{1}{2}$ per cent annual rise in their gross national product to the export of punch presses, combines, vehicles and other such developmental machinery to underdeveloped regions.

Communications:

In this session, Harry Ashmore, editor of the Encyclopedia Britannica, Professor Dallas Smythe of the University of Illinois and Denis Healey developed the thesis that, whereas instant and almost ubiquitous communications were now available through the use of satellites, moon-reflections and other technical devices, the intent and content of, and the responses to, information *as variously interpreted* would remain the crucial determinants of international consensus or dissent, and thereby of war or peace.

Economic Disparities:

In the Thursday morning session Ramanohar Lohia of Hyderabad took exception to the statements of the Conference economists (as, with easy charm, he questioned nearly every other statement at the Conference), to the effect that free world trade would solve any immediate problems;

indeed, asked Lohia, how could this be equitably arranged when a laborer in India had to work an average of 20 hours for a total wage of 20 cents to produce as much as an American could in 60 minutes? And who, apart from a few families in India with an income of up to $20,000 per day, could buy the American goods? Nor had United States aid helped; on the contrary it had done little but further enrich the rich while preventing the spontaneous industrial development of the masses of India, who in turn had been kept from revolution by the caste system, and had thus remained oppressed for 1500 years. What was needed—entoned Lohia for calculated shock effect—was a Marxian-Leninist concept of universal brotherhood, and a Cuba without Russia on the Indian Subcontinent.

David Horowitz, Governor of the Bank of Israel, then presented perhaps the most scholarly, factual and realistic address of the entire Conference. He agreed with Lohia that economic as well as imperialistic colonialism must be abandoned as dead, and that other means must be found to rectify the confusions and disparities in the world order, i.e., the admixture of idealogic struggles and slogans with material aid; the fact that a fourth of the countries with economic influence have three-fourths of the world's income; that two-thirds of the world's population is on marginal or submarginal subsistence; that the life expectancy of this large segment of mankind (including that in India) is less than 35 years; that the concepts of communism will continue to appeal to the oppressed and depressed masses; that if the population explosion continues at the present rate of doubling every 42 years, these masses may number six billion in the year 2000; that medical progress, which favors both longevity and natality, may further increase this number; that the farming populations of the world will be caught in the lethal scissors of falling agrarian and rising industrial prices; that despite the World Bank, the Colombia Plan, etc., goods will continue to flow *toward* industrialized nations; and finally, that although current safeguards will mitigate the previously severe reactions of unemployment and recession, in most countries world economic disparities would continue to cause political unrest, military maneuvers, and possibly a war that might truly end all human warriors. Nor could we prevent such eventualities by outmoded concepts of self-corrective "business cycles," or colonial extensions of national industrial systems (Britain has been better off without her colonies), or Marxian predictions of proletarian impoverishment followed by a concerted and effective workers' revolution or, for that matter, the Soviet delusion of a universal economy without incentive and competition. Instead, to achieve world peace, we must drop meaningless political shibboleths (including those of capitalism versus communism) and proceed to plan and implement, with adequate knowledge and media of exchange already at hand, a more equitable world economic and social order.

Stanley Sheinbaum, consultant to the Center for the Study of Democratic Institutions, cited some additional economic gaucheries more specifically committed by the United States, e.g., "devoting most of our energies to a Rich Man's Club called the Western Alliance;" treating undeveloped regions (e.g., Laos and the Congo) as "nations" even though they had little or no political cohesion or economic identity; expressly forbidding our Department of Agriculture to help other countries develop crops that might compete with ours; and finally, exporting large quantities of inappropriate and sometimes useless goods, often to the wrong people, and then attempting to use such "foreign aid" as a military weapon.

CULTURAL DIFFERENCES

That afternoon Professor Richard McKeon of the University of Chicago regretted the passing of the "virtues of the Greeks" and E. H. Carr of Cambridge, called for a continued respect for cultural and individual differences in a world that must never become stereotyped by excessive "communication" and "integration".

THE WORLD OF MAN

In my own address to the Conference on its final day, I suggested that perhaps some of its discussions had involved us in one of the less pardonable of logical sins—the one Whitehead had called the *reification of abstractions*. In effect, *men* conceived, constructed and operated for their differing purposes various systems of law, economics, technology, government—and, for that matter, war—yet our discourses at times seemed to imply that these human concepts and maneuvers had somehow become transformed into independent deities that had acquired wills and powers of their own with which to rule their creators. But man was still master of his own fate, regardless of how he wished to obscure this in awesome myths; it was therefore with men, not with anthropomorphized abstractions that we had to deal. True, this was not always easy: apropos of Mr. Healey's kind offer to refer some of the world's leaders to me, I could cite the probably apocryphal story of the putative patient who entered the psychiatrist's office dressed in a tiger skin, with boiled spinach draped over his ears and a fried egg in his hair, and announced, while waving his torch majestically: "Doctor, I would like to consult you about my brother!" And yet, despite wide variations among individuals and cultures, certain human aspirations were so nearly universal that they could unify mankind if properly understood and utilized. These were: first, every man's desire for health and longevity (or covertly, immortality) as a primary basis for technologic power; second, his needs for friends and allies on progressively larger scales; and third, man's penchant for developing diversely exploratory but essentially merging systems of comforting philosophy and hopeful faith. Anthropologists, sociologists and psychologists, in centuries of study, had accumulated many useful understandings of man's motivations, values and conduct, and psychiatrists daily utilized such operational insights to help confused and troubled men direct their behavior into more intelligent, humanitarian and thereby eventually more successful channels. In fact, those who could appeal directly to most of humanity—among whom could be included such unlicensed subspecialists as Louis Armstrong, David Oistrakh, Danny Kaye or the Bolshoi Ballet—had already demonstrated their capacity to promote international rapport despite the machinations of their political and military betters. In any case, we who were less adept but perhaps more variously articulate now stood ready to offer our knowledge, experience and skill to future conferences, and to join with our colleagues in other fields of science, art and statesmanship in a concerted effort to resolve the present crisis in man's affairs.

My comments were favorably received, and were included in Chairman Hutchins' closing summary. The majority of the Conference participants then boarded a cruise ship on which, between stopovers to visit the mutely eloquent ruins of the Minoan, Greek and Byzantine cultures, the discussions continued. At one of these the dissatisfactions not only among many of the scholars, but among the industrialists and financiers who had attended the preceding Conference sessions became manifest, and most explicitly so in the complaint that, although the formal papers and discussions had been scholarly and literate, they had rarely clarified or defined basic issues, had led to no plans for practical action, and had seemed to end in academic futility. At this juncture, after various preliminary conversations, particularly with Lyle Spencer, President of Scientific Research Associates, and Professor Dallas Smythe of the University of Illinois, I submitted the following proposal:

A Proposal to Help Avert World Suicide

Nearly all informed and thoughtful men and women believe that unless the rapidly mounting tensions between the United States and the Soviet Union are reduced, a nuclear war will result that would not only wipe out all that America cherishes but would destroy civilization and humanity itself. It is therefore of the utmost urgency that every conceivable step be taken toward the restoration of confidence and, eventually, friendship between these two great nations. However, in view of their current attitudes of mutual mistrust and belligerence, any proposal must have the following characteristics to be effective:

First, it must be made with complete sincerity and credibility.

Second, it must not pose a further economic or military threat to either nation.

Third, it must have instant and universal appeal.

Fourth, it must be politically and administratively feasible, and therefore practicable within a short period.

Fifth, if proposed by the United States, it should redound to our credit under nearly all conceivable interpretations and circumstances.

It is now painfully evident that, largely because they did not fulfill these criteria, many of our former overtures toward peace with the USSR have unfortunately jeopardized our relationships with other nations, seriously imperiled our health through atomic fallout, and brought us to the brink of a global Armageddon. This has been true of our previous modes of rapprochement, our proposals for partial disarmaments by weapons or zones, our tragically futile investments in bomb shelters, and our direct recourse to threats of nuclear retaliation. An approach entirely different in spirit, appeal and effectiveness is therefore essential in the current crisis.

THE PLAN

One such proposal, in essence, is that we offer to send to Russia, as soon as possible, large numbers of students, mostly from the ages of seventeen to twenty, for the purpose of broadening their education and promoting new and mutually advantageous understandings between our two countries. At the same time, we shall invite the Soviet Union to send comparable numbers of their students to live in our homes and attend our schools for similar purposes. The numbers considered may range annually from ten thousand to any larger number of properly qualified young people, and the periods from one to two years.

The universally significant impact of this proposal would be to certify unmistakably to all the civilized world that we had no intention of unleashing nuclear destruction on a nation that was playing host to our own sons and daughters. Simultaneously, we would be inviting the Russians to show the same sincerity and humanity—a request they could not ignore in the open and compelling court of world opinion. If the Soviets refused, we would gain the desirable advantage of an expression of good will; if they accepted, one path would be open that might lead to world peace.

In the latter case, the following steps would still require thorough consideration and carefully planned action:

Enabling Legislation by Congress authorizing exchange visas for properly qualified students.

Financing: Private funds could be solicited from individuals and foundations already interested in ensuring an equitable world peace.

Organization: The American Friends Service Committee or a similar organization could be employed as a nucleus, or new groups could be formed in various cities under a central coordinating agency in Washington or elsewhere.

Selection of Students: This would be on the basis of scholastic excellence, character and adherence to ideals of human justice and freedom, and we would hope for similar candidates from the Soviets.

Many other problems would remain: Preparation in languages, coordination of educational levels, adequate supervision and protection, and similar matters; however, initial surveys have indicated that none would present great difficulties. On the contrary, these surveys have revealed relatively little absolute opposition versus a consensus of acceptance by both youths and parents ranging from qualified endorsement and support to immediate and enthusiastic offers of participation. The successful Franco-German student exchange program, both at university and high school levels, also provides evidence that this type of plan can prove dramatically effective.

Be it therefore resolved that an Executive Committee be formed to expedite further investigations of essential aspects of this project with a view to early action. All men and women of good will are welcome to cooperate.

COMMITTEE ON YOUTH FOR TOMORROW
October 30, 1961

The reactions to this proposal could properly be characterized as electric: nearly all subsequent discussions revolved about it—with the minor exception of two United States congressmen aboard who contended that "we ought to maintain U.S.-Soviet tensions for the sake of Berlin." (One actually posed the incredible question: "would anyone really risk the Western Alliance just to save civilization?") Nearly everyone was enthusiastic, and several of the men of means, some with world-wide business connections, offered to finance the initial stages of the movement. Professors Coing and Ellul, in addressing one session, offered an illuminating account of how such an interchange of students and teachers had already sprung up spontaneously among French and German high schools and universities, and had contributed immensely to the growing rapport between these two countries; indeed, each was currently revising its history books to eliminate passages expressive of their previous traditional enmity. A survey of American mothers and teenagers aboard ship revealed an almost unanimous desire to participate in a similar arrangement between the United States and Russia as soon as possible.

An Executive Committee was therefore constituted to implement the plan when the group returned to the United States along the following lines:

(1) Securing influential sponsorship among educators and statesmen

(2) Facilitating enabling legislation in Congress

(3) Coordinating our efforts with various foundations and other agencies in allied fields

(4) Organizing the plan on a national and international basis

It is not here relevant to detail the subsequent minor vicissitudes and predominant successes of the plan, except perhaps to state that within a week after our return from the Conference it had been endorsed by the President of the American Association for the Advancement of Science, the President-elect of the American Psychiatric Association, the Secretary of the American Friends' Service Committee, the Vice-President of the American Broadcasting Company, the President of the Peace Research Institute, representatives of the State Department and the White House Staff, and other national leaders in education, science and statesmanship. Among these was Ambassador James J. Wadsworth, our recent representative at the United Nations, who not only obtained General Eisenhower's recommendation to his People to People Movement, but offered to see Khrushchev to implement the proposal. *Mirabile dictu,* the plan also received initial clearance from the Russian Embassy, which put the Committee in touch with citizen's organizations of scientists and educators with similar objectives in the USSR. Mayor Richard J. Daley has suggested that Chicago schools be available for student exchanges not only with the USSR, but with its associated People's Republics, and similar pilot arrangements have been explored in New York and California.

In psychiatric essence, then, these and other developments have indicated that man, if need be, can confront unflinchingly the dreadful visage of the impending end of humanity, and that from this nightmarish encounter they can emerge with clearer thoughts and with firmer resolutions to discard their personal prejudices and parochialisms so that they may join in endeavors essential to the good of humanity.

Dynamic group autotherapy on no lesser scale will now suffice.

Name Index*

(Principal References in *Italics*)

*Thanks are due to Miss Sevilla Laird for aid in the preparation of this index.

282

Subject Index*

(Principal References in *Italics*)

*Thanks are due Dr. Thaddeus Kostrubala for aid in preparing this index.